Commonly used drugs dose modifi...

Drug			
Amlodipine			...lose
Amoxicillin			...D
Atorvastatin			...ose
Buprenorphine SL	Standard dose but with caution	Standard dose but with caution	Standard dose but with caution
Ceftazidime	0.5–1g q24h	As for CKD stage 5 (post-HD)	0.5–1g q24h
Cefuroxime	750mg–1.5g q12–24h	750mg–1.5g q24h (post-HD)	750mg–1.5g q24h
Ciprofloxacin	50% standard dose	As for CKD stage 5	50% standard dose q8h
Citalopram	Avoid	Avoid	Avoid
Co-amoxiclav (PO)	375 mg q12h	As for CKD	As for CKD
Diltiazem	Standard dose	Standard dose	Standard dose
Erythromycin	Standard dose	Standard dose	Standard dose
Fentanyl	SC: pre-procedure or breakthrough 12.5–25mcg q1–4h	As for CKD stage 5	As for CKD stage 5
Fluconazole	50% standard dose	Standard dose post-HD on dialysis days only	As for CKD stage 5
Fluoxetine	Standard dose q24–48h	Standard dose or q24–48h	Standard dose or q24–48h
Imipenem	250mg (or 3.5mg/kg whichever is lower) q12h	As for CKD stage 5	As for CKD stage 5
Morphine	Avoid	Avoid	Avoid
Omeprazole	Standard dose	Standard dose	Standard dose
Sildenafil	Commence with 25mg	As for CKD stage 5	As for CKD stage 5
Simvastatin	Maximum 10mg	As for CKD stage 5	As for CKD stage 5
Tramadol	50mg q12h	As for CKD	As for CKD
Warfarin	Standard dose	Standard dose	Standard dose

OXFORD MEDICAL PUBLICATIONS

Oxford Handbook of
Dialysis

Published and forthcoming Oxford Handbooks

Oxford Handbook of
Dialysis

FOURTH EDITION

Jeremy Levy
Consultant Nephrologist
and Adjunct Professor of Medicine
Imperial College Healthcare NHS Trust, London, UK

Edwina Brown
Consultant Nephrologist
and Honorary Professor of Renal Medicine
Imperial College Healthcare NHS Trust,
London, UK

Anastasia Lawrence
Senior Renal Lecturer Practitioner
and Honorary Senior Lecturer
Imperial College Healthcare NHS Trust & Buckinghamshire
New University, London, UK

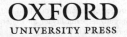

OXFORD
UNIVERSITY PRESS

OXFORD
UNIVERSITY PRESS

Great Clarendon Street, Oxford, OX2 6DP,
United Kingdom

Oxford University Press is a department of the University of Oxford.
It furthers the University's objective of excellence in research, scholarship,
and education by publishing worldwide. Oxford is a registered trade mark of
Oxford University Press in the UK and in certain other countries

© Oxford University Press 2016

Published in the United States of America by Oxford University Press
198 Madison Avenue, New York, NY 10016, United States of America

British Library Cataloguing in Publication Data
Data available

Library of Congress Control Number: 2015941610

ISBN 978–0–19–964476–6

Printed and bound in Turkey by Promat

Foreword

Dialysis is at the same time one of the most exciting aspects of the care of kidney patients, yet to the beginner also the most mysterious and daunting. Unfamiliar concepts, impressive technology, new jargon, expert patients—all of these can make for anxious times for the young doctor, nurse, or other health worker joining the multiprofessional team which cares for people with end-stage renal disease.

This Oxford Handbook provides much solace for the beginner. It provides plenty of easily navigable practical advice across every aspect of dialysis and its related challenges, with sufficient theoretical background to make sense of the day-to-day clinical decision-making. And all in a true handbook—both small enough and light enough to fit in most pockets.

Since I was a tyro nephrologist much has changed in the world of dialysis. For one thing there are many more patients, and many are older and frailer. There has been greater creativity in strategies to improve clinical outcomes and increase independence for the hospital environment—frequent home haemodialysis, and assisted peritoneal dialysis are just two examples. And we need a proper understanding of the complex end-of-life issues which arise for more patients on dialysis and their carers.

This new edition addresses these recent issues and many more with advice which is both authoritative and practical, as well as refreshing all the content familiar to the readers of earlier editions.

Although its authors are all from the UK, this book has global value, espe cially in the several parts of the world where the provision of dialysis has been inadequate for many reasons, but is now rapidly expanding. When there is such rapid expansion, the education and training needs of the local clinical team in ensuring high-quality dialysis care, can easily outstrip locally available resources. In such situations this Oxford Handbook will be an invaluable pragmatic educational tool.

I wish this book had been available when I started out in nephrology. It would have saved me many anxieties, and I am sure would have improved the care I was able to give.

John Feehally
University of Leicester, UK

Preface

Welcome to the fourth, completely updated, edition of the *Oxford Handbook of Dialysis*, which we hope you will find useful. It has been 7 years since the last edition, and amazingly 15 years since the first edition, and in that time there have been many developments in dialysis and in treating patients with end-stage kidney disease. We now have much better evidence for various interventions (although renal medicine remains relatively poorer at generating high-quality evidence than other areas of medicine), and for the first time now some good trial data to support choices in treating patients, ranging from managing their anaemia or bone disease through to haemodialysis strategies.

We have therefore updated every section of the book which now covers all haemodialysis techniques, haemodiafiltration, nocturnal and home dialysis, frequent dialysis, peritoneal dialysis in all its forms, plasma exchange, the medical, nursing, and psychosocial aspects of managing patients with end-stage kidney disease, nutrition, the acute management of renal transplantation particularly with reference to dialysis patients, palliative and end-of-life care in renal disease and use of analgesics, a completely new section on renal replacement therapy in acute kidney injury, updated drug dosing guidelines including new drugs, and summaries of the most recent guidelines from Europe (European Best Practice Guidelines), the UK Renal Association, the USA (KDOQI and KDIGO) and Australasia. Bone disease, anaemia, cardiovascular disease, infections, pain, and the widespread complications of chronic kidney disease are all discussed, with practical guidance and management, presented in a compact and easy-to-use format.

We have added new sections on home haemodialysis, frequent haemodialysis, new intradialytic monitoring techniques, new peritoneal dialysis fluids, encapsulating peritoneal sclerosis, sleep disorders, management of patients with stroke, care of dying patients with kidney disease or on dialysis, and a new section on acute kidney injury. New drugs such as the new epoetins and phosphate binders are included. We have ensured that the sections on nursing and nutrition for dialysis patients have been written by the appropriate experts, experienced renal nurses and dieticians respectively, and both completely refreshed and updated.

We hope we ensured the book remains easy to use and read, which has always been one of our primary aims, but also comprehensive, focussed, and practical, and clearly aimed at the whole multiprofessional team of colleagues looking after patients on dialysis. We hope this book will have a home in every renal unit, dialysis centre, intensive care unit, renal ward, and be close to hand for every nephrologist, intensivist, renal trainee, renal nurse, dietician, technician, and pharmacist, and that it helps improve the care of patients with kidney disease.

Contents

Contents

Contributors

Rania Betmouni
Department of Pharmacy
Hammersmith Hospital
London, UK

Lina Johansson
Specialist Renal Dietitian
Imperial College Healthcare
NHS Trust
London, UK

Wendy Lawson
Lead Pharmacist
Infectious Diseases Imperial College
Healthcare NHS Trust London, UK

Symbols and abbreviations

➔	cross-reference
~	approximately
↔	normal
↑	increased
↓	decreased
→	leading to
♂	male
♀	female
ACEI	angiotensin-converting enzyme inhibitor
AGE	advanced glycation end-product
AKI	acute kidney injury
ALP	alkaline phosphatase
ALT	alanine aminotransferase
ANA	antinuclear antibody
ANCA	antineutrophil cytoplasmic antibody
APD	automated peritoneal dialysis
aPPT	activated partial thromboplastin time
ARB	angiotensin II receptor blocker
AST	aspartate aminotransferase
AVF	arteriovenous fistula
AVG	arteriovenous graft
AVP	arginine vasopressin
β_2m	β_2 microglobin
β_2mA	β_2 microglobin amyloidosis
bd	twice daily
BP	blood pressure
BVM	bag-valve-mask
C_{crea}	creatinine clearance
CABG	coronary artery bypass grafting
CAD	coronary artery disease
CAPD	continuous ambulatory peritoneal dialysis
cfu	colony-forming units
CNS	central nervous system
CPR	cardiopulmonary resuscitation
CRP	C-reactive protein
CRRT	continuous renal replacement therapy

CVC	central venous catheter
CVP	central venous pressure
CVVH(F)	continuous venovenous haemofiltration
CVVHDF	continuous venovenous haemodiafiltration
DEXA	dual energy X-ray analysis
DNAR	do not attempt resuscitation
DOPPS	Dialysis Outcomes and Practice Patterns Study
DTPA	diethylenetriamine pentaacetic acid
eGFR	estimated glomerular filtration rate
EPO	erythropoietin
EPS	encapsulating peritoneal sclerosis
ESA	erythropoietin-simulating agent
ESKD	end-stage kidney disease (also known as ESRD/ESRF)
FBC	full blood count
FDA	Food and Drug Agency
GBM	glomerular basement membrane
GDP	glucose degradation product
GFR	glomerular filtration rate
GGT	gamma-glutamyltranspeptidase
GI	gastrointestinal
GP	general practitioner
Hb	haemoglobin
HBsAg	hepatitis B surface antigen
Hct	haematocrit
HD	haemodialysis
HDF	haemodiafiltration
HDL	high-density lipoprotein
HLA	human leucocyte antigen
HUS	haemolytic uraemic syndrome
IBW	ideal body weight
ICU	intensive care unit
IDH	intradialytic hypotension
Ig	immunoglobulin
IHD	ischaemic heart disease
INR	international normalized ratio
IP	intraperitoneal
IPD	intermittent peritoneal dialysis
iPTH	intact parathyroid hormone
ISPD	International Society of Peritoneal Dialysis
IV	intravenous

IVIG	intravenous immunoglobulin
JVP	jugular venous pressure
KDOQI	Kidney Disease Outcomes Quality Initiative
LDL	low-density lipoprotein
MI	myocardial infarction
MRSA	meticillin-resistant *Staphylococcus aureus*
MW	molecular weight
NCDS	National Cooperative Dialysis Study
NICE	National Institute of Health and Care Excellence
nPCR	normalized protein catabolic rate
NSAID	non-steroidal anti-inflammatory drug
NSP	non-starch polysaccharide
od	once daily
PCR	protein catabolic rate
PD	peritoneal dialysis
PDC	personal dialysis capacity
PET	peritoneal equilibration test
PMP	per million population
PO	per os; orally
PTA	percutaneous transluminal angioplasty
PTFE	polytetrafluoroethylene
PTH	parathyroid hormone
Qa	access blood flow rate
Qb	blood flow rate
RAS	renin–angiotensin system
RBV	relative blood volume
RCT	randomized controlled trial
RLS	restless leg syndrome
RO	reverse osmosis
RRT	renal replacement therapy
RVD	renovascular disease
SBE	subacute bacterial endocarditis
SC	subcutaneous
SLE	systemic lupus erythematosus
tds	three times daily
TMP	transmembrane pressure
tPA	tissue plasminogen activator
TSAT	transferrin saturation
TTP	thrombocytopenic thrombotic purpura
U&E	urea and electrolytes

UF	ultrafiltration
UFH	unfractionated heparin
UKM	urea kinetic modelling
US	ultrasound
VDRA	vitamin D receptor agonist
VISA/GISA	vancomycin (glycopeptide) intermediate *Staphylococcus aureus*
VRE	vancomycin-resistant *Enterococcus*
VRSA	vancomycin-resistant *Staphylococcus aureus*
WBC	white blood cell
WTE	whole time equivalent

The new patient with renal failure

Incidence and prevalence of kidney disease

End-stage kidney disease (ESKD) is loss of renal function requiring treatment with any form of chronic dialysis or transplantation. Dialysis for acute kidney injury (AKI) is not considered ESKD unless renal function fails to recover. Data on the incidence and prevalence of renal failure are collected by various registries around the world, and in most countries the incidence is increasing. Mean incidence of ESKD across Europe rose from 79 to 117 new patients per million population (PMP) per year between 1990 and 2000, and to 123 PMP by 2010. The highest incidence reported in Europe is from Turkey. (See Table 1.1.)

UK renal registry data

In the UK, 108 new patients PMP were dialysed in 2012 (annual acceptance rate). Median age was 64.6 years (66.1 for white and 57.8 for non-white incident patients). Diabetes now is the single most common renal diagnosis, at 26% for incident (but not prevalent) patients.

United States Renal Data System (USRDS) data

In the USA, 349 new patients PMP/year were dialysed in 2011. Mean age was 62.7 years. Diabetes was the cause of ESKD in 44.7% of patients. There is great ethnic variation, with incidences of 940 for African Americans and 453 for Native Americans—3.4 and 1.6 times greater respectively than the rate of 280 found among the white population.

Table 1.1 International comparisons (2011) from USRDS Atlas of ESRD 2013

ESKD	Incidence (PMP per year)	Prevalence (PMP)
Argentina	156	797
Australia	110	893
Belgium	188	1184
Canada	161	1172
Chile	197	1236
Denmark	111	851
Finland	85	803
France	149	1091
Hong Kong	157	1152
Israel	188	1120
Japan	295	2309
Malaysia	209	980
New Zealand	119	906
Portugal	226	1662
Russia	43	196
Spain	121	1075
Taiwan	361	2584
Turkey	238	868
UK	113	871
USA	362	1924

Definition and prevalence of chronic kidney disease

The Kidney Disease Outcomes Quality Initiative (KDOQI) developed a classification of chronic kidney disease (CKD) in 1997. This classification was refined in 2012 in the CKD guidelines published by KDIGO (Kidney Disease Improving Global Outcomes) to include albuminuria as a predictor of outcome. (See Tables 1.2 and 1.3.)

The prevalence of CKD in the USA has most recently been determined by NHANES (National Health and Nutrition Examination Survey) 1999–2006:

• Stage 3a: 4.6% population
• Stage 3b: 1.6% population
• Stage 4:   0.4% population
• Stage 5:   0.1% population
• Albuminuria A2: 5.4% population
• Albuminuria A3: 1.3% population.

Tables 1.2 Classification of CKD by GFR (KDIGO 2012)

Stage	Description	GFR (mL/min/1.73m²)
1	Kidney damage with normal or high GFR	>90
2	Mild decrease in GFR	60–89
3a	Mild to moderate decrease in GFR	45–59
3b	Moderate to severe decrease in GFR	30–44
4	Severely decreased GFR	15–29
5	Kidney failure	<15 or dialysis

Table 1.3 Albuminuria categories in CKD (KDIGO 2012)

Category	Albumin excretion rate (mg/24h)	Albumin:creatinine ratio (mg/mmol)	Terms
A1	<30	<3	Normal to mildly increased
A2	30–300	3–30	Moderately increased
A3	>300	>30	Severely increased

Referral to a nephrologist
- The figures for prevalence are probably an underestimate.
- Over 19 million of the adult US population have some form of CKD.
- A population survey in the UK (of a predominantly white population) using chemical pathology central records and a serum creatinine of >180µmol/L for men and 135µmol/L for women to define CKD, found a prevalence of 5554 PMP (or 0.55% of the population) for CKD.
- Prevalence increased hugely with age, from 78 PMP in those <40 years to 58,913 PMP in those >80 years.
- A similar survey in Northern Ireland found 1.3% of the population (having a blood test) had a creatinine >150µmol/L, rising to 10.5% of patients with diabetes.
- Nephrologists cannot see all patients with CKD as defined above! Guidelines have been drawn up to try and identify those patients who need referral, those that need ongoing care by nephrologists, and those that can be managed in the community.

When patients should be referred to a nephrologist
- Suspected acute kidney injury
- Estimated glomerular filtration rate (eGFR) <30mL/min/1.73m^2
- eGFR <60mL/min/1.73m^2 and falling >5 mL/min/year or 10mL/min/5 years
- Proteinuria—protein:creatinine ratio >100mg/mmol
- Microscopic haematuria
- Fall in GFR on starting angiotensin-converting enzyme inhibitor (ACEI) or angiotensin II receptor blocker (ARB) >15%
- Possible systemic illness
- Haemoglobin (Hb) <11g/dL
- Electrolyte, calcium, or phosphate disturbance
- Refractory hypertension.

Causes of end-stage kidney disease

The most informative renal dialysis and transplant registries are:
- The USRDS (collects data on >90% of all patients undergoing dialysis in the USA).
- The European Dialysis and Transplant Association (EDTA; data voluntarily supplied from units in 40 countries across Europe; 70% of the patients live in France, Germany, Italy, Spain, or the UK).
- The Australia and New Zealand Dialysis and Transplant Registry (ANZDATA; contains data on all patients in Australia and New Zealand who have received dialysis or a transplant since 1980).
- The UK Renal Registry: collects data on almost all patients on dialysis in the UK. (See Table 1.4.)

Arteriopathic renal diseases

Include hypertension, malignant hypertension, renal artery stenosis or occlusion. Hypertensive diseases represent 26% of all primary diagnoses in the USRDS, but <10% in Europe.

Glomerulonephritis

The most common cause of renal failure in Australia and New Zealand (23% of all patients) and common in Europe (up to 25%), but only the third major cause the USA (17%). Only two-thirds of these have a defined histological diagnosis. In some registries, patients can be labelled as likely GN (not biopsy proven).

Diabetes

The most common cause of renal failure in the USA and many other countries (Australia, New Zealand, Mexico, and others). In the USA, ~40% of new patients starting dialysis had diabetes. The proportion of patients with diabetes has doubled over the last 20 years. Surprisingly low prevalence in the UK ESKD population but increasing. Over the last couple of years the relative increase in diabetic patients reaching ESKD seems to have slowed.

Table 1.4 Causes of ESKD across the world (most recent data usually 2011/12). Percentage of all patients in each registry with each diagnosis

Primary renal disease	ANZDATA	UK	USRDS
Glomerulonephritis (GN)	23	19	17
Diabetes	35	16	39
Hypertension/renovascular	15	9	26
Infective or obstructive nephropathies (inc. reflux)	3	11	4
Cystic or congenital disease	6	10	7
Miscellaneous	12	18	3
Unknown	6	17	4

Infective and obstructive nephropathy

Includes reflux, pyelonephritis, chronic interstitial nephritis, urolithiasis, and congenital and acquired obstructive nephropathies. Common cause of renal replacement therapy (RRT) in Europe and UK, but rare in other registries.

Familial disease

Predominantly adult (autosomal dominant) polycystic kidney disease but also includes oxalosis, Fabry's disease, cystinosis, Alport's syndrome, and tuberose sclerosis.

Miscellaneous

Analgesic and gouty nephropathy, cortical necrosis, tuberculosis (TB), human immunodeficiency virus (HIV) nephropathy, sickle cell disease, radiation nephritis, sarcoidosis, and traumatic renal loss. Specific toxins such as lead, cadmium, lithium, and ciclosporin are more regionally confined. Also includes acute interstitial nephritis. Neoplasms are a rare cause of ESKD, but include myeloma, amyloidosis, light chain deposition disease, and renal tract tumours.

Causes of acute kidney injury

The most common causes of AKI occurring in hospitals are pre-renal disease (volume depletion, dehydration, cardiac failure or sepsis) and acute tubular necrosis (ATN; ischaemia or nephrotoxins). The distinction between pre-renal, intrinsic renal and post-renal causes for AKI is useful in excluding possible causes of acutely impaired real function. (See Box 1.1.)

Many of these are treatable, with excellent recovery of renal function:

• ATN, rhabdomyolysis, and toxic nephropathy usually recover over a period of days to a few weeks.
• Obstruction can be relieved surgically or percutaneously, and renal function returns often within a couple of days.
• Most causes of rapidly progressive GN (RPGN) can be successfully treated with immunosuppression. Almost all patients with antineutrophil cytoplasmic antibody (ANCA)-associated disease will recover renal function, even with severe renal failure, while those with moderate renal failure caused by anti-glomerular basement membrane (GBM) disease will also recover.
• Acute interstitial nephritis, acute pyelonephritis, and accelerated hypertension also have a good prognosis (at least in the short term).
• Myeloma cast nephropathy, haemolytic uraemic syndrome (HUS), and atheroembolism have poorer outcomes, with significant numbers of patients failing to recover renal function.

Box 1.1 Causes of hospital-acquired AKI (but huge variations between individual hospitals)

• ATN	45%
• Pre-renal	21%
• Acute on chronic renal failure (usually ATN)	13%
• Urinary tract obstruction	10%
• GN or vasculitis	4%
• Acute interstitial nephritis	2%
• Atheroembolic disease	1%.

ICU AKI

In ICUs, 10–30% of patients develop AKI, with high mortality rates (30–70%). Many of these patients have multiorgan failure, rather than isolated renal failure, and a significant number of survivors require long-term RRT. Prognosis is usually dependent on the co-morbid conditions and number of organs failing, rather than the presence of renal failure per se.

Modality of renal replacement therapy worldwide

In the USA, 91.3% of patients with ESKD receive in-centre haemodialysis (HD), 1.3% home HD, and 7.4% peritoneal dialysis (PD), with marked geographic variation. The number of new patients starting PD per year has fallen in the USA from a peak of 9407 in 1995 to 6875 in 2005, but with a slight subsequent increase to 7387 in 2011.

Home HD is becoming more popular in many countries but rates vary considerably; it is most common in New Zealand (18%), Australia (9%), and Canada (4%), but in many countries comprises <1% of the dialysis population. PD is most widely used in Hong Kong (74% of ESKD patients), New Zealand (33%), Canada, Australia, and Denmark. Renal transplantation remains the most successful form of RRT. Rates vary from 61 PMP in Norway, 57 PMP in the USA, 53 PMP in Spain, 44 PMP in the UK, 38 PMP in Canada, 27 PMP in New Zealand, and 9 PMP in Hong Kong. (See Table 1.5.)

Cost of ESKD

In the USA, the total direct medical payment for ESKD exceeds US$21 billion. This is expected to double by 2020. Figures from other countries are difficult to obtain. A dialysis patient costs US$34,000 as an outpatient per year, or US$77,000 per year, including hospital admissions. In the UK, total costs for dialysis patients are ~£35,000/year, mostly for dialysis itself and transport (to and from the dialysis unit). Comparable figures for Spain are ~38,000 euro/year, and for Australia ~$Au 200,000 (~100,000 euro).

Table 1.5 HD popularity worldwide

	In-centre HD	Home HD	PD
USA	91	1	7
UK	82	3	15
Australia	72	9	19
Canada	79	4	17
Chile	95	0	5
Denmark	75	5	20
Finland	77	4	19
France	89	1	10
Hong Kong	24	1.5	74
Israel	94	0	6
Japan	97	0	3
New Zealand	49	18	33
Portugal	94	0	6
Russia	92	0	8
Taiwan	90	0	10
Turkey	92	0	8

Patient survival with ESKD

Survival rates of patients starting RRT continue to improve year on year. In the UK, 87% of patients survive 1 year (after the first 90 days). 6% of patients die within the first 90 days. 5-year survivals range from 87% for those aged 18–34, 67% for those aged 45–54, and 29% for those aged 65–74.

USRDS data exclude the first 90 days of care and exclude patients who die within this time. Over the last decade, the overall 1st year death rate for patients has not changed significantly and is ~23 deaths per 100 patient years. 1-year survival is ~80% overall. 5-year survival, however, continues to rise and is 35% overall for all dialysis modalities.

In the USA, patients starting dialysis aged 15–19 have an estimated 17 remaining years of life compared with 61 years for the general population; for those aged 30–34 years these figures are 11 and 47 years, respectively; for those aged 50–54 years, 6 and 27 years, respectively; and for those aged 60–65 years, 4.5 and 21 years, respectively. Survival is increased in American black people and worse in diabetics. Dialysis does not prolong life!

Co-morbidity

Increasingly common in new patients with ESKD; overall 55% of patients in the UK were reported to have one or more co-morbidities: 29% diabetes, 24% ischaemic heart disease, 17% angina, 13% peripheral vascular disease, 10% cerebrovascular disease or previous cerebrovascular accident, 7% chronic obstructive pulmonary disease (COPD), and 12% cancer. Diabetes is reported in 25% of ESKD patients in Australia, 36% in Germany, and 44% in the USA.

Cause of death in ESKD

Overall, cardiac arrest, acute myocardial infarction (MI), and other cardiac causes account for half of the reported deaths in ESKD patients. Infection is the next major cause (25%) and cerebrovascular disease is the third largest cause of death (6%). One in five dialysis patients withdraws from dialysis before death in the USA because of failure to thrive or medical complications. Withdrawal is more common in older, white dialysis patients. Withdrawal rates in the USA are higher than in most other countries, possibly because of the initial acceptance of patients with marginal benefit from dialysis. In the UK, 35% patients die from cardiac disease, 20% from infection, 13% from stopping dialysis, 9% from malignancies, and 7% from cerebrovascular disease.

Presentation of renal disease

Patients with renal failure present with the relatively non-specific symptoms of renal impairment (see ➔ Presenting clinical features of ESKD, p. 14), with symptoms attributable to an underlying systemic disease, e.g. vasculitis, systemic lupus erythematosus (SLE), myeloma, hypertension, or because a doctor has found an elevated urea or creatinine, or performed urinalysis. The key task of the nephrologist is to identify the underlying disease, and to distinguish possibly recoverable AKI from ESKD.

Other roles of the nephrologist include:
- establishing the precise degree of renal impairment
- detecting and correcting reversible factors
- correcting and minimizing the complications of renal failure
- detecting and treating coincidental and co-morbid diseases
- assessing social circumstances
- assessing the patient's understanding of the disease and its prognosis
- planning follow-up, management, and potential future dialysis and transplantation needs
- providing a clear explanation to the patient and family.

Reversible causes of AKI must be promptly diagnosed and treated:
- ureteric or bladder outflow obstruction
- anti-GBM disease or vasculitis (especially ANCA associated)
- other causes of RPGN (SLE, crescentic primary GN)
- acute interstitial nephritis
- accelerated hypertension
- renal vascular disease
- acute pyelonephritis (especially in diabetics, transplant recipients)
- drug-induced renal failure
- ATN
- rhabdomyolysis
- myeloma cast nephropathy.

Presenting clinical features of ESKD

In approximate order of frequency:
- Anorexia
- Nausea and vomiting
- Fatigue and weakness
- Pruritus
- Lethargy
- Peripheral oedema
- Dyspnoea
- Insomnia
- Bleeding tendency
- Pulmonary oedema
- Apathy
- Muscle cramps
- Feeling cold
- Raynaud's phenomenon
- Metabolic flap
- Nocturia, polyuria
- Headache
- Pericarditis
- Fever
- Cough
- Diarrhoea
- Constipation
- Seizures
- Hiccough
- Restless legs
- Growth retardation is very common in children.

Sexual dysfunction (loss of libido, impotence, and infertility) is rarely volunteered spontaneously, but is extremely common (in men and women). It may be caused by the renal failure itself or a variety of prescribed drugs.

Neuropathy, cognitive impairment, confusion, coma and proximal myopathy are now very rare features of ESKD.

Additional features in AKI
- Visible haematuria
- Loin pain
- Haemoptysis
- Rash
- Neuropathy
- Infections
- Predisposing factors, e.g. hypotension, drug use, hypovolaemia.

Examination findings in ESKD

Often depend on the length of history of CKD, and time of referral to nephrologist. Early referral can often prevent these signs developing by appropriate and timely interventions (e.g. erythropoietin (EPO) therapy, control of Ca and PO_4 balance, blood pressure (BP) control).

- Skin pigmentation or excoriation
- Anaemia
- Hypertension
- Postural hypotension
- Oedema
- Left ventricular hypertrophy (LVH)
- Peripheral vascular disease
- Arterial bruits
- Respiratory crackles
- Pleural effusions
- Palpable kidneys (polycystic) or liver
- Abdominal scars
- Peripheral neuropathy
- Proximal myopathy
- Corneal calcification
- Retinal fundal examination (hypertension or diabetes).

Urine may show a variety of changes depending on the cause of renal failure (haematuria, proteinuria, casts).

See Table 1.6 for investigations for patients with ESKD.

Table 1.6 Baseline investigations in patients with ESKD	
Sodium	Usually normal, but may be low with water overload
Potassium	Raised—often with precipitant, e.g. diet, ACEIs, transfusion, surgery, gastrointestinal (GI) bleed, potassium-sparing diuretics
Bicarbonate	Low
Chloride	Normal in renal tubular acidosis
Urea	Affected by protein intake, hydration, liver disease
Creatinine	Affected by muscle mass and increasing tubular secretion with advancing renal impairment
Albumin	Reflects urinary losses, protein intake and hepatic synthesis. Low levels (<40) at start of RRT strongly associated with poor prognosis
Calcium	May be normal, low, or high depending on parathyroid activity
Phosphate	Rises late in CKD. Ca–P product predictor of metastatic calcification

Table 1.6 (Contd.)

Alkaline phosphatase	Raised in hyperparathyroidism or osteomalacia (bone isoenzyme)
Aspartate aminotransferase and bilirubin	Normal unless liver disease
Glucose	Undiagnosed diabetes (type II) common, especially in Asian populations
Parathyroid hormone (PTH)	Raised progressively in renal impairment
Cholesterol and triglycerides	Both may be raised—cardiovascular disease major cause of morbidity and mortality
Hb	Usually low (less commonly in polycystic disease). Exclude other haematinic deficiency or haemoglobinopathy as necessary
Ferritin, iron, transferrin saturation	Large iron stores required for effective use of EPO. Relative iron deficiency nearly universal
White cells	Usually normal unless SLE, drugs, etc.
Platelets	Usually normal unless drugs, hypersplenism, aplasia
Clotting	Usually normal except prolonged bleeding time
Blood grouping	For cross-matching as necessary, and for transplant purposes
Human leucocyte antigen (HLA) tissue typing	As pre-transplant investigation
Cytotoxic antibodies	Especially in women and those who have received blood transfusions
Hepatitis serology	Define baseline hepatitis B virus (HBV) and hepatitis C virus (HCV) status. Vaccinate non-immune patients (HBV). Hepatitis B serum antigen (HBsAg)-positive patients should have eAg and eAb status defined
Cytomegalovirus (CMV) serology	Pre-transplant assessment
HIV	All patients should be counselled and screened pre-transplant, and in some units pre-dialysis
ECG	For LVH and ischaemia
Echocardiography	If indicated for ventricular function, hypertrophy, ischaemia, chamber dilatation
Chest X-ray (CXR)	Cardiomegaly
Bone X-rays (hands, spine)	If evidence of hyperparathyroidism
Renal ultrasound	To confirm diagnosis or exclude treatable acute on chronic cause

Other tests as necessary, e.g. complements, antinuclear antibody (ANA), lupus anticoagulant, ANCA, anti-GBM antibodies, thyroid function, cryoglobulins, protein electrophoresis.

Assessment of kidney function at/near end stage: serum biochemistry

Serum creatinine

Serum creatinine is an unreliable marker of renal function in ESKD.

- Produced from the breakdown of creatine phosphate in muscle at a constant rate ($\circlearrowleft$ 15–25mg/kg body weight/day, $\circlearrowright$ 10–20mg/kg per day).
- Excreted predominantly by filtration without reabsorption.
- Tubular secretion also plays a part in creatinine excretion.
- For most patients serial plasma creatinine measurements can be used to monitor change in renal function (deterioration or improvement). However, early in the development of renal impairment, plasma creatinine may not increase as GFR declines because of increased tubular secretion of creatinine. This process becomes saturated at a plasma creatinine of ~140–170µmol/L. Thereafter, a further decline in GFR will manifest as a rise in serum creatinine.
- Near ESKD, increasing uraemia will often be associated with a decline in dietary intake, and further rises in serum creatinine will not occur as GFR falls. In fact, low serum creatinine is associated with higher mortality.
- Finally, creatinine generation rates decline with advancing renal failure.

Other factors affecting serum creatinine include:

- dietary meat intake
- drugs inhibiting tubular creatinine secretion (cimetidine, trimethoprim, cobicistat among others, can increase serum creatinine by up to 50µmol/L)
- interference with colorimetric creatinine assays (especially ketones, cefoxitin, and flucytosine) increases the reported value by up to 40µmol/L
- women, children, the elderly, and those with reduced muscle bulk also have reduced creatinine generation rates, and hence will have a lower serum creatinine for a given GFR
- protein and creatine supplements.

Blood urea

A less useful measure of renal function because:

- rate of production is not constant (increasing with high-protein diets, tissue breakdown, steroids, and haemorrhage, and low in liver disease and low-protein diets)
- 40–50% of filtered urea is reabsorbed in the proximal tubule
- volume depletion will enhance urea reabsorption together with salt and water retention in the proximal tubule (under the action of arginine vasopressin (AVP)).

Urea clearance can be a useful measure, but underestimates GFR.

Assessment of kidney function at/near end stage: reciprocal creatinine plots

Serial creatinine measurements can be graphed as their reciprocal against time (usually on a logarithmic scale). Many patients will show a linear decline in renal function when expressed in this manner, which can be useful in assessing the rate of decline in renal function. The method has all the same potential problems as isolated measurement of serum creatinine, but has the advantage of a graphical output that may help both patient and doctor appreciate the decline in function with time. Individual patients have varying slopes of their reciprocal creatinine plots. (See Figs 1.1 and 1.2.)

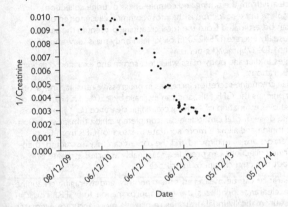

Fig. 1.1 Decline in renal function over time as demonstrated by a reciprocal creatinine plot.

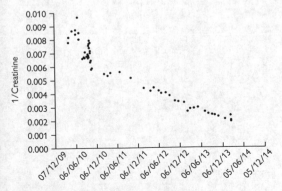

Fig. 1.2 Decline in renal function over time as demonstrated by a reciprocal creatinine plot.

Assessment of kidney function at/near end stage: creatinine clearance

Can be determined from a timed urine collection (usually 24h) and contemporaneous plasma sample:

$$Creatinine\ clearance\ (mL/min) = \frac{Urine\ volume \times Urine\ [creatinine]}{Plasma\ [creatinine] \times 1440}$$

- Errors arise from tubular secretion of creatinine (overestimates GFR by 10–15%), from variability in the assay for creatinine (10–15%), and particularly from the timing and completeness of urine collection.
- Incomplete urine collection is the most common cause for error, and can be estimated from the total creatinine present in the sample. Men usually excrete 175–220μmol/kg lean body mass/day, and women130–175μmol/kg per day.
- Changes in diet and body mass will affect serum and excreted creatinine concentrations.
- Tubular creatinine secretion increases in progressive renal failure (acute or chronic) as the GFR falls, and can increase by >50%. This can lead to a gross overestimation of GFR by creatinine clearance (C_{crea}) measures. A single dose of oral cimetidine can completely inhibit tubular secretion of creatinine and allow a more accurate measure of GFR from C_{crea}.
- If the errors are all minimized and the patient carefully instructed, then 24h urine collections can provide a reasonably accurate estimate of GFR, but this rarely happens in practice.

Urea clearance can be measured simultaneously, and averaging creatinine and urea clearance produces the best approximation for GFR. This can be done automatically in laboratories to provide more accurate estimates of GFR.

Assessment of kidney function at/near end stage: eGFR and calculated creatinine clearance

Estimating GFR by calculation from serum creatinine has become the most common method for measuring renal function (eGFR) and, although there are concerns about the accuracy of this in some circumstances, overall eGFR represents a major benefit in identifying reduced GFR. Although alternative methods of estimating GFR have been developed, e.g. from cystatin C, creatinine-based equations remain the standard method for estimating GFR clinically (KDIGO CKD guidelines 2012).

MDRD (modification of diet in renal disease) and CKD-EPI formulae for eGFR

For patients with known renal disease the MDRD formula is more accurate, estimates GFR rather than C_{crea}, and includes factors for race and serum albumin. It is corrected for body surface area (BSA). It is less accurate in patients with either very poor levels of renal function or near normal function.

In SI units:

$$GFR/1.73m^2 = 170 \times PCr\ (\mu mol/L) \times 0.0113^{-0.999}$$
$$\times Age^{-0.176} \times (Urea(mmol/L) \times 2.8)^{-0.17} \times Albumin^{0.318}$$
$$\times [0.762\ if\ female] \times [1.18\ if\ black].$$

In conventional units:

$$GFR/1.73m^2 = 170 \times PCr(mg/dL)^{-0.999} \times age^{-0.176}$$
$$\times Serum\ Urea\ Nitrogen\ (mg/dL)^{-0.17} \times Albumin^{0.318}$$
$$\times [0.762\ if\ female] \times [1.18\ if\ black].$$

A simple variant using only serum creatinine, age, and sex is almost as accurate:

$$GFR/1.73m^2 = 186.3 \times (SCr\ (\mu mol/L) \times 0.0113)^{-1.154}$$
$$\times (age)^{-0.203} \times 0.742\ (if\ female).$$

These formulae will overestimate C_{crea} in patients on low-protein (or low-meat) diets, but are otherwise reasonably accurate. They are not of value in patients with rapidly changing renal function.

The CKD-EPI study equation may be slightly more accurate especially at higher levels of GFR:

$$GFR/1.73m^2 = 141 \times min(Scr/\kappa,1)^\alpha \times max(Scr/\kappa,1)^{1.2090} \times 0.993^{Age} \times 1.018 \text{ [if female]} \times 1.159 \text{ [if black]}$$

where Scr is serum creatinine (mg/dL), κ is 0.7 for females and 0.9 for males, α is −0.329 for females and −0.411 for males, min indicates the minimum of Scr/κ or 1, and max indicates the maximum of Scr/κ or 1.

The formulae are available through many websites, e.g. ℠ www.renal.org, www.nephron.com, www.hdcn.com.

Cockroft–Gault formula

This was developed to calculate C_{crea} based on plasma creatinine. It has all the potential problems for all formulae based on serum creatinine. In conventional units:

$$CCr \ (mL/min) = \frac{(140 - Age \ (years)) \times weight \ (kg)}{72 \times PCr \ (mg/dl)}$$

For women multiply by 85 (not 72).

In SI units:

$$CCr \ (mL/min) = \frac{1.23 \times (140 - Age \ (years)) \times weight \ (kg)}{PCr \ (\mu mol/l)}$$

For women multiply by 1.04 rather than 1.23.

Calculated C_{crea} is often more reliable than 24h urine collections due to the inaccuracies in the urine collection itself. The calculation is still based on serum creatinine and will thus be inaccurate in patients with low muscle bulk, and has not been fully validated in children, pregnancy, and the very elderly. It is not accurate in normal renal function and cannot be used to estimate true GFR accurately in this setting.

This method is reasonably reliable in mild renal impairment but overestimates GFR by up to 100% as GFR falls to 10mL/min. The eGFR calculated from the MDRD equation is a better alternative. The only exception may be in drug dosing since the eGFR is normalized for BSA while conventionally the Cockroft–Gault calculation is not, and includes patient body weight which might be relevant in drug distribution.

Assessment of kidney function at/near end stage: other methods

Pre-dialysis Kt/V

Kinetic methods may be a more reliable measure of renal function in patients close to dialysis, but are not familiar to non-nephrologists. Mean normalized urea clearance (daily Kt/V) can be calculated using a 24h urine collection for measurement of urea clearance (multiply × 7 = Kt for a weekly figure), and estimating V from the patient's height and weight. Alternatively, Kt/V can be calculated using the same computerized models as in dialysis patients on the basis of a 24h urine urea quantitation and plasma urea. Using conventional criteria for institution of dialysis, many patients have a daily pre-dialysis Kt/V of ~0.15 when dialysis is begun, which would be considered underdialysis in a patient established on HD (daily Kt/V ~0.5). Using Kt/V as the measure of renal function in patients with CKD will generally prompt earlier initiation of dialysis and also provides a better measure of nutritional status by the simultaneous calculation of normalized protein catabolic rate (nPCR). Dialysis should be considered when the weekly Kt/V <2.0 or nPCR <0.8.

Isotopic measures

More accurate measures of GFR use [^{51}Cr]EDTA, [^{99m}Tc]DTPA, or [^{125}I] iothalamate clearance, and overestimate GFR by only a few mL/min (very little secretion). They require IV injection of radiolabelled compound, and subsequent blood sampling to measure rate of loss of isotope from blood. DTPA clearance can be determined by external gamma camera counting over the kidneys to estimate the proportion of the isotope taken up by the kidneys after a given time. In severe renal failure, isotopic methods are more reliable measures of renal function than serum creatinine or C_{crea}. Non-isotopic indicator decay methods include iohexol clearance.

Cystatin C

An endogenous cysteine protease inhibitor produced by almost all nucleated cells at a constant rate, regardless of volume status, inflammation, or drug interactions. Measurement reflects GFR more accurately than serum creatinine. Routine assays are still not available.

Complications of renal failure: symptomatic

Complications of renal failure include immediate symptomatic problems and more long-term effects on rate of deterioration of renal function or future morbidity and mortality. (See Table 1.7.)

Symptomatic complications

Cardiovascular disease

This is the major complication of renal disease; many more patients will die from a cardiovascular event than develop ESKD.

- Long-term follow-up studies of general health in the USA (National Health and Nutrition Examination Survey (NHANES) II) have shown that cardiovascular mortality is almost doubled in people with GFR <70mL/min, i.e. even with very moderate renal impairment.
- Presence of microalbuminuria (in diabetics and non-diabetics) doubles cardiovascular mortality.
- Overt proteinuria (>300mg/24h) trebles or quadruples risk of cardiovascular events and death.
- There is an increased mortality in patients known to have cardiovascular disease if renal impairment also present.

Table 1.7 Major complications of renal failure

Symptomatic	Cardiovascular disease
	Anaemia
	Renal bone disease
	Malnutrition
	Growth retardation in children
	Fluid overload
	Pericarditis
Metabolic and/or risk factor for future event	Hypertension
	Lipid abnormalities
	LVH
	Vascular calcification and stiffness
	Hyperkalaemia
	Acidosis
	Secondary hyperparathyroidism
	Hyperphosphataemia
	Inflammatory state

- Large epidemiological studies have shown that risk of cardiovascular events increases as GFR falls below 60mL/min, with risk increased 2- to 4-fold for stages 4 and 5 CKD. One study has shown that the risk of a cardiac event is increased 100-fold for a 40-year-old man on dialysis compared with what is expected if renal function is normal.

Risk factors for cardiovascular disease in renal patients

Many are the same as in the general population, although some may be more common in patients with renal disease, e.g. hypertension, lipid abnormalities, diabetes, male sex, and LVH.

Anaemia

Contributes towards the tiredness experienced by patients with renal failure. Also predisposes to LVH (an independent cardiovascular risk factor). Data from several national registries show that patients starting dialysis with a higher Hb survive longer.

- Hb can start to fall when GFR declines to 30–40mL/min.
- Failure of EPO production is the major cause of renal anaemia, although it is essential to check other haematinics (iron, plasma vitamin B_{12}, and red cell folate levels). Haemoglobinopathies, such as thalassaemia, should also be considered.
- Many patients will respond to oral iron treatment.
- Recent trials of early use of EPO in pre-dialysis patients have suggested an increased mortality in patients with Hb >13g/dL.
- UK National Institute for Health and Care Excellence (NICE) guidelines state a Hb target of 10.5–12.5g/dL.
- US KDOQI guidelines state a Hb target of 11–12g/dL and no greater than 13g/dL.
- Use of IV iron and EPO to achieve these targets is discussed in Management of renal failure: treatment of anaemia, p. 42.

Complications of renal failure: renal bone disease

Caused mainly by hyperparathyroidism and osteomalacia. Develops at a relatively early stage of renal failure when the GFR starts to fall below 30–40mL/min. The underlying cause is decreased production of 1,25 dihydroxy vitamin D by the failing kidney. This results in decreased intestinal calcium absorption and hypocalcaemia. Low plasma calcium and 1,25 vitamin D levels both cause increased secretion of PTH. Retention of phosphate also stimulates PTH secretion. Early manifestations of hyperparathyroidism are biochemical: hyperphosphataemia, hypocalcaemia, and raised plasma PTH levels. Symptoms develop later and consist of bone and joint pains, and pruritus. Closely linked with the development of cardiovascular disease. See ⊃ Treatment of renal bone disease, p. 492, for management. (See Fig 1.3.)

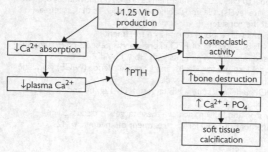

Fig. 1.3 Mechanisms underlying renal bone disease.

Complications of renal failure: malnutrition

Poor nutrition

This is a predictor of poor outcome at the start of dialysis. It develops as patients become anorectic. Patients spontaneously reduce their protein intake as well as their overall calorie intake, and some become severely cachectic. There are various biochemical markers of nutrition, but the most easily measured is plasma albumin. Low albumin may also reflect ongoing inflammation rather than nutritional status. Restrictive diets, persistent heavy proteinuria, coexisting disease, and increasing age are all risk factors for malnutrition.

Growth retardation

This is a major complication of renal failure in children; the younger the child when renal failure develops, the more severe the growth retardation. At early ages, reduced growth rate is predominantly due to poor nutrition; around puberty, retardation is due to insensitivity to the action of growth hormone.

Complications of renal failure: fluid overload

This is both a complication and a mode of presentation of severe renal failure.
- Clinical features are ankle oedema, pulmonary oedema, pleural effusions, and ascites. (See Table 1.8.)
- Clinical examination findings will depend on the degree of fluid retention:
  - if mild—ankle oedema alone
  - in more severe fluid overload—more extensive oedema and pulmonary oedema
  - high BP (can differentiate from fluid overload of heart failure).
- Patients with coexisting cardiac disease will be at increased risk of developing pulmonary oedema with fluid overload.
- The simplest way to monitor changes in fluid control is by body weight. An increase in weight by 1kg equates to retention of 1L of fluid. This is only true over short periods of time, or if the body weight is constant. If the patient is anorectic and losing flesh weight, he/she could become fluid overloaded with little change in total body weight.
- Measurement of bioimpedance can provide an accurate measure of fluid overload but is not routinely available.
- Chest ultrasound imaging where available for 'comet-tails' or 'lung rockets' can provide an accurate marker of increased extravascular lung water.

Table 1.8 Clinical features of fluid overload

Symptoms	Shortness of breath
	Paroxysmal nocturnal dyspnoea
	Ankle swelling
Signs	Raised jugular venous pressure (JVP)
	Basal crepitations
	Generalized oedema
	Increasing weight
	Rise in BP

Complications of renal failure: metabolic

Lipid abnormalities

Occur in all patients with heavy proteinuria. The main abnormality is a raised plasma cholesterol level, which occurs as hepatic synthesis is increased. Lipoprotein (a) levels start to rise as soon as microalbuminuria appears as the first manifestation of renal disease in diabetics. The hyperlipidaemia of renal disease contributes to the high incidence of cardiovascular disease and may play a role in the progression of renal damage. Patients without proteinuria may have relatively increased serum triglycerides, and dysregulation of normal apolipoprotein metabolism. (See Fig 1.4 and Table 1.9.)

Hyperkalaemia

A potentially fatal complication of renal failure. As potassium is predominantly an intracellular ion, a small shift of potassium from the intracellular to extracellular space will cause a rise in plasma potassium.

Acidosis

Invariably occurs with severe renal failure but is found at an earlier stage in tubulointerstitial renal diseases. Unless severe (when hyperventilation occurs), acidosis itself will not cause symptoms. Bone disease, muscle catabolism (leading to negative nitrogen balance), poor nutrition, and growth retardation in children are all exacerbated by acidosis. Acidosis also predisposes to hyperkalaemia, and is associated with a faster decline in renal function.

Inflammation

Is part of the MIA syndrome (malnutrition, inflammation, atherosclerosis), which is a feature of the normal ageing process, but is exacerbated by renal failure. Markers of inflammation (C-reactive protein (CRP), interleukin-6) increase with age and decreasing GFR, and are associated with vascular disease and malnutrition.

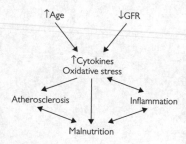

Fig. 1.4 Metabolic complications of renal failure

Table 1.9 Causes of hyperkalaemia in renal failure

Increased potassium intake	Dietary intake
	Potassium supplements (oral or IV)
	Absorption from blood (haematoma or GI bleed)
Shift of potassium from cells	Acidosis
	Muscle breakdown
	Released from red blood cells after transfusion
Decreased renal excretion	Worsening renal failure
	Potassium-sparing diuretics
Decreased secretion in collecting duct (i.e. ↓ aldosterone action)	Spironolactone
	ACEIs
	ARBs
	Ciclosporin
	Tacrolimus

Complications of renal failure: cardiovascular

Pericarditis

Occurs only in severe renal failure. Chest pain is not invariable and the diagnosis is made by detecting a pericardial rub. The pericardial effusion is usually haemorrhagic and may be large enough to cause tamponade. Pericarditis is now a rare complication as dialysis is commenced earlier.

Hypertension

Almost invariable in renal disease, even when there is minimal deterioration in renal function. Detection of hypertension is often the initial presentation of renal disease. Control of hypertension is vital to minimize cardiovascular risk and LVH. Hypertension control is the most effective method of slowing the rate of progression of most types of renal disease.

Left ventricular hypertrophy

Develops because of hypertension and anaemia. LVH is an independent risk factor for cardiovascular disease and poor survival on dialysis.

Vascular calcification

More common in ESKD than in patients with other causes for vascular disease, and includes the heart valves. Associated with stiffening of arteries. Multiple predisposing factors, including hyperparathyroidism, inflammation, hyperphosphataemia, calcium loading in the form of calcium-containing phosphate binders, and use of vitamin D metabolites.

Management of renal failure: aims

The aims of management of renal disease are:
- diagnosis and treatment of reversible causes
- slow rate of progression of renal damage
- minimize cardiovascular risk
- BP control slows the rate of progression of renal damage and minimizes cardiovascular risk
- control dyslipidaemia—minimizes cardiovascular risk and may slow down rate of progression of renal damage
- identify and treat complications—particularly anaemia and hyperparathyroidism (can occur even in stage 3 CKD when GFR is in the 30–40mL/min range)
- prevention of symptoms—mainly those due to fluid overload or uraemia
- start planning and education for dialysis or conservative care
- start planning and education for transplantation if appropriate.

Management of renal failure: blood pressure control

This is the cornerstone of management of CKD. Factors to consider are:
- What level is control?
- Which drugs to use?
- Achievement of control.

What level of BP is control?

Most guidelines for BP control have had targets that are often difficult to achieve in practice. More recent guidelines have recognized that targets should be graded depending on age. The most recent UK guidelines for the first time recommended 24h ambulatory recording in all patients, with evidence for cost saving. (See Table 1.10.)

NICE/British Hypertension Society guidelines 2011
- Aim for target clinic BP <140/90 mmHg in people aged <80 years
- Aim for target clinic BP <150/90 mmHg in people aged ≥80 years
- When using ambulatory or home BP monitoring, aim for target average BP during person's waking hours of:
  - <135/85 mmHg for people aged <80 years
  - <145/85 mmHg for people aged ≥80 years.

Table 1.10 Guidelines for BP control in CKD

Renal Association (2011)	BP <140/90 mmHg
	If diabetes or proteinuria >1g/24h,
	BP target lowered to <130/80 mmHg
KDIGO (2012)	BP <140/90 mmHg
	If diabetes or proteinuria >1g/24h,
	BP target lowered to <130/80 mmHg
	Treat elderly patients with caution; consider age, co-morbidities, and possible adverse events such as postural hypotension and drug side effects

Management of renal failure: which drugs for BP?

Which antihypertensive drugs should be used?

Some drugs may have an additional renoprotective effect in addition to lowering BP.

- ACEIs or ARBs minimize the effect of angiotensin II on the kidney, reduce proteinuria, and cause dilatation of the efferent arteriole with increased blood flow. They also reduce the growth factor activity of angiotensin II in the kidney.
- Both ACEIs and ARBs have been shown to reduce proteinuria more than any other class of drugs.
- There is evidence in diabetic and non-diabetic renal disease that the addition of an ACEI for BP control results in a slower rate of deterioration in renal function, particularly when proteinuria is present.
- ARBs have also been shown to reduce the rate of decline of renal function in diabetic nephropathy (in type II diabetes mellitus (DM)).
- ACEIs and ARBs have been used in combination to provide maximal suppression of the renin–angiotensin system (RAS) and maximal reduction in proteinuria, but studies have shown that this approach results in more side effects such as hyperkalaemia and AKI with no benefit regarding renoprotection, especially in patients with diabetes. *ACEIs and ARBs should therefore no longer be routinely prescribed together.*
- Both ACEIs and ARBs are contraindicated for patients with known renovascular disease (RVD) and should be used with caution in patients at risk of having RVD. They both block efferent arteriolar constriction caused by angiotensin II, and the resultant efferent arteriolar dilatation leads to a drop in glomerular perfusion and hence a decrease in GFR.
- Hyperkalaemia can be a complication of either drug, particularly if they are used in combination.
- Calcium antagonists cause afferent arteriolar dilatation with increased blood flow through the kidney. They also inhibit the action of many growth factors in the kidney. Their effect on proteinuria is variable and not as marked as with ACEIs.
- Calcium antagonists have not been shown to have a direct renoprotective effect, but remain a very important group of drugs to achieve BP control.
- Use of diuretics enhance actions of ACEI and ARBs on BP lowering and reduction of proteinuria, but may cause deterioration in renal function. May also worsen metabolic control of glucose, lipids, and uric acid.
- Spironolactone may be a useful additional drug at higher levels of renal function, but has to be used with caution as renal function deteriorates because of risk of hyperkalaemia—best avoided if patient also on an ACEI and an ARB.

Management of renal failure: how to achieve blood pressure control

This involves careful monitoring of the patient and selection of appropriate drugs. Compliance is a major problem, so drugs chosen should have minimal side effects and preferably need to be taken only once a day, with long duration of action to achieve full 24h BP control (but reduce dose if renally excreted when renal function declines). The following are useful guidelines for controlling BP in renal disease:

* In diabetics, and non-diabetics with proteinuria >1g/24h, use an ACEI or ARB unless the patient is at risk of having RVD. Use an ARB if the patient develops a cough on an ACEI.
* Dose of ACEI or ARB should be increased to full dose (if tolerated) to provide maximal reduction of proteinuria (independent of BP lowering).
* If BP not controlled, the logical next choice is to use a drug raising renin levels as this will enhance the action of the ACEI or ARB:
  * note: thiazides are not effective in patients with low GFR
  * loop diuretics (bumetanide, furosemide) should be used with caution, as GFR will decrease further if patient becomes volume depleted; a modest rise in plasma creatinine, however, may have to be accepted if this is the only means of achieving BP control
  * calcium antagonists are well tolerated in patients with renal failure; as well as causing vasodilatation, they enhance renin release.
* α-Blockers, e.g. doxazosin, are useful as third-line drugs to achieve control.
* β-Blockers are sometimes needed and are particularly useful if the patient also has angina. They should be used with caution in diabetic patients requiring insulin and in patients with peripheral vascular disease.
* Frequent monitoring of BP is essential:
  * ambulatory BP monitoring (ABPM) and home monitoring of BP by the patient often give a more accurate measure of BP control than clinic BP readings
  * this is particularly important in trying to achieve the low levels of BP required in renal disease, as there is a risk of overtreatment and symptomatic hypotension
  * upper arm cuff monitors are reasonably accurate for home monitoring and are relatively cheap.
* Encouraging patients to monitor their own BP often improves control, as the patient is more involved with their treatment. Once a week checks are sufficient, but it is sensible to do these at different times of the day.
* Home BP readings have been shown to correlate better with decline in renal function than clinic readings.

NICE/British Hypertension Society recommendations

These guidelines have recently been revised as a result of head-to-head trials showing that β-blockers were usually less effective than the comparator drug at reducing major cardiovascular events, in particular stroke.

Use of β-blockers

Evidence from recent trials have resulted in recommendations that β-blockers are not a preferred initial therapy for hypertension. They may, however, be considered in younger people, particularly:

- those with an intolerance or contraindication to ACEI or ARBs
- women of childbearing potential (use of ACEIs and ARBs is contraindicated if a woman is trying to conceive)
- patients with evidence of increased sympathetic drive
- if a second drug is then required, add a calcium channel blocker rather than a thiazide-type diuretic to reduce patient's risk of developing diabetes
- if BP is well controlled with regimen which includes a β-blocker, there is no absolute need to replace it with another agent.

Algorithm for treatment of hypertension

	<55 years*	≥55 years, or black patient
Step 1	A	C or D
Step 2	A + C or A + D	
Step 3	A + C + D	
Step 4	Add: further diuretic therapy or	
	α-blocker or	
	β-blocker	

A = ACEI or A2RB; C = calcium-channel blocker;
D = thiazide-type diuretic

* For patients with CKD, includes patients with proteinuria >1g/24h or diabetes, though this is not addressed in these guidelines.

Management of renal failure: slowing the rate of decline

Other means of slowing the rate of deterioration of renal function are:

- *Blood glucose control in diabetics:* there is evidence in both type 1 and type 2 diabetes that tight control of blood glucose has a beneficial effect on the rate of deterioration of renal function. In type 2 diabetes, this can be achieved with both oral agents and insulin. Metformin should be used with care and at reduced dose in patients with renal impairment (eGFR <60mL/min), but the benefits (cardiovascular and metabolic) probably outweigh the risk until eGFR is <30mL/min. Metformin should be stopped once eGFR is <30mL/min (risk of lactic acidosis).
- *Lipid control:* there is evidence from animal studies, and some evidence in patients, that lowering plasma cholesterol and the use of low fat diets slow the rate of decline of renal function.
- *Optimizing fluid balance:* fluid depletion affects renal function adversely as it causes hypotension and poor renal perfusion.
- *Low-protein diet:* whether protein restriction slows the rate of progression of renal failure remains controversial. Compliance is difficult, particularly if patients are also restricting fat intake, and in diabetics. There is also a major concern over protein malnutrition, particularly if the renal disease is very slowly progressive (long-term use of diet).
- *Correcting acidosis:* there is recent randomized controlled trial (RCT) evidence that oral sodium bicarbonate slows rate of decline of renal function.
- *Use of EPO:* some data that rate of decline of renal function may be slower in patients using EPO, though this needs to be confirmed in a sufficiently powered RCT.

Management of renal failure: lipids and fluid balance

Lipid control

The increased risk of cardiovascular disease in renal failure is partly due to the increased frequency of hyperlipidaemia. Other risk factors include raised lipoprotein (a) and homocysteine. Although there are no clinical studies demonstrating the benefits of lipid control in renal disease, general recommendations are to minimize risk factors and aim for plasma cholesterol <5.0mmol/L. This is achieved by:

- diet—all patients with renal disease should be given advice about 'healthy eating'
- drug therapy—particularly statins (dose depends on renal function because of risk of myositis); fibrates are contraindicated in advanced renal disease
- ezetimibe can safely be added to a statin to enhance cholesterol lowering
- folate supplementation may reduce homocysteine levels, but trials fail to show any effect on cardiovascular outcomes.

Optimizing fluid balance

Fluid overload

All patients should be assessed for fluid overload whenever seen. This can be corrected by the use of diuretics, and salt and fluid restriction. Larger doses of diuretics are needed as renal function worsens, but renal function can deteriorate during diuresis because of the reduction in blood volume and hence renal perfusion. Patients with advanced renal failure can be precipitated on to dialysis when treated with diuretics. Patients with cardiac failure can often only maintain adequate renal perfusion when oedematous, with some degree of pulmonary oedema.

Fluid depletion

Worsens renal function because of reduced renal perfusion. Any patient with renal impairment, normal BP (not on hypotensive drugs), and no oedema is probably fluid depleted. If necessary this can be managed with oral sodium supplements (slow sodium or sodium bicarbonate). IV saline is indicated in the presence of postural hypotension.

Management of renal failure: treatment of anaemia

Anaemia causes significant morbidity in patients with renal failure.

• Detection of anaemia and its treatment is one of the principal goals of good pre-dialysis management.
• Anaemia may be considered a result of uraemia if GFR <30mL/min (<45mL/min in diabetics) and no other cause is identified.
• If Hb <12g/dL in men and postmenopausal women, or <11g/dL in premenopausal women, check ferritin, transferrin saturation, vitamin B_{12}, and red cell folate.
• Aim for serum ferritin ≥200mcg/L.
• Iron replacement: should initially be with oral iron, but if ferritin remains below target, or if more rapid response needed (Hb <10g/dL) arrange for IV iron.
• Once serum ferritin ≥200mcg/L for at least a month, EPO, darbepoetin alfa, or an erythropoietin-stimulating agent (ESA) should be commenced if:
  • Hb <10.5g/dL
  • Hb 10.5-11.5/dL *and*
    —symptomatic angina or claudication
    —exertion significantly limited by shortness of breath
    —patient does job dependent on manual labour or exertion.
• Target Hb for pre-dialysis patient on EPO is 10.5-12.5g/dL and <13g/dL, i.e. same as for patients on dialysis.

US KDIGO guidelines have recently been much more cautious in recommending EPO institution but advising individualized decision-making based on balance of potential benefit with risk of stroke or worsening hypertension, and *not* recommending EPO if Hb >10g/dL, and if used aiming to maintain Hb <11.5g/dL.

Once EPO or darbepoetin alfa or an ESA is started, management is the same as for patients on dialysis.

Management of renal failure: calcium and phosphate

Hyperparathyroidism

The principles are the same as for patients on dialysis. It is important to avoid hypercalcaemia, which can cause acute deterioration in renal function because of fluid depletion and calcium precipitation in the kidney.

Hyperphosphataemia

This is caused by phosphate retention and hyperparathyroidism. Management involves:
- dietary phosphate restriction
- use of phosphate binders: calcium carbonate, calcium acetate (less calcium absorbed so lower risk of hypercalcaemia), sevelamer, and lanthanum carbonate—for more details, see ➜ Maintenance of normal phosphate levels, p. 494.

Management of renal failure: metabolic complications

Hyperkalaemia

Plasma potassium needs to be monitored regularly. Hyperkalaemia does not cause warning symptoms before fatal arrhythmia occurs. Management consists of the following:

- Monitoring of drug treatment—avoid potassium supplements and potassium-sparing diuretics (amiloride, triamterene, spironolactone); careful use of ACEIs and ARBs, especially in combination.
- Low potassium diet.
- Oral ion-exchange resins (e.g. Resonium A®, which exchanges sodium for potassium, or Calcium Resonium®, which exchanges calcium for potassium). Resonium A® should not be used in patients with fluid overload. Expensive if used long term, not very palatable, and can cause constipation. Can be dissolved in lactulose to avoid constipation.
- Fludrocortisone may help lower serum potassium by increasing colonic potassium excretion.
- IV insulin and glucose if plasma potassium is >6.5mmol/L, given as a bolus of 50mL of 50% glucose or better 125mL of 20% dextrose with 10–12 units of short-acting insulin. Blood glucose must be monitored carefully for several hours afterwards. Plasma potassium should be repeated 1h later—if still high, an insulin and glucose infusion may be needed (same concentration, run at 5mL/min).
- Oral or IV sodium bicarbonate if the patient is acidotic but not fluid overloaded.
- β-Agonists such as salbutamol given by inhaler or nebulizer can lower serum potassium by 0.6–1mmol/L, but can worsen tachycardias.
- HD if plasma potassium remains high despite these methods—very unusual except with advanced renal failure.

Acidosis

- Plasma bicarbonate should be maintained in the normal range with oral sodium bicarbonate to prevent exacerbation of bone disease and increased muscle catabolism.
- Start at dose of sodium bicarbonate 500mg bd and titrate upwards until plasma bicarbonate is in normal range:
  - 1g sodium bicarbonate provides 10mmol sodium.
- Correction of acidosis will lower plasma potassium.
- Use of oral sodium bicarbonate often limited by the increased sodium intake which makes control of fluid overload and BP more difficult.

Poor nutrition

Appropriate nutritional advice should be given to all patients with renal failure as low plasma albumin and malnutrition are poor prognostic factors for long-term survival on dialysis. There is an increasing awareness that starting dialysis early (i.e. GFR <10mL/min, rather than when the patient is very symptomatic with GFR <5mL/min) avoids the anorexia and poor nutrition associated with severe renal failure.

Management of renal failure: prevention of symptoms

The level of GFR at which symptoms develop varies from individual to individual. Generally, symptoms are less pronounced when renal failure progresses slowly over several years. Most patients remain asymptomatic until GFR is <20mL/min. Older patients and diabetics tend to develop symptoms at relatively higher GFRs. Initial symptoms include increasing tiredness and exhaustion on exertion, and patients later become overtly anorectic. Family or friends may notice changes before the patient.

Management should prevent and treat these symptoms and enable patients to maintain their usual lifestyle and employment. This can be achieved by:

- correction of anaemia by the use of an erythropoietic agent
- counselling and education—depressive symptoms are very similar to those of uraemia, and patients can become anxious or depressed by the thought of dialysis
- protein restriction—prevents the accumulation of nitrogenous waste products and makes the patient feel better (less uraemic); however, protein intake usually falls spontaneously in advancing renal failure because of anorexia, and additional protein restriction may worsen malnutrition
- control fluid balance—fluid overload causes shortness of breath, and fluid depletion causes hypotension, both of which will exacerbate tiredness
- starting dialysis early when symptoms restrict the patient's lifestyle, even if GFR is still ~10mL/min. US (KDOQI) guidelines are to start dialysis when GFR is 15mL/min, but this is not the practice in the UK or most of Europe, and is probably not acceptable to many patients; there is no evidence that a very early start to dialysis leads to better survival.

Assessment of patients for dialysis: early referral

Patients who require dialysis within 3 months of referral to a nephrologist are at increased risk of morbidity and mortality compared with those under long-term specialist care. Up to 30% of patients begin RRT <6 months after referral to a nephrologist; this is particularly true for older patients. Advantages of early referral include:

- ability to slow rate of progression of renal deterioration
- control of BP and lipids minimizes cardiovascular risk thereby reducing 'co-morbidity load' when patient eventually starts dialysis
- use of ACEIs and statins, both of which may have beneficial effects over and above BP lowering and cholesterol control
- timely treatment of anaemia and use of EPO
- prevention of bone disease by proper management of serum phosphate and calcium, and PTH
- early dietary interventions including 'healthy lifestyle' advice to minimize cardiovascular morbidity
- hepatitis B vaccination can be carried out pre-dialysis when the immune response is greater
- patient can be educated about dialysis
- most appropriate modality of dialysis can be chosen
- psycho-educational interventions can delay time until dialysis needed;
- access for dialysis can be planned in advance—emergency access for HD and PD has more complications
- protection of forearm veins
- increases compliance with treatment
- enables pre-emptive transplantation (mostly from living donors)
- dialysis can be commenced 'early' before become symptomatic; patients are fitter and long-term outcome may be improved
- higher quality of life and better physical functioning.

Late referral to a nephrologist also represents a loss of chance for the patient and loss of money for society.

Assessment of patients for dialysis: when to start

Patients can be placed on the UK deceased donor transplant list once their GFR is <15mL/min and dialysis is thought likely to be needed within the next 6 months. Ideally, information about the various dialysis options should be introduced within a year of the projected need to start dialysis. Some patients are content just to 'know' that they will need dialysis at some point in the future, but do not want any more details until closer to the time. Some do not want to know the details because they are frightened. Such patients may come to false conclusions, e.g. they can no longer go on holiday for fear they may be caught abroad needing urgent dialysis. Some patients will have to make major career decisions, e.g. whether to accept a post abroad. There are also patients who are 'in denial', i.e. know that they will need dialysis, but think it will never actually happen to them, so deny all symptoms and end up starting dialysis when they are really sick. Finally, a few patients will decide that dialysis is not for them—time will be needed to counsel them and their families or friends appropriately.

Assessment of patients for dialysis: factors to be assessed

The assessment period helps to determine which modality of RRT is best suited for the patient, assuming that there is no resource limitation affecting dialysis supply.

Treatment modalities for ESKD

- HD:
  - centre
  - satellite
  - home
- PD:
  - continuous ambulatory PD (CAPD)
  - automated PD (APD)
  - assisted PD (aPD)
- Transplantation:
  - deceased donor
  - living related donor
  - living unrelated donor (usually emotionally related)
- Conservative management:
  - best supportive care.

Factors that need to be assessed

- *Age:* not a barrier to dialysis—both PD and HD can be used successfully in the elderly. The elderly are at greater risk from co-morbid illnesses, physical disabilities, and social isolation; all need to be taken into account when determining the optimum modality of dialysis.
- *Eyesight:* although there are aids enabling poorly sighted individuals to carry out PD, these are only suitable for very motivated patients with social support.
- *Mobility:* if hospital transport is needed for HD, hours spent away from home are greatly extended. PD, however, is not suitable for patients with poor mobility unless there is appropriate social support to help with exchanges or carry out APD.
- *Manual dexterity:* poor dexterity makes PD difficult unless family members can help.
- *Housing:* PD is only possible if there is room to store supplies, and a clean area close to running water (for hand washing), where exchanges can be performed. If assessment is made early, it may be possible to change or alter accommodation to suit PD requirements.
- *Family or social support:* dialysis is stressful, whichever modality is used. Many PD patients benefit from support at home particularly if they are disabled or have other medical problems. Family support is also important for enabling compliance with dietary restrictions, and for transport to hospital for clinic visits and HD sessions.
- *Attitude to chronic illness:* very variable both between individuals and between different cultural and ethnic groups. Some patients are determined to live as normal a life as possible on dialysis, while others take on the sick role and depend on family support, without much objective evidence of their need to do so.

- *Work:* all attempts should be made to enable dialysis patients to remain in work. Many patients in full-time employment opt for PD (particularly APD) or HD at home or overnight in hospital. Depending on the flexibility of their employer, some patients on HD dialyse during the day, usually in a late afternoon or early evening shift. The increase in satellite units means that HD can be organized nearer to the patient's home or place of work, thereby decreasing travelling time.
- *Diabetes:* many patients with diabetes have coexistent vascular disease. Patients with active retinopathy are at risk of vitreous haemorrhage, and should be warned of the increased risk with the use of heparin on HD. There is no good evidence that HD or PD is more suited to the diabetic patient.
- *Coexistent vascular disease:* patients with ischaemic heart disease are at risk of angina or MI during hypotensive episodes that can occur on HD. Hypotension is more frequent on HD in patients with poor left ventricular function. Vascular access can be difficult to establish in patients with arterial disease.
- *Respiratory disease:* there is no evidence that the presence of intra-abdominal fluid in PD causes deterioration in pulmonary function in lung disease. Such patients tend to tolerate excess fluid less well and can become short of breath when only mildly fluid overloaded.
- *Abdominal examination:* a prerequisite to proceeding with PD. PD is contraindicated if likelihood of adhesions from previous surgery, particularly in the pelvis. Presence of colostomy, ileostomy, or ileal conduit contraindicate PD, but a feeding gastrostomy does not. Hernias should be repaired before catheter insertion. An inoperable hernia may be a contraindication to CAPD, but reduced volume overnight APD or intermittent PD (IPD) may be possible if HD is not an option. Retroperitoneal surgery, e.g. nephrectomy, aortic surgery, should not be a contraindication to PD, as subsequent adhesions are unlikely. PD should be delayed until 3 months after aortic aneurysm repair to ensure that fibrous tissue has grown over the graft.
- *Compliance:* patients known to be poor compliers tend to do badly with a home-based treatment such as PD, unless they become motivated by the fear of changing to a modality of dialysis they do not want. Often such patients choose PD as they want to retain their independence and would cope equally poorly with the routine of HD.
- *Use of immunosuppressive drugs:* patients taking immunosuppressive drugs at the start of dialysis (e.g. for SLE, vasculitis, or a failing transplant) have an increased risk of infections related to central venous catheters (CVCs) or peritonitis, and infections are more severe. Steroids in particular delay wound healing, hence a longer time should be allowed for planning dialysis access whether for PD or HD.
- *Hepatitis B status:* hepatitis B-positive patients must be isolated if on HD. This has resource implications, and some patients may feel isolated if dialysed separately from the main unit. These difficulties are not encountered on PD.

Assessment of patients for dialysis: when not to dialyse

Apart from patient choice, there are no hard and fast rules. Some practitioners would argue that all patients should be treated unless they explicitly refuse. This is not a universal view. Predictors of poor outcome are:
- dementia, unless there are family members who are dedicated to helping with treatment and care
- severe peripheral arterial disease
- hypotensive heart failure
- severe mental illness, so the patient has no awareness of the treatment and is unable to comply
- malignant disease with poor prognosis.

However, any experienced dialysis doctor or nurse will have treated patients doing better or worse than expected. If the patient is being assessed some time before needing dialysis, the option of not dialysing should be discussed if the prognosis is thought to be very poor. 'Not dialysing' does not mean 'no care', but rather full conservative and supportive management. However, it can be difficult to identify such patients, and a trial of dialysis for 1–2 months could be considered to establish whether the overall condition of the patient improves. Decisions not to dialyse must be taken after full discussion with the entire care team, the family, and almost always the patient, unless mentally incompetent. If a patient decides not to undertake dialysis, family members need to be informed. All discussions and decisions should be recorded in the notes, so that dialysis is not commenced should the patient come to hospital terminally ill due to renal failure.

Patients who present with severe renal failure needing immediate dialysis are the most difficult to assess. Severely uraemic patients can be confused and very ill. Increasing dementia in an elderly patient may be due to progressively severe renal failure. The decision not to dialyse can therefore only be made if it becomes obvious that the physical or mental state of the patient is not improving after some time on dialysis.

Supportive care in ESKD

With increasing awareness of the poor outcome on dialysis for older patients with multiple co-morbidities, the option of no dialysis is increasingly becoming a standard component of pre-dialysis education. Around 10–20% of pre-dialysis patients in UK renal units select conservative management after careful discussion with pre-dialysis kidney teams.

Patients who opt for conservative or supportive management (rather than dialysis) continue to need regular follow-up from the renal team. Symptoms can be treated and quality of life enhanced, although death is clearly inevitable at some point. For elderly patients with significant co-morbidities, however, length of life may not be increased by dialysis, and quality of life may suffer (high incidence of sepsis, hospital admissions, repeated interventions for vascular access, greater likelihood of dying in hospital rather than at home).

- Optimal management of BP will minimize rate of further deterioration of renal function, and reduce the risk of a cardiovascular event such as MI or stroke.
- Treatment of anaemia with IV iron and erythropoietic agents will greatly enhance quality of life.
- Correction of hypocalcaemia to prevent fits.
- Symptom control:
  - *tiredness*: treatment of anaemia
  - *nausea*: low-protein diet and use of antiemetics such as metoclopramide
  - *shortness of breath and oedema*: cautious use of diuretics; if patient becomes volume depleted, renal function will deteriorate further, thereby exacerbating uraemic symptoms
  - *pain*: mostly due to co-morbidities such as peripheral vascular disease or arthritis; non-steroidal anti-inflammatory drugs (NSAIDs) should be avoided, and codeine-containing drugs should be used with caution.
- Death is inevitable, so the patient's and family wishes should be established:
  - patient should be referred early to the local palliative care team for appropriate inpatient and community management
  - primary care and community palliative care services should be utilized so that patient can die at home if he/she/family wishes.
- Often patients will die from their co-morbid disease, e.g. cardiac or vascular disease, malignancy, etc.

Assessment of patients for dialysis: role of pre-dialysis nurses

Specialist nurses have taken on a major role in most units for the pre-dialysis assessment and education of patients with severe CKD, and often other tasks.
- As part of the multidisciplinary care for patients with CKD.
- Patient education.
- Home visits combined with education, assessment, and family involvement.
- Family education.
- Management of renal anaemia, iron, EPO dosing and titration.
- Contribution to control and management of hypertension.
- Control and management of calcium and phosphate (with dieticians).
- Prevention of renal bone disease.
- Avoiding malnutrition (with dieticians).
- Dialysis access planning.
- Transplant planning
- Social and psychosocial support.
- Formal counselling.
- Patients' information evenings.
- Liaison with employers, educational institutions.

Checklist for assessing patients in a low clearance clinic

Cardiovascular

- Assess for: hypertension (BP/LVH); atheroscleros[is] (vascular) ...
  in the dialysis department or home
- Right for renal transplantation
- BP control in terms of fluid (AVF) impact on morbidity ...
  in ESKD

- If good control, weight the cardiovascular risk in the low ...
  patients so to highlight them in a later identification and planning
  of surgery ... if there are cardiovascular problems ...
  ... (anaemia), and fluids, antibodies against kidney antibodies ...
  Design and assessment for transplantation ... transplant candidate
  or home haemodialysis
- Check renal transplant ... if ... needs a preventative option

Biochemistry

- If measuring bicarbonate: ... for dialysis to reach acidosis drivers ...
- Needs to maintain ... Hcp, calcium, phosphate, PTH, ... Amount of ...
  bone ... maintaining acceptable ... profiles
- Calcium, phosphate, maintain at ... PO4, ... mmol/L, ... detection of
  evidence of ... biological abnormality if calcium biochemical... may also be ...
  ... in ... levels
- Restrict ... calcium ... intravenous ... and ... emulate and ... if higher ...
  bone turnover ...
- Calcium intake ... if ... ... if ... ... in ... kidney transplantation or preventive
  PTH ... and ... if non-calcium avoidance
- Other ... ... in ... ... high ... ... or ... ... oedema

Anaemia

- If non ... and Hb ... term > 20% ... ... or ... is not adverse or
  absorb ... iron ... given ... ... in appropriately iron status ...
- Check vitamin B₁₂ and folate, and ... folic acid and ... vitamin supplement
  as needed
- Consider ... erythropoiesis agents Hb > 110g/L or symptom, including Hb
  (reticulocyte), iron profile, and vitamin status as monthly

Transplantation

- Assess if all patients once eGFR < 20 ... ...
  ... infection and ... not age ... ... limit ... transplantation
- ... ... and ... with hatch cloth, ... X-ray, ECG, echocardiogram ...
  carotid Doppler ... and ... depth on symptoms and ... renal ...
- Assess ... renal ... peripheral vascular disability, ...
- Ask ... patient during ... to be considered, and to highlight if any ...
  ... cancer, and ... for the transplant ...
- Refer to the nephrologist from ... ...
- ... cross ... ... if any ... held on ... related transplantation ...
- Living donor assessment, ... to ... ... and ... BMI screen

Checklist for assessing patients in a low clearance clinic

Dialysis plans
- Assess medical suitability (PD/HD/either). (See Table 1.11.)
- Refer to dialysis education nurse.
- Refer to renal social worker.
- HD: book arteriovenous fistula (AVF) surgery 3–6 months prior to ESKD.
- PD: book catheter insertion before patient too symptomatic—allows patient to be maintained on residual renal function rather than having temporary HD if there are catheter-related problems.
- Check HBsAg, anti-HBsAg antibodies, anti-HCV antibodies.
- Consent and test for HIV if potential transplant candidate.
- Immunize against HBV.
- Check antibody response 7–8 months post vaccination.

Biochemistry
- Deteriorating biochemistry may indicate need to start dialysis.
- Refer to dietician early (especially if K >5mmol/L, PO_4 >1.6mmol/L, hyperlipidaemia, obese, or losing weight).
- Calcium carbonate/acetate to achieve PO_4 1.3–1.8mmol/L (consider sevelamer or lanthanum carbonate if calcium high, diabetes or vascular calcification present).
- Alfacalcidol/calcitriol to achieve Ca 2.2–2.6mmol/L and PTH 2–3 times normal.
- Calcimimetics (cinacalcet) may play an important role in controlling PTH, Ca, and PO_4 when routinely available.
- Oral sodium bicarbonate if bicarbonate <24mmol/L (watch BP, oedema).

Anaemia
- IV iron to achieve ferritin >200mg/L—most patients do not tolerate or absorb oral iron, which is therefore not particularly efficacious.
- Check vitamin B_{12} and folate, add folic acid and B_{12} vitamin supplements as needed.
- Consider erythropoietic agent if Hb <10g/dL or symptomatic (and BP controlled, iron replete, no other cause for anaemia).

Transplantation
- Consider in all patients once GFR <20mL/min.
- Co-morbidity and not age is factor limiting transplantation.
- Assess cardiac and respiratory fitness (CXR, ECG, consider pulmonary function tests, stress test, echocardiogram, and coronary angiography).
- Assess urinary tract, peripheral vasculature, obesity.
- Assess patient desire, understanding, and psychological state.
- Discuss pros and cons of transplantation.
- Refer to transplant education nurses.
- Discuss possibility of living related or unrelated transplant donors.
- Blood group, tissue type, serum for cytotoxic antibodies, CMV status.

Table 1.11 Haemodialysis vs peritoneal dialysis—the relative advantages and disadvantages of HD and PD are related to the inherent differences between the two modes of dialysis

	HD	PD
Dialysis characteristics	Intermittent	Continuous
	3 ×4h on machine, usually in hospital	Daily: 4 exchanges/day or cycling machine at night
Dialysis procedure	Mostly dependent on nurses and technicians	Carried out by patient in own home
	Session times dependent on availability in unit; can be at antisocial hours	Dialysis can be fitted round patient's lifestyle
	Independent of patient's ability to learn or carry out technique	Dependent on patient or family member performing dialysis
Transport time	Extends time needed for dialysis sessions If hospital transport needed, transport time greatly increased	Treatment done at home
		Transport to hospital only needed for clinic or emergency visits
Travel/holiday	Arrangements need to be made with a local HD unit prior to travel—payment often needed	PD fluid can be delivered to most parts of world with prior notice—cost usually included in contract with company providing dialysate
	Patient has to dialyse at times offered by unit	Patient carries on doing dialysis independently
	Some units will not accept patient if hepatitis B, hepatitis C or HIV +ve	
Dialysis adequacy	Dependent on blood flow, dialysate flow and membrane characteristics	Dependent on peritoneal membrane permeability and exchange number and volume
	Adequacy easily increased by increasing hours on dialysis or size of membrane	Residual renal function plays important role Increased adequacy achieved by increasing exchange volume and number, often with aid of APD

(continued)

Table 1.6 (*Contd.*)

	HD	PD
Ultrafiltration (UF)	Reasonably predictable	Less predictable—poor UF can be cause for conversion to HD
	Regulated by degree of negative pressure in dialysate compartment	Regulated by increasing concentration of glucose in dialysate or by use of glucose polymer solution
	Pre-set at beginning of dialysis on the machine	Dependent on membrane permeability—poor UF with high permeability
	Amount that can be removed limited by cardiac status; greater risk of hypotension with poor cardiac function	UF often declines with time on dialysis
Access for dialysis	Need to allow 2–3 months for fistula to develop before useable	Access easy to establish. PD catheter can be used immediately, but advisable to allow to heal for 2 weeks
	Fistulae can be difficult to create in diabetics or patients with arterial disease	
	Acute access with CVCs have high complication rate: infection, thrombosis, venous stenosis	
Infectious complications	Septicaemia associated with catheter infections can be life threatening. Complications of catheter infections often dangerous, e.g. SBE, septic arthritis, epidural abscess	Catheter exit site infection—rarely serious. Peritonitis—if serious, usually resolves after catheter removal; rarely fatal
Cardiovascular complications	Risk of hypotension with fluid removal—increased if poor cardiac function. Arrhythmias can occur as plasma potassium falls during dialysis. Angina, MI, and stroke can be precipitated by hypotensive episode. Fluid overload can occur if poor UF	Safer for patients with poor cardiac function, severe ischaemic heart disease, or cerebrovascular disease
Anaemia	Frequent—caused by reduced EPO levels and increased GI blood losses related to use of heparin	Less severe—prolonged red cell survival and less GI blood loss
	70–80% require EPO	30–50% require EPO

Table 1.6 (*Contd.*)

	HD	PD
Psychosocial	Not suitable for patients with needle phobia. Body image problems with fistula, particularly young women	Hb usually rises spontaneously for first few months on PD. Body image problems with PD catheter—may prevent patient from accepting PD
	As dialysis carried out by others, not dependent on patient's physical or mental ability	Dependent on patient or family member being able to learn and comply with technique. 'Burnout'—occurs after long period of time on PD
	Can be inconvenient for family or social support as patient may have to dialyse at antisocial hours and require help with transport	Care of dependent family member can be easier if dialysis carried out at home and life not disrupted by 3 times per week hospital visits
Contraindications	Inability to achieve vascular access. Severe ischaemic heart disease. Severe heart failure	Presence of colostomy, ileostomy, or ileal conduit. Intra-abdominal adhesions. Inoperable hernia
Survival	Survival on PD and HD similar for first 3–4 years	Survival on PD and HD similar for first 3–4 years
	High technique survival—low drop out to PD (because of lack of vascular access)	Relatively high drop out rate (to HD) because of peritonitis, poor UF, or inadequate dialysis when residual renal function lost
	Experience with long-term patient survival for 20 years plus	Little experience of long-term survival. Risk of encapsulating peritoneal sclerosis with long term (>5 years) PD

Choosing which dialysis modality

Ideally, selection of dialysis modality should be driven by patient choice, unless there is a medical or social contraindication to a particular modality. Unfortunately, resource availability (limited HD facilities or lack of HD nurses) often limits patient choice (very variable across the world). There is also prejudice against PD driven either by local medical or nursing misinformation, or by a healthcare reimbursement system that favours HD (in some countries). (See Table 1.12.)

Table 1.12 Contraindications to HD or PD

	Dialysis modality contraindicated
Absolute contraindications	
Colostomy, ileostomy, ileal conduit	PD
Intra-abdominal adhesions	PD
Very poor housing	PD
No spare space in home	PD
Poor personal hygiene	PD
Morbid obesity	PD
Thrombosed central veins	HD
Severe angina	HD
Hypotensive heart failure	HD
Relative contraindications	
Frailty/dementia	PD (unless assistance from family member or carer)
Long distance from HD unit	HD
Severe vascular disease	HD
Active diabetic retinopathy	HD

Concept of integrated care

Rather than thinking of one modality of treatment vs another, it is best to think of the patient's life span on renal replacement treatment. A single patient may well utilize all modalities so it is sensible to use each to its optimal benefit. (See Table 1.13.)

Thinking of the patient pathway through the various treatment modalities:
- optimal time to use PD is when there is residual renal function, i.e. when starting dialysis or when transferring back to dialysis after transplantation
- use of PD at onset of dialysis delays need for vascular access, which is preserved for later on when PD is no longer suitable.

Table 1.13 Concept of integrated care

Modality	Strength	Weakness
PD	Increased patient freedom	Risk of underdialysis when patient becomes anuric
	Arm vessels not used for vascular access	Increase in membrane permeability and loss of UF with time on PD
	Longer preservation of residual renal function	
HD	Long-term technique survival	Limited by availability of vascular access
	Suitable for patients unable to perform own dialysis	Availability dependent on local resources
Transplantation	Longer patient survival than on dialysis	Limited by lack of kidneys
		Depends on patient's age and co-morbidities.

Education for dialysis

Should be commenced once GFR approaches 20mL/min and/or within the year preceding need. It is a time-consuming process so is best done away from a busy clinic, by a dedicated nurse or counsellor. Home visits by an educator often extremely useful. It requires:

- involvement of family members and social support network, as appropriate
- information about kidney function
- knowledge about symptoms to expect as kidney failure gets worse
- information about pros and cons of HD and PD
- information about pros and cons of pre-emptive transplantation, transplantation after dialysis starts, use of living donors, and how the deceased waiting list works
- developing an understanding of how each modality would impact on the patient's lifestyle, particularly with regard to work needs, hours of work, and need for travel, both for holiday and for work
- an assessment as to whether a patient's home is suitable for PD or home HD (especially storage area)
- an assessment of the support the patient can reasonably expect from family and social networks
- providing opportunities for the patient to visit PD and HD units
- providing opportunities for the patient to talk to other PD or HD patients (if necessary)
- developing an understanding that RRT is not usually restricted to just one modality, but follows different pathways involving several modes of treatment
- developing an understanding that outcomes of RRT treatment are mostly related to associated co-morbidities and that lifespan is reduced
- enabling a patient to make a decision not to have a dialysis by giving realistic information about likely benefits of dialysis and how dialysis procedure will affect quality of life
- providing information to a patient about end of life and how it can be managed if the patient is opting for or interested in conservative care.

Dialysis modality decision-making

There is considerable variability in the use of different dialysis modalities between individual renal units. This may be partly due to different patient populations and social factors, but the predominant reason is thought to be due to variability in patient education, physician bias, and the involvement of patients in decision-making. Studies have shown that around 80% of patients want to be involved in the decision of choice of dialysis modality, yet 30–80% of patients in surveys report no involvement.

Models of decision-making

- *Patriarchal*: decision is made by healthcare team with no patient involvement.
- *Informed decision-making*: patient is given information and asked to make decision; ability of patient to do so will depend on their comprehension of information given.
- *Shared decision-making*: probably optimal method as this involves discussion between patient and healthcare team.

Shared decision-making

Enables patient to make decision about treatment choices depending on risks and benefits and how these are affected by lifestyle choices.

- *Clinician* shares diagnosis, cause of disease, prognosis, treatment options, and outcome probabilities.
- *Patient* shares experience of illness, social circumstances, attitude to risk, values, and preferences.
- This process therefore enables patient to be involved in treatment decisions.
- Clinicians have to accept that patient may make 'wrong' decision or one that clinician does not agree with.
- There are many challenges:
  - time-consuming
  - not part of healthcare culture—perception that patients do not want this and doctors/nurses are not appropriately trained
  - patients also need to be more assertive and demand to be involved in decisions
  - appropriate information and patient education need to be developed—decision aids, translation into different languages.

Choice of dialysis modality: case histories

Case 1

G.F. is a 42-year-old man with immunoglobulin A (IgA) nephropathy. He had been an erratic attender at the renal clinic though aware his renal function was deteriorating. He presented with increasing tiredness and some nausea. Blood tests confirmed he had reached ESKD. Several family members were keen to offer him a kidney. After discussion, G.F. selected PD as this could be fitted round the shift patterns of his job as a bus driver. Six months later he had a successful transplant from his brother.

Case 2

A.G. is an 83-year-old woman who lives on her own. Her only living relative is a niece who lives 200 miles away; most of her friends have died. When told that she had ESKD, her initial reaction was to say that she did not want dialysis. However, she was frightened of dying and was pleased to think that she could feel less tired. She therefore agreed to a trial of dialysis. She had no social support, and was very anxious. It was therefore felt that she would do better on HD. Dialysis was started using a Tesio® CVC line as access. Unfortunately, this became infected and two further catheters did not function well. During this time she developed angina at rest. She was not fit for an anaesthetic to create a fistula, and HD became increasingly difficult because of angina. The option of stopping dialysis was again discussed, but she decided to try assisted APD with a healthcare assistant visiting her at home.

Case 3

D.W. is a 47-year-old man with severe learning problems needing institutionalized care. He initially presented as an emergency with undiagnosed renal failure. Fortunately, there was some improvement in renal function, allowing time for many discussions with him and his carers. It was clear that the care home would not be able to carry out PD. By the time he needed dialysis, he had some understanding of what was involved. He has now been on HD for several years. Initially, he needed to be brought to hospital with a carer, but was then able to come on hospital transport on his own.

When to start dialysis in ESKD

When dialysis was first available, it was only offered to patients who were uraemic and at risk of imminent death. Since then, the threshold at which dialysis is started has steadily fallen. The UK Renal Association guidelines are to start dialysis when the GFR is <10mL/min. The potential advantages of starting dialysis earlier are:

- improved rehabilitation—patient usually still able to work
- fewer complications starting dialysis as patient is fitter
- patient does not become ill if there are delays in starting dialysis (e.g. poorly draining PD catheter, poorly functioning vascular access)
- avoids poor nutritional state associated with more severe renal failure—a low plasma albumin when starting dialysis is a poor prognostic factor
- avoids emergency need for dialysis—decline of renal function is very variable so that patients who appear to be quite stable can suddenly present as an emergency.

Dialysis is started in some patients to enable specific treatments or interventions which would carry high risk with severe renal failure. Examples are:

- coronary interventions pre-transplantation
- major surgery, e.g. abdominal surgery for malignancy
- parenteral nutrition because of fluid volume and risk of fluid overload.

Trials, however, have not shown any survival advantage of earlier starts to dialysis and there are many disadvantages to starting dialysis too early:

- All types of dialysis will adversely affect patient's lifestyle.
- Dialysis is an active medical intervention and therefore is associated with complications which can cause considerable morbidity and even death.
- Loss of residual renal function associated with fluid removal and hypotension on haemodialysis could adversely affect survival.
- Many older frail patients can tolerate relatively low GFR particularly if rate of decline of GFR is slow; avoiding starting dialysis too soon means that some will die from their co-morbidities rather than face the burden of dialysis at the end of their life.
- Before starting dialysis, therefore, it is important to consider whether:
  - symptoms are due to uraemia or co-morbidities, and can they be controlled by alternative means
  - symptoms are likely to be improved by dialysis
  - overall prognosis of patient related to co-morbidities
  - whether there has been an acute decline in kidney function which is potentially reversible, e.g. related to hypotension, intercurrent infection etc. If degree of uraemia is not life-threatening (GFR >6mL/min/1.73m^2, potassium, acidosis, and fluid status controllable medically), delaying starting dialysis gives time for kidney function to improve.

How to persuade the patient to start dialysis

This can be surprisingly difficult. Patients, understandably, do not want to start dialysis and many would rather put it off as long as possible. Even intelligent patients given detailed education can remain in a state of denial. This is most frustrating for the medical team who want to shield the patient from developing an acute and potentially life-threatening complication such as pulmonary oedema or hyperkalaemia. The patient should be encouraged to continue attending the renal clinic so that he/she can be monitored regularly, and can eventually be persuaded to start dialysis.

It is sometimes useful to use expressions such as 'You are in the grey area—dialysis will make you feel better; you have the advantage of being able to start at a time which is convenient for you. You do not want to wait until the black area where dialysis is needed as an emergency and therefore with many more complications'.

There are some patients who fail to attend any clinic and eventually present as an emergency.

Clinical indications for starting dialysis in ESKD

Plasma creatinine

No absolute figure can be given as this depends as much on muscle mass as on renal function. An elderly woman may have to start dialysis with a plasma creatinine of <300μmol/L, while a 25-year-old man may not start until his plasma creatinine is 800μmol/L. Ethnicity is also important; Asians tend to have low muscle mass while Afro-Caribbeans have a high muscle mass. Low creatinine can be associated with poor outcome since it reflects malnutrition and low muscle mass.

GFR

Difficult to measure at low levels of renal function. C_{crea} tends to overestimate GFR because of tubular secretion. Radioisotope measurements such as [^{51}Cr]EDTA are more accurate, but expensive and often not routinely available. Estimated GFR using the MDRD formula is now widely used and is reasonably accurate at low levels. The problem with using eGFR or plasma creatinine is that renal function can remain stable for long periods, therefore it is important to consider the rate of decline and patient symptoms additionally. This is particularly true in the elderly who may have a low muscle mass and therefore lower plasma creatinine.

Symptoms

Tiredness and anorexia develop once the GFR is <10mL/min. However, tolerance of renal impairment is very variable, with some patients (especially the elderly or diabetics) becoming markedly symptomatic with GFRs of ≥10mL/min, while others remain well with GFRs as low as 5mL/min. Patients may also be in a state of denial, and only present as an emergency.

Weight loss

Any evidence of weight loss indicates the need to start dialysis, as poor nutrition is such a poor prognostic factor.

Fluid overload

Only a relative indication. Initial management should be with diuretics (with caution to avoid a decline in renal function). If function worsens, or the patient remains fluid overloaded despite high dose diuretics, dialysis ought to be commenced.

Hyperkalaemia

Another relative indication as it can usually be managed medically.

Pericarditis

A very late complication of renal failure and rarely seen today. It remains an absolute indication for starting dialysis.

The acutely presenting patient or 'crashlander'

Around 30–40% of patients start dialysis in an unplanned manner. Many studies and registry data show that such patients have a worse outcome in terms of both morbidity and mortality. To improve outcomes, it is therefore important to consider why patients with ESKD should present 'acutely', how this can be avoided or minimized, and how management of these patients may be improved to avoid complications.

Reasons for 'crashlanding'

- Acute deterioration in renal function in a patient with CKD; this can occur due to:
  - fluid depletion of any cause; remember that trivial fluid losses, e.g. increased sweating in hot weather, can cause profound hypotension and drop in GFR if angiotensin system blocked
  - decreased cardiac function—coronary event, arrhythmias, heart failure
  - urinary obstruction, e.g. stone, tumour, blood clot
  - exposure to nephrotoxic agent, e.g. X-ray contrast, drugs such as NSAIDs, aminoglycosides
  - sepsis of any cause.
- CKD not recognized by other healthcare teams so patient not referred to nephrologist.
- Patient not known to medical teams—more common with older patients who explain non-specific symptoms as 'getting old'. Not unknown for younger patients to tolerate symptoms without seeking medical help.
- Foreign patients who present acutely ill—some know that they have CKD and hence this is the reason for leaving their own country, but some are genuinely unaware of diagnosis.
- Patients in denial of diagnosis or of need for dialysis so do not attend clinic or refuse to start dialysis until crisis occurs, e.g. pulmonary oedema, vomiting, etc.
- Delays in forming access for dialysis so no available fistula or PD catheter when symptoms or biochemistry dictate that dialysis should be started.

Avoiding acute starts

- Use of eGFR and guidelines for when to refer to renal clinics should improve detection of CKD in the community—though at the risk of overloading nephrology services with stable mild CKD.
- Avoidance of nephrotoxic agents and drugs in patients known to have CKD.
- Advising patients on ACEIs and ARBs to drink more in hot weather.
- Appropriate fluid replacement in patients when fluid depleted.
- Pre-dialysis education and counselling to help patients come to terms with and choose the treatment modality that suits their lifestyle.
- Adequate resources for timely placement of vascular and peritoneal access.

Reasons for poor outcome

- Patients often ill with multiple co-morbidities, septic, etc.
- Use of CVCs for access to start HD often out of hours—increased complication rate as staff may be inexperienced.
- High risk of line sepsis when using temporary catheters, particularly femoral catheters.
- Risk of femoral vein thrombosis or occluded central neck veins.
- Often fluid and electrolyte problems could have been managed medically and without need of acute dialysis with its attendant risks.

Long-term outcome for 'crashlanders'

- Higher mortality than patients starting dialysis in a planned manner.
- Patients tend not to have same quality of education as those in pre-dialysis clinics—or given no education.
- They therefore tend to remain on HD and are not given option of transferring to or starting on PD.

Use of PD

- PD can be safely used and may well be optimal mode of dialysis if poor cardiac function with risk of hypotension on HD.
- Avoids use of temporary venous access with all its complications.
- PD catheter can be used immediately if incisions are kept small—APD regimen with small volume exchanges should be used.
- Most patients who present acutely do not actually need urgent dialysis—though there is a tendency to do so. This gives time to discuss option of PD with patient and family.

Psychosocial effects of starting dialysis in ESKD

Initial reactions to a diagnosis of ESKD include shock, grief (loss, helplessness, and despair), denial, and finally acceptance. Patients also become aware (though often not initially) that dialysis is not curative.

Psychosocial factors, especially depression and social support, may be associated with mortality in dialysis patients, poor adequacy of dialysis, low serum albumin, and low Hb. They may also interfere with a patient's access to medical care, their compliance with dialysis and drug treatments, their nutritional status and eating habits, and with hypothalamic–pituitary and immune functions. Conversely, psychosocial adaptation is crucial for long-term survival.

Assessing psychosocial morbidity in ESKD is problematic, and most instruments are confounded by medical co-morbidity common in these patients, the case mix and the effects of a physical intervention (dialysis) on patient responses.

Common effects include:
• depression
• anxiety
• behavioural changes
• short temper
• poor concentration
• lack of motivation
• anger
• denial.

Psychosocial effects of starting dialysis in ESKD: depression and anxiety

Depression

Incidence varies from 5% to 60%. True clinical depression is much less common than 'feeling sad'. Depression is related to loss of kidney function, physical and cognitive abilities, sexual function, and of their role in family, work, and community life, and is initially triggered by the severe medical illness the patient has suffered. Symptoms include:

- depressed mood
- loss of interest
- change in appetite (increased or decreased)
- sleep disturbance
- fatigue
- aches and pains
- difficulty concentrating
- loss of libido
- suicidal ideation
- feelings of worthlessness or guilt
- psychomotor agitation or retardation.

Some of these can of course be a consequence of uraemia. Depression scores are reduced with higher dialysis adequacy. Daily dialysis provides excellent psychological rehabilitation. Post-dialysis fatigue is also associated with depression.

Treatment involves awareness, early assessment, counselling, and drug treatment as appropriate:

- Tricyclic antidepressants can worsen hypotension, and have significant anticholinergic side effects, and can cause cardiac conduction disturbances.
- Selective serotonin reuptake inhibitors can cause GI disturbance, tremor, headache, and nervousness, but are generally better tolerated than tricyclics. Although cleared by the liver, the dose is generally reduced. Fluoxetine has been most widely used in ESKD, but also paroxetine and citalopram
- Selective norepinephrine reuptake inhibitors such as venlafaxine should probably be avoided as they are renally excreted, with active metabolites also potentially renally excreted, which can cause fits.
- Monoamine oxidase inhibitors are best avoided in ESKD.

Anxiety

Reported in 50–70% of ESKD patients, and is related to social status, work, long-term health, early mortality, financial circumstances, and dialysis access. Usually managed by counselling, cognitive or behavioural therapy, and stress reduction techniques.

Dementia is an increasing problem in the ESKD population and can present as depression or anxiety.

Psychosocial effects of starting dialysis in ESKD: others

Body image

Is closely associated with self-esteem and easily perturbed in ESKD. Can result in a variety of emotional reactions. Often viewed very differently by staff (a 'good' fistula may be disfiguring to the patient).

Social support

Has been strongly related to survival in most chronic illnesses. Family problems are common in ESKD. Lack of social support is an important factor in failure of CAPD and transfer to HD. May be viewed negatively in the form of dependency and lack of independence.

Sexual dysfunction

Very common in ESKD. Up to 65% of patients never have intercourse, and half of these would like to do so. Associated with anxiety and depression, and also with hyperprolactinaemia, hyperparathyroidism, vascular disease, neuropathy, antihypertensive drugs, diabetes, and possibly zinc deficiency. For young patients the issue of fertility often arises.

Non-compliance

Found in 2–50% of patients. Often due to differing beliefs (of the patient) in the effectiveness of the treatment, lack of knowledge and education, or unpleasant side effects. Associated with increased risk of death. Can often be overcome by improved communication and patient education. Also related to the relationship between the patient and staff (patients who don't like their nurses are less compliant). Increasingly referred to as concordance.

Quality of life measurement

Essentially subjective. Scoring systems need to be disease-targeted, with appropriate control populations. Quantitated using KDQOL (kidney disease quality of life) primarily. Other measures include Karnofsky index, Beck depression inventory, Illness Effects Questionnaire, Sickness Impact Profiles, and SF-36 health survey. Elderly patients generally have the same outcome measures as younger patients. Quality of life improves when patients have the freedom of choice of modality of dialysis.

Others

ESKD affects patients' ability to travel, have holidays, and obtain life insurance, loans, and mortgages. These issues are often not raised with medical staff, but may be of great concern to the patient. Dialysis units should be able to help patients with these issues rapidly, and without giving conflicting advice. The effects of ESKD on the patient's family are also important, both for their own physical and mental health, and for that of the patient.

Mental and physical well-being of dialysis staff can also affect, and be affected by, that of the patients.

Haemodialysis

Principles of haemodialysis

Dialysis removes nitrogenous (and other) waste products, and corrects the electrolyte, water, and acid–base abnormalities associated with renal failure. Dialysis does not correct the endocrine abnormalities of renal failure, nor prevent cardiovascular complications. It requires the use of a semipermeable membrane that will allow the passage of water and small molecular weight (MW) solutes, but not large molecules (e.g. proteins). (MW of urea = 60, creatinine = 113, vitamin B_{12} = 1355, albumin = 60,000, IgG = 140,000 Da.) The first dialysis membranes were simple sausage skins (cellulose), but, increasingly, synthetic materials are being used.

Dialysis

This refers to the diffusion of solutes across a semipermeable membrane down a concentration gradient. The rate of diffusion is greatest when the concentration gradient is highest. This is the main mechanism for the removal of urea and creatinine, and for the replenishment of serum bicarbonate. Diffusion is proportional to the temperature of the solution (which increases random molecular movements), and inversely proportional to the viscosity and size of the molecule removed (large molecules diffuse slowly). Increasing blood flow through a dialyser (i.e. delivery of solute) increases the clearance, particularly of small MW solutes (urea, creatinine), by maintaining a high concentration gradient. Membrane characteristics can also determine rate of diffusion—high-flux membranes are thin and have large pores, and thus have a low resistance to diffusion. Diffusion is hindered if 'unstirred' layers of fluid can accumulate on either side of a dialysis membrane. This can be minimized by maintaining high flow rates, and by the design of the dialyser. Protein-bound solutes will not be removed by diffusion as the carrier proteins do not pass through the membrane. Only the free (unbound) fraction will be dialysed.

Ultrafiltration

This is the convective flow of water and dissolved solutes down a pressure gradient caused by hydrostatic or osmotic forces. Water is easily driven through the semipermeable membrane, and small solutes are 'dragged' along. Large molecules will not pass through the membrane. In HD. it usually occurs as a result of the negative pressure generated in the dialysate compartment by the dialysate effluent pump (transmembrane pressure, TMP). The rate of ultrafiltration (UF) depends on the pressure gradient. Dialysis membranes differ in their permeability to water and solutes, and can be low- or high-flux membranes. Membrane permeability is measured as the UF coefficient, KUf, in mL/h/mmHg, and can vary from 2 to 50 (5–10 indicates moderate water permeability; >10 indicates high water permeability).

Diafiltration

This is the simultaneous use of dialysis and UF to provide solute and water clearance.

Principles of haemodialysis in practice

Principles of haemodialysis in practice

At its simplest, a dialysis machine simply pumps blood and dialysate through the two compartments of a dialyser.

- The dialysate is a solution of purified water, sodium, potassium, magnesium, calcium, chloride, dextrose, and bicarbonate or acetate.
- The blood and dialysate are kept separate within the dialyser by a semipermeable membrane. As the dialysate contains no waste products of metabolism (urea, creatinine, etc.), these will diffuse from blood into dialysate.
- Diffusion is maximized by maintaining high flow rates (of blood and dialysate), and by pumping the two solutions in opposite directions (countercurrent flow).
- Convective clearance can be added by generating a TMP within the dialyser. Continuous RRT (CRRT) relies mainly on convective mechanisms for solute removal, and often does not have any dialysate at all. In conventional HD, small MW molecules are not removed to any great extent by convection, but almost entirely by diffusion. In contrast, large MW molecules (e.g. β_2-microglobulin (β_2m) or vitamin B_{12}) are removed more effectively by convection than diffusion. This has led to an increasing use of UF methods in HD to increase removal of larger MW molecules (haemodiafiltration (HDF) or high-volume haemofiltration).

A HD machine is made more complex by the addition of a number of safety devices, pump controllers, pressure and flow monitors, air leak detectors, patient BP monitors, the ability to change the composition of the dialysate, and increasingly systems to monitor blood chemistry, access flow, and delivered dialysis dose, and provide data to remote controllers and databases. (See Fig. 2.1.)

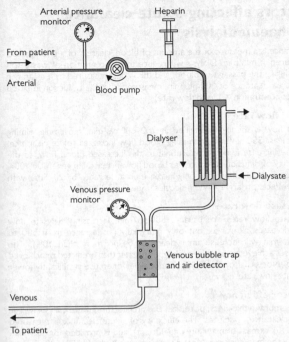

Fig. 2.1 Basic haemodialysis circuit.

Factors affecting solute clearance on haemodialysis

Clearance is a measure of the amount of blood 'cleared' of a given solute, measured in mL/min. Dialysis will reduce the concentration of waste solutes during the passage of blood, and this is best measured by a clearance (e.g. urea clearance of 100mL/min, measured from the reduction in blood urea concentration × blood flow rate).

Blood flow rate

Blood flow is usually maintained at 200–600mL/min, most units aiming for at least 350mL/min. Increasing blood flow increases solute clearance, but the increase is not proportional to the increased blood flow, as the efficiency of diffusion is reduced as blood flow increases. In general, a 100% increase in blood flow may only increase urea clearance by 20–50%, with lesser effects on larger MW molecules. (See Fig. 2.2.)

Dialysate flow rate

Dialysate flow rates are usually ~500mL/min. Increasing dialysate flow rate increases clearance, but only marginally (an increase from 500 to 800mL/min will increase urea clearance by no more than 10%). The increases achieved in practice are slightly greater than predicted or achieved in vitro. Nocturnal or daily dialysis modalities often use significantly lower dialysate flow rates.

Dialyser efficiency

The membrane thickness, pore size, and architecture of the dialyser will all affect clearance of solutes. The efficiency of solute clearance is measured by the KoA (mass transfer urea coefficient), and is provided for each dialyser by the manufacturer. Most dialysers have a KoA of ~300–500mL/min, increasing to >700mL/min for high-efficiency dialysers. Changing to a higher KoA dialyser has a greater effect on urea clearance than increases in blood or dialyser flow rates. Increases in blood flow have a greater effect on clearance in high efficiency dialysers.

Molecular weight of solute

Larger molecules diffuse slowly, and hence have reduced clearances. Increasing blood flow has less effect on clearance of larger molecules than on smaller molecules.

Time

Length of a dialysis session is the single most important determinant of solute clearance. Changes in other parameters are almost always introduced to minimize the amount of time a patient needs to spend on dialysis. Small solute clearance can often be maintained during short dialysis by using high-flux membranes, high blood flows, etc., but the long-term outcomes remain unclear, especially as extracellular volume control is usually inadequate (persistent hypertension), and large molecule clearance is not maintained.

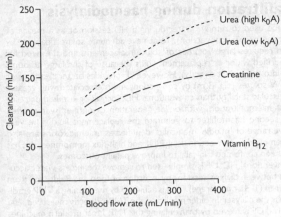

Fig. 2.2 Effect of increasing blood flow on solute clearance.

Ultrafiltration during haemodialysis

UF can be used to remove water during a HD session or as a means of solute clearance (by convection). To achieve adequate solute clearance by filtration requires large volumes of solute replacement, and the need for highly purified water or replacement fluids (because of the large amounts infused into the patient directly). However, UF provides better clearance of large MW solutes (e.g. $\beta_2 m$) by convection, and is associated with greater cardiovascular stability than conventional HD. Increasing use is thus being made of haemofiltration, with online generation of purified water, often using a second haemofilter to generate the replacement fluid. The very extensive range of 'middle' molecules identified as uraemic toxins are also better removed by convection using HDF and high-flux membranes: this has not yet been confirmed clinically to improve patient outcomes.

In conventional HD, UF is simply used to remove the excess water accumulated between dialysis sessions by ingestion of food and fluids, and from metabolism (1–4L on average). This is achieved by maintaining a TMP gradient across the dialyser. In older machines, the TMP is directly measured, and the desired UF achieved by manipulating the TMP. Most modern machines use volumetric control, whereby the inflow and outflow volumes from the dialyser are measured directly and continuously, and the amount of UF delivered determined from the difference.

Methods of ultrafiltration during haemodialysis

Pressure control

The pressure in the blood compartment is usually +50–100mmHg, depending on the blood flow rate (but will be higher if there is venous stenosis). The pressure in the dialysate compartment can be lowered by reducing the dialysate inflow rate with a clamp when the pump is on the outflow line. Negative pressures of up to −500mmHg can be achieved in this way. Pressures greater than this can lead to rupture of the dialyser. Pressures are usually measured in the blood and dialysate outlet lines. Pressure within the dialyser blood compartment will be slightly higher than that measured at the outlet, and some machines measure the inlet pressure too.

The amount of TMP needed to remove a given volume of excess water can be calculated from the KUf of the dialyser (provided by the manufacturer), and the machine is programmed to calculate the necessary TMP to achieve a desired UF rate.

Volumetric control

This is a much more accurate method of UF control, and increasingly important with the use of higher flux membranes. Small errors in the measurement of TMP (under pressure control) may cause huge volume changes. In addition, the KUf of dialysers can change during a dialysis session as a result of protein deposition, partial blood clotting, and changes in haematocrit (Hct). Almost all modern dialysis machines use volumetric control. Volumetric control systems measure the UF rate directly by quantifying the volume of dialysate passing through the dialyser, and are therefore not susceptible to such problems. UF rate can be adjusted by altering the flow rates.

High-efficiency and high-flux haemodialysis

High-efficiency dialysis

This is defined by a high clearance rate of urea (>210mL/min), and a high urea KoA (mass transfer coefficient × surface area) of the dialyser (>600mL/min). The KUf (UF coefficient) of the dialyser may be low or high, and the membrane synthetic or cellulosic. At low blood flow rates (<200mL/min) the urea clearance of both high- and low-efficiency dialysers is the same, and the potential advantage of the former is not exploited. High-efficiency dialysis requires large surface area membranes, high KoA, high blood flow and dialysate flow, and bicarbonate dialysate (not acetate).

It requires excellent access to provide high blood flows (which might not be not achieved with standard percutaneous catheters). Higher dialysate flow (>500mL/min) increases the solute clearance only with blood flows >200mL/min.

High-flux dialysis

This refers to the rate of water transfer across the dialysis membrane, and is usually synonymous with use of a high-permeability membrane (β_2m clearance >20mL/min). Requires volumetric UF control to avoid accidental catastrophic volume depletion. Middle and large molecule clearance is better because of larger membrane pore size. Dialysers can be synthetic or cellulosic. Ultrapure, pyrogen-free dialysate and bicarbonate buffering are necessary because of the risk of backfiltration from dialysate into blood.

Some evidence from short-term studies (mostly small numbers and not prospective) suggests that high-flux dialysis with biocompatible membranes may lead to better preservation of residual renal function, fewer inflammatory responses, higher serum albumin, better nutritional status, less dyslipidaemia, lower β_2m levels, and less dialysis amyloidosis. The large randomized prospective HEMO study did not demonstrate any benefit of high-flux membranes (see ➲ The HEMO study, p. 174) on morbidity or mortality overall, although in the subgroup of patients on dialysis for >3.7 years cardiovascular mortality was reduced in patients on high-flux dialysis, and a Cochrane review based on almost 4000 patients treated with high- vs low-flux dialysis suggested ~15% reduced mortality in patients on high-flux dialysis. The Membrane Permeability Outcome (MPO) study also showed no survival benefit overall, but the subgroup of patients with serum albumin < 40g/L or with diabetes did have improved outcomes using high-flux dialysers.

Haemofiltration and haemodiafiltration

Haemofiltration provides solute clearance solely by convection, as solutes are dragged down a pressure gradient with water. Large volumes of filtrate are removed and need to be replaced (>40L each session). HDF combines dialysis with large volume UF, i.e. convective and diffusive removal of solutes using a high-flux membrane.

Replacement fluid must be ultrapure, with minimal endotoxin contamination, as fluid is administered directly into the patient, necessitating ultrapure water. Highly permeable large (high-flux) membranes, high blood flows, and accurate control of volume replacement are also necessary.

The procedure has historically been much more expensive than conventional dialysis, but the cost difference has been reduced with falling costs of haemodiafilters and online production of pure replacement fluids from dialysate concentrates and water using two or three ultrafilters within the dialysis machine, usually for incoming water, after proportioning and immediately before the patient.

The volume of UF is usually 60–150L/week for pure haemofiltration, and 9–50L/session in HDF. Replacement solutions can be infused either before (pre-dilution) or after the dialyser (post-dilution), and some dialysers accommodate mid-dilution. Pre-dilution reduces the clearance delivered by UF, which should be increased to deliver equivalent clearances. Post-dilution can lead to haemoconcentration in the dialyser and protein fouling of the membrane. Dialysate flow rates need to be increased since the substitution fluid is diverted from the dialysis fluid, and rates of 700–1000mL/min are needed. (See Fig. 2.3.)

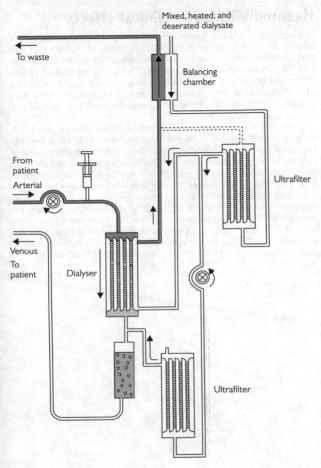

Fig. 2.3 Haemodiafiltration circuit using online ultrafiltration for production of ultra-pure dialysate and replacement fluids.

Haemodiafiltration clinical effects

Haemofiltration provides better removal of large MW solutes (e.g. β_2m, advanced glycation end-products (AGEs)), improved clearance of low MW uraemic toxins, and better cardiovascular stability and BP control than HD. Inflammatory markers are improved. It may be especially beneficial to patients likely to be on dialysis for a long time, without the likelihood of a transplant, or larger patients in whom it is impossible to achieve adequate Kt/V with HD. Intradialytic symptoms are often reduced with haemofiltration techniques.

Short-term studies have shown increased serum albumin and Hb in patients on HDF, reduced pruritus, reduced EPO dose despite improved Hb, increased delivered Kt/V, reduced need for carpal tunnel decompression surgery for amyloid, lower phosphate binder requirements, and improved nutritional indices. Residual renal function may be better preserved with HDF. HDF can cause increased losses of water-soluble vitamins.

Despite these observations in cohort studies, several clinical trials have failed to show beneficial effects on overall or cardiovascular mortality and hospitalization. A major problem may have been patients achieving low convection volumes. Subgroups analysis has suggested that patients achieving more than ~15–21L ultrafiltration do have significantly improved mortality. Patients undertaking HDF should probably aim for UF volumes of more than ~21L.

Dialysers

A dialyser (or filter) consists of a rigid polyurethane shell containing hollow fibres (capillaries) or sheets (parallel plates) of the dialysis membrane. Two ports allow blood and two ports allow dialysate to pass through the dialyser. The hollow fibres or parallel plates maximize the surface area of contact between blood and dialysate. In hollow fibre dialysers, blood flows through the capillaries. In parallel plate devices, blood and dialysate flow between alternate sheets.

There is little to choose between the two structures. Hollow fibre devices may have slightly lower priming volumes, and are easier to reuse, but may clot slightly more easily and may retain ethylene oxide (if used as a sterilant). Hollow fibre dialysers are much more commonly used in most countries.

An ideal dialyser should have:
• high clearance of small and medium MW toxins
• adequate UF
• negligible losses of proteins and amino acids
• non-toxic composition
• minimal activation of cells or thrombotic pathways
• minimal blood volume
• reliability
• reusability
• low cost.

No single dialyser meets all these needs.

Technical specifications

- Priming volumes vary from 40 to 150mL (not including blood lines—~150mL).
- Surface areas vary from 0.5 to 2.2m^2.
- KUf from 2.5 to 85mL/h/mmHg. Cellulose (and most modified cellulose) membranes have KUf <10. (KUf <4 is moderate permeability, and >8 high. High-permeability membranes require volumetric control of UF to ensure safe use.)
- KoA urea varies from 200 to 1200mL/min (<300 represents a low efficiency dialyser, >600 a high-efficiency dialyser).
- Specification sheets also provide clearances for urea and vitamin B$_{12}$ (and sometimes creatinine, phosphate, and inulin) at blood flows between 200 and 400mL/min, and sieving coefficients for albumin (should be 0) and β$_2$m.
- Molecular weight cut-offs range from 3kDa to >15kDa, and almost 65kDa for some newer high-flux dialysers.
- Dialysers are sterilized by gamma irradiation, ethylene oxide, or steam. Steam and irradiation pose least risk to patients, as ethylene oxide must be thoroughly rinsed out prior to use and can cause reactions; it is now rarely used.
- Must be pre-rinsed with >2L of rinsing solution prior to connection to the patient to prevent release of fragments from the dialysis circuit (sometimes termed 'spallation'—the leaching of solid or soluble compounds into the body), and remove other potential contaminants or sterilants from manufacture.

Dialysis membranes

Can be made from cellulose, modified cellulose, or synthetic materials. Modified cellulose has various chemicals substituted for the hydroxyl groups on the native cellulose. Cellulo-synthetic material is formed by the addition of a synthetic compound to cellulose, resulting in a change in the surface and increased biocompatibility. Fully synthetic membranes are being increasingly used such that cuprophan manufacture was discontinued in 2006. Novel membranes are being developed in which further agents are bonded to the surface, e.g. vitamin E. (See Table 2.1.)

Cellulose membranes can cause complement and leucocyte activation, while synthetic membranes have the greatest biocompatibility. Re-use of cellulose (without use of bleach as a cleanser) greatly increases biocompatibility due to absorption of proteins on to the membrane. Cellulose membranes are low flux. Modified cellulose membranes can be low or high flux, biocompatible (cellulose triacetate) or incompatible (cellulose acetate). Synthetic membranes can also be low or high flux, but are all biocompatible. Solute removal by synthetic and modified cellulose membranes is similar, although β_2m clearance is greater with synthetic membranes. The clinical significance of this is as yet unclear, although for patients unlikely to receive a transplant but survive long term, the reduced β_2m accumulation may translate into less dialysis amyloid. Generally, membranes used for haemofiltration (either continuous or high flow) are synthetic. There are some data suggesting vitamin E-coated membranes (e.g. Excebrane®) cause less oxygen free radical formation, and may be even more biocompatible. AN69® has been modified by binding polyethyleneimine (AN69ST®). This binds heparin, allowing substantial reductions in heparin needed to prevent circuit clotting (priming alone is sufficient).

Table 2.1 Dialysis membranes

	Material	Alternative names
Cellulose	Cuprammonium rayon	Cuprophan®
	Cuprammonium cellulose	
	Regenerated cellulose	
Modified or substituted cellulose	Cellulosynthetic	Hemophan®
	Cellulose acetate	
	Cellulose diacetate	Dicea®, Diaphan®
	Cellulose triacetate	
	Cellulose hydrate	
Synthetic	Polysulfone, polyethersulfone	Biosulfane®, PS, Helixone®
	Polyacrylnitrile	PAN, AN69®, SPAN®
	Polymethylmethacrylate	PMMA
	Polyamide	Polyflux®
	Polycarbonate	Gambrane®

Reactions to membranes

These are not always due to the membrane itself, but can be due to the sterilant, associated drugs, complement activation, or unknown mechanisms. Sometimes called 'first use' reactions, but can occur with re-use (see ➲ Complications during dialysis, p. 140, for more detail).

Type A reactions

These occur within minutes of starting dialysis, with dyspnoea, wheeze, a feeling of warmth, urticaria, cough, hypotension, collapse, or cardiac arrest. They are predominantly due to immune reaction to ethylene oxide, and patients can have elevated IgE antibodies to ethylene oxide-altered proteins. Also occur in patients taking ACEIs and dialysed with AN69® (or more rarely other PAN membranes). AN69® may increase bradykinin levels or activate bradykinin, even in patients not taking ACEIs, and ACEIs block the inactivation of bradykinin. Type A reactions also occur with endotoxin-contaminated water or dialysates, and occasionally to heparin.

Type B reactions

These are more common but much milder, often occur 20–40min after starting dialysis, and usually cause back and chest pain. Cause unknown and incidence declining.

Rarely other reactions have been reported.

- A syndrome of acute deafness and blindness was reported in the 1990s in patients treated with aged cellulose acetate dialysers >11 years old. No patient recovered and all had died in 1 year. Thought to be due to degraded membrane products.
- In 2002 a number of patients died after using Baxter Althane (cellulose diacetate) dialysers. Cause of death was from residual perfluorocarbon within the dialysers. This is a volatile hydrophobic fluid completely insoluble in water, which led to massive gas formation in the right side of the heart and pulmonary capillary blockade. The perfluorocarbon had been used for repair of leaking hollow fibres during manufacture.

Biocompatibility of membranes

Biocompatibility of membranes

Membranes can have varying effects on the cells and proteins to which they are exposed. A biocompatible membrane elicits the least inflammatory response in patients exposed to it; it does not cause complement, kallikrein, or cellular activation, has minimal interactions with proteins, and is not thrombogenic (low thrombin generation and release of platelet factor 4). The design of the dialyser and the precise nature of the membrane can affect its biocompatibility. Hydroxyl groups in cellulose activate the alternative pathway of complement and subsequently neutrophils. Substituted cellulose and synthetic membranes generally cause less complement activation, but also strongly bind complement proteins and prevent their efflux into the circulation.

Improved biocompatibility had been associated with:
- reduced amyloid deposition
- fewer hypersensitivity reactions
- less intradialytic hypotension (IDH)
- slower loss of residual renal function after beginning dialysis
- reduced infections
- improved nutritional status
- reduced protein catabolism
- improved lipid profiles
- possibly with better long-term morbidity and mortality.

However, data are conflicting, outcome trials comparing dialysers are lacking, and the clinical relevance of increased biocompatibility remains controversial. Despite this, current European guidelines recommend large pore, high-flux, biocompatible membranes especially for patients likely to be on dialysis for >3.7 years. (See Table 2.2.)

Table 2.2 Biological responses induced by interactions with dialysis membranes

Blood component	Biological response
Complement	Alternative pathway activation
	Anaphylatoxin production
Coagulation system	Factor XII activation
	Intrinsic pathway activation
	Increased tissue plasminogen activation
Cytokines	Some have increased serum levels
Erythrocytes	Haemolysis rarely
Neutrophils	Leucopenia
	Increased adhesion molecule expression
	Degranulation
	Release of reactive oxygen
Lymphocytes	Activation
	Impaired T-cell proliferation
Monocytes	Increased interleukin-1
	Decreased responsiveness
Platelets	Activation
	Increased adhesion
	Thrombocytopenia
	Increased platelet factor 4 and ADP release

Biocompatibility and acute and chronic kidney disease

Biocompatibility and acute kidney injury

In theory, biological reactions to membranes may worsen the catabolic state of AKI and aggravate the pro-inflammatory state (especially in multiorgan failure and sepsis). Neutrophil activation would also worsen injury both locally in the kidney and systemically. Several RCTs have been performed comparing bioincompatible (usually low-flux cellulose) and biocompatible membranes in AKI, with conflicting results. Convincing evidence for lower mortality and better and faster renal recovery is currently lacking. Large randomized prospective studies have not shown any differences in outcome between patients treated with cuprophan and PMMA membranes, or between polysulfone (high or low flux) and cellulose diacetate. The severity of the underlying disorder and the skill of the nursing and medical staff probably outweigh the nature of the dialysis membrane in the prognosis and outcome of patients with severe AKI. Future trials are likely to be difficult as CRRT generally uses synthetic membranes and is increasingly used in patients with AKI.

Biocompatibility and chronic kidney disease

There are no randomized trials of morbidity or mortality comparing biocompatible and incompatible membranes in maintenance dialysis. Several uncontrolled studies have suggested improved outcomes with synthetic membranes; however, whether the effect is due to biocompatibility, increased delivery of dialysis, increased haemofiltration, or increased permeability of the membranes is unclear. The Tassin group in France continued to use cellulose membranes for many years and reported excellent morbidity and mortality (with long hours and superb BP control), and randomized studies from Italy demonstrate no benefit of polysulfone over cellulose after 2 years of follow-up. β_2m clearance is increased by most synthetic membranes (especially polysulfone, PAN, and AN69®), due to increased convective and diffusive clearance and adsorption to the membrane. Synthesis of β_2m may also be reduced with biocompatible membranes due to reduced activation of mononuclear cells. Clinical studies have produced conflicting results, with β_2m levels either unchanged or reduced, and a single study suggesting reduced radiological changes of dialysis-related amyloid in patients using AN69®.

Dialysis machines: key features

In principle, these simply consist of a blood pump, dialysate delivery system, and safety monitors. Increasingly sophisticated monitors (blood, dialysate, and patient) and sensing software are incorporated to provide real-time management and a continuous record of individual dialysis sessions. The NxStage® machine (developed for home dialysis programmes) is slightly different (see ➔ Home dialysis machine technology, p. 241) since there is no blood air interface, and a disposable cartridge containing the circuit and volumetric balancing.

Blood pump

Usually roller (peristaltic)—usual blood flow rate 200–600mL/min.

Bubble trap

Minimizes risk of air within the circuit returning to the patient, when combined with a distal air detector.

Heparin administration

Usually provided by the dialysis machine via a syringe pump.

Dialysate delivery

Machines either mix (proportion) dialysate and bicarbonate with pure water individually for the patient, or a single machine performs this centrally before distributing the pre-mixed dialysate to several dialysis machines. Dialysate concentrate is usually liquid (and may contain acetate), while bicarbonate is usually added via a second concentrate either as a solid (to be mixed with water) or as a liquid. Bicarbonate is almost universal now. Individual preparation of dialysate provides greater flexibility, while central proportioning can be cheaper. Water/dialysate must be heated to ~37°C and degassed (to remove dissolved gases). The dialysate pump may allow generation of a negative pressure for UF. (See Fig. 2.4.)

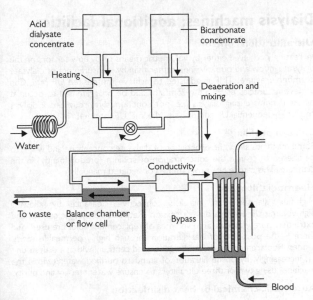

Fig. 2.4 Dialysate delivery in HD machines.

Dialysis machines: additional facilities

Ultrafiltration control

Increasingly achieved either by volumetric means or by flow sensors on the dialysate inflow and outflow lines, rather than by measurement of dialysate chamber pressure. TMP is adjusted to achieve the desired UF rate. Can achieve accuracies of 99.5% (~25mL/h) and be programmed to occur at different times during dialysis (i.e. not continuously throughout a dialysis session)—sequential UF and dialysis. Maximal UF rates ~4L/h.

Sodium profiling

Some machines allow the proportion of dialysate concentrate and water to be altered to change the concentration of sodium (predominantly) in the dialysate. This can be pre-programmed or initiated manually.

Haemodiafiltration

High-flux dialysers can increase convective clearance by allowing high-volume UF during a dialysis session. Requires volumetric control and extremely pure water as large volumes of replacement fluids are used, and there is the possibility of backfiltration through highly permeable membranes. Replacement fluids can be generated centrally within a dialysis unit or, increasingly, by online filtration of standard purified water (within the machine) using two or three ultrafilters to ensure water sterility and purity.

Automatic chemical or heat disinfection

This can be pre-programmed or manual.

Single- or double-needle dialysis

Almost all machines allow either option. Single-needle dialysis has the advantage of a single venepuncture, but is usually less efficient, and has increased risk of recirculation. A 'Y' connector allows arterial blood to be pumped into the machine, and venous blood to be returned to the patient through the same needle, but not at the same time. A defined volume of blood is withdrawn through the arterial circuit, before the previously dialysed blood is returned to the patient. Requires specialized tubing with an expansion reservoir, as blood withdrawal and return are not synchronous, and usually needs two blood pumps.

Dialysis machines: monitors

Blood circuit monitoring

Air detectors
These are placed distally in the venous circuit together with a bubble trap. Often ultrasonic. Linked to a blood line clamp to stop blood returning to the patient, if air is sensed.

Pressure monitors
These are often placed just before the blood pump (arterial) and after the dialyser (venous). The arterial monitor records excess negative pressure due to poor flow through the access, and can detect line disconnection (when the pressure approaches zero) and poor access flows (increasingly negative pressure); the venous monitor records excess pressure due to increased resistance to venous return. Both monitors are linked to alarms (when predefined pressure limits are exceeded) and can stop the blood pump and clamp the lines.

Dialysate monitoring

Blood leak
This detects rupture of the dialyser. Usually by infrared or photodetector monitoring. Sensitivity <0.5mL of blood/min.

Temperature
Continuously monitored to ensure correct dialysate temperature. High temperatures can cause haemolysis. Cold solutions can cause hypothermia. When monitor alarms, dialysate is diverted to waste. Can be used to reduce patient's body temperature (usually by 0.5–1°C), to reduce hypotension, and improve UF.

Conductivity
The electrical conductivity of the dialysate is used to monitor the correct proportioning of concentrate with water. Many machines will use conductivity to allow alterations in the sodium concentration of the dialysate (sodium profiling). When monitor alarms (high or low conductivity), dialysate is diverted to waste.

Pressure
Some machines monitor the pressure in the dialysate outflow line to calculate TMP.

Online Kt/V
By monitoring the urea concentration in the dialysate outflow line, the actual amount of dialysis delivered during each session can be determined. Can also be done by measuring ionic dialysance in the dialysis circuit as a surrogate for urea clearance or measures of ultraviolet absorbance. Provides real-time reporting of delivered dialysis (urea) clearance.

Dialysis machines: patient monitors

BP
Some machines monitor arterial pressure automatically.

ECG
Can be monitored by the machine (e.g. for remotely monitored dialysis).

Blood volume monitors
These monitor the Hct or protein concentration in the arterial blood line by optical or ultrasonic sensors as a surrogate for blood volume (as water is removed from the blood, blood volume falls, and red blood cell and protein concentration increase). They can measure relative blood volume (RBV) reliably and reproducibly, and allow automatic feedback. Reduction in blood volume generally precedes hypotension, hence intervention prior to hypotension can be judged by the reduction in RBV and can reduce the UF rate, increase the dialysate sodium concentration, or infuse normal or hypertonic saline. Most software relies on expert systems, which 'learn' the most appropriate time and mode of intervention for an individual patient. Can also measure absolute Hct and oxygen saturation.

Monitoring fluid balance
Blood volume monitors can analyse the effects of a short period of rapid UF on blood volume to determine the hydration status of a patient. The rate of refilling of the vascular compartment can give a measure of extravascular fluid.

Access recirculation
Can be measured by the change in temperature in the arterial blood line after reducing or increasing the dialysate temperature (by 2.5°C) for a few minutes (thermodilution), or by injecting 5mL of isotonic or hypertonic saline and measuring change in conductivity. Non-invasive.

Access blood flow
Can be measured by saline injection techniques during Hct monitoring or change in Hct due to a short period of UF.

Delivered Kt/V
Can be calculated from online measurement of urea (or total toxin) removal or change in dialysate conductivity.

Dialysate

Dialysis solutions are usually prepared from concentrates and contain either acetate or bicarbonate as a buffer. Acetate use is now rare worldwide. The precise composition can be varied if needed, and increasing use is being made of individualized dialysate prescription. This is achieved by modern dialysis machines permitting the accurate proportioning of water and dialysis concentrate, and monitoring the final concentration of solutes (by electrical conductivity). Alternatively, concentrates are diluted centrally within a dialysis unit and the prepared dialysate is distributed to several dialysis machines for direct use. Central proportioning does not allow individualized prescription of dialysate.

Acetate-containing dialysate were widely used, as a single concentrate can be easily manufactured containing all the elements needed but have been mostly superseded by bicarbonate-containing concentrates. They are more physiological, provide better control of acidosis, and produce fewer complications and side effects during dialysis. During manufacture and storage, however, solute precipitation can occur, hence magnesium and calcium are separated from the bicarbonate to prevent precipitation of carbonate crystals. Most of the solutes are contained within the dialysate concentrate, while bicarbonate and sodium are provided as a solid or liquid separately, to be mixed within the dialysis machine at a late stage. Small amounts of acetic or lactic acid are included with the calcium and magnesium to combine with bicarbonate during mixing and generate carbonic acid (from CO_2). This lowers the pH of the final solution to 7–7.4 and ensures solubility of the salts. It is also possible to make up dialysate from three concentrates—electrolytes and glucose, sodium chloride, and bicarbonate, to allow for finer control of the individual components. (See Table 2.3.)

Table 2.3 Usual composition of dialysate

Sodium	132–155mmol/L
Potassium	0–4mmol/L
Calcium	1.25–1.75mmol/L
Magnesium	0.25–0.75mmol/L
Chloride	90–120mmol/L
Acetate	30–45mmol/L (only in acetate-based dialysates)
Bicarbonate	27–40mmol/L
Dextrose	0–5.5mmol/L
pH	7.1–7.3

Sodium

Previously, low-sodium dialysates were used to minimize hypertension. This is complicated by a high incidence of cramps and disequilibrium symptoms, hypotension, and even hypertension induced by stimulation of the renin–angiotensin pathways. Higher sodium concentrations minimize muscle cramps, nausea, vomiting, and hypotension, and concentrations of up to 150mmol/L have been used. High sodium may, however, increase thirst and promote hypertension in the long term by salt and water overload.

Sodium profiling

Sodium profiling (or ramping or modelling) refers to the use of variable sodium dialysate concentrations during an individual dialysis session to attempt to minimize hypotension. (See Fig. 2.5.)

- Generally, high dialysate sodium is used in the initial phase of dialysis, and reduced later.
- High initial sodium maintains plasma osmolality during the period of maximum rate of urea diffusion (early in dialysis), thus supporting plasma refilling from the interstitium.
- The dialysate sodium concentration can subsequently be reduced.
- A number of controlled trials have demonstrated the benefit of sodium profiling in intradialytic symptom control, especially for the reduction of cramps and better vascular stability.
- Continuous conductivity measurement of dialysate is used to monitor sodium concentration.
- The major risk is sodium accumulation if the dialysate sodium is not reduced sufficiently during dialysis or the initial concentration is too high, leading to increased thirst, fluid overload, and hypertension. This can be a major problem if sodium concentrations are not individualized to the patient's pre-dialysis serum sodium concentration. Hence the importance of accurate measurement of dialysate sodium.
- This technique should be used carefully.

Dialysate sodium (mmol/l)		
From	To	
150	130	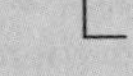
150	130	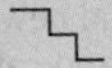
148	138	
155	135	

Fig. 2.5 Examples of sodium profiling regimens.

Other electrolytes and glucose

Potassium

For maintenance HD there is rarely a need to change the dialysate potassium from 1.5 to 2mmol/L. In AKI with oliguria, rhabdomyolysis, or the need for multiple blood transfusions, lower (or no) potassium dialysates may sometimes be needed, but should be used with great caution since plasma potassium can fall quickly at the start of dialysis. Some patients require higher potassium, or careful dietary advice, if they have persistent hypokalaemia from diarrhoea or vomiting, or daily dialysis.

Calcium

Water softening, deionizers, and reverse osmosis (RO) have removed the problem of hard water-induced hypercalcaemia. Sufficient calcium is necessary to reverse the hypocalcaemia present in most patients without hyperparathyroidism. Conversely, low-calcium dialysates (1.25mmol/L) are needed in patients with uncontrollable hyperparathyroidism and hypercalcaemia. Reducing dialysate calcium is an important method to help manage hyperparathyroidism (when combined with vitamin D therapy and phosphate binders).

Glucose

May help prevent disequilibrium by maintaining osmotic pressure during the rapid removal of urea, and help buffering.

Quality

High-quality dialysate is especially important with the use of highly permeable membranes and high-volume haemofiltration.

Acid–base: acetate and bicarbonate

Correction of acidosis is a crucial component of dialytic therapy. Hydrogen ions cannot be removed by dialysis because of their low concentration in plasma water as a result of buffering. Alkali is therefore added to the dialysate to diffuse into the blood. Historically, bicarbonate-containing solutions were frequently infected and unstable, and acetate was introduced as a stable alkali equivalent. Acetate is metabolized to acetyl coenzyme A both in peripheral tissues and in the liver, capturing a single hydrogen ion. Subsequent decarboxylation releases the hydrogen ion into the respiratory chain.

Bicarbonate was reintroduced in the 1980s using new mixing and delivery techniques, and new dialysis machines became capable of mixing separate bicarbonate- and calcium-containing solutions. Bicarbonate cartridges are now widely used; powder is continuously dissolved into a concentrated solution, which the machine proportions prior to mixing with dialysate.

Acetate has been associated with cardiovascular instability during dialysis, and with acetate accumulation when used with higher flux dialysers. Controlled studies have demonstrated clear benefits of bicarbonate for intradialytic symptoms, morbidity, and BP control. Acetate is now rarely used.

Water purification

Water purification

Patients are exposed to 300–400L of dialysate per week with conventional HD (20,000L/year), and more with high-flow haemofiltration. In HD, dissolved substances can diffuse across the membrane, and backfiltration occurs with use of high-flux membranes. In high-flow haemofiltration, large quantities of replacement solutes are directly infused into the patient, together with whatever contaminants are present in the water. (See Tables 2.4 and 2.5.)

An episode of fatal microcystin poisoning was reported from Brazil where water contaminated with blue-green algae (cyanobacteria) was inadequately purified. Patients suffered acute neurotoxicity and subacute hepatotoxicity. An episode of acute poisoning with fluoride occurred in 1994 in a dialysis unit from a deionization unit, and aluminium poisoning from inappropriate concrete lining in a water pipe supplying a dialysis unit in Curacao.

Treatment and toxicity

Water treatment is a multistage process involving:
- microfilters (which remove particulate material)
- activated carbon (adsorbs chloramine, organic contaminants, chlorine, and acts inefficiently as a filter)
- sometimes chelation
- further microfilters (≤1μm pore size)
- water softeners (which remove calcium and magnesium, iron and manganese, by ion exchange for sodium cations)

Table 2.4 Potential water contaminants

Particulates	Dissolved substances	Microorganisms
Clay	Aluminium	*Bacillus* spp.
Sand	Calcium	*Micrococcus* spp.
Silica	Magnesium	*Corynebacterium* spp.
Iron	Chloramines	*Staphylococci* spp.
	Copper	*Streptococci* spp.
	Fluoride	*Escherichia coli*
	Nitrate	*Pseudomonas* spp.
	Sulphate	*Flavobacter* spp.
	Zinc	*Aerobacter* spp.
	Microbial pyrogens	*Xanthomonas* spp.
	Endotoxin	*Klebsiella* spp.
		Enterobacter
		Mycobacteria
		Clostridium spp.

Table 2.5 Contaminants causing toxic effects

Contaminant	Effect
Aluminium	Microcytic anaemia, encephalopathy, dementia, bone disease (osteomalacia)
Calcium (magnesium)	Nausea, vomiting, headache, weakness, hypertension
Copper	Nausea, headache, haemolysis, hepatitis
Zinc	Anaemia, nausea, vomiting, fever
Sodium	Hypertension, pulmonary oedema, thirst, confusion, headache, fits, coma
Lead	Neurological disorders
Chloramine	Haemolysis, anaemia, methaemoglobinaemia
Fluoride	Osteomalacia, pruritus, nausea, arrhythmias
Nitrate	Cyanosis, methaemoglobinaemia, nausea, hypotension
Sulphate	Nausea, vomiting, acidosis
Microbial pyrogens, endotoxin	Nausea, vomiting, fever, hypotension, shock, enhanced dialysis amyloid formation

- reverse osmosis (RO)(membrane filtration and deionizing using a membrane with a cut-off ~300Da)
- sometimes deionizers and ultraviolet radiation treatment or nanofiltration.

Water needs to be stored and distributed to individual dialysis machines while retaining its purity and lack of microbial contamination. For high-flow haemofiltration, ultrapure water is required, and is usually produced by further UF steps either centrally or online within the dialysis machine (using hollow-fibre haemofilters), or by sequential deionization or further RO treatment. Biofilm must be prevented from forming in pipework and storage tanks.

European standards for microbial purity of dialysis water allow <100 bacteria cfu/mL, and <0.25IU/mL endotoxin (<200cfu/mL and 2.0IU/mL in the USA). Ultrapure water must have <0.1cfu/mL and endotoxin <0.03IU/mL. Use of ultrapure water in itself reduces CRP levels in patients, lessens anaemia, improves ESA responsiveness and may improve nutritional status. European Best Practice guidelines recommend ultrapure water for all dialysis modalities (conventional and high flux).

For maximum recommended levels of contaminants in dialysis water (from the Renal Association guidelines), see Table 2.6.

Table 2.6 Water contaminants

Contaminant	Maximum recommended concentration(mg/L = ppm)	Initial test frequency (unless available from water supplier)
Aluminium	0.01	3-monthly
Calcium	2 (0.05mmol/L)	3-monthly
Total chlorine	0.1	Not less than weekly
Copper	0.1	3-monthly
Fluoride	0.2	3-monthly
Magnesium	2 (0.08mmol/L)	3-monthly
Nitrate (as N)	2 (equates to 9mg/L NO_3)	3-monthly
Potassium	2 (0.05mmol/L)	3-monthly
Sodium	50 (2.2mmol/L)	3-monthly
Bacteria (total viable count)	100cfu/mL	Not less than monthly
Endotoxin	0.25IU/mL	Not less than monthly
Ammonium	0.2	3-monthly
Arsenic	0.005	3-monthly
Cadmium	0.001	3-monthly
Chloride	50	3-monthly
Chromium	0.014	3-monthly
Lead	0.005	3-monthly
Mercury	0.0002	3-monthly
Sulphate	50	3-monthly
Barium	0.1	As indicated
Beryllium	0.0004	As indicated
Silver	0.005	As indicated
Thallium	0.002	As indicated
Tin	0.1	As indicated
Zinc	0.1	As indicated

Vascular access: overview

Vascular access patency is crucial for patients with ESKD. 25% of hospital admissions for dialysis patients are for access problems, and access failure is a major cause of morbidity. Without early referral or planning, up to 75% of new patients beginning HD require admission for temporary access placement, with increased morbidity, infections, and even mortality.

Dialysis units should develop vascular access strategies to minimize the complications associated with poor access. This should include:
• maximizing AVF use (as the preferred access for most patients)
• planning AVF formation at an early stage in patients with CKD
• reducing the incidence of infections and thrombosis
• actively (prospectively) detecting access at risk for thrombosis and failure.

Synthetic grafts have a significantly increased risk of thrombosis, infections, and need for interventions, and their use should be minimized. Primary AVFs have higher long-term patency than prosthetic grafts in patients of all ages (>60% better at age 40) and 10% of the infection rate. (See Table 2.7.)

Timing of access placement

Early patient referral to nephrologists and early formation of permanent access minimizes complications and is associated with lower morbidity and mortality. Consideration for fistula formation should begin within 1 year of anticipated need for dialysis, and primary AVF should be created at least 6–12 months prior to anticipated need. Synthetic grafts can be inserted 1 month before needed. Temporary or tunnelled access should only be inserted at the time of need.

Table 2.7 Prevalence of access type

	Catheters	AVF	Grafts
UK	22%	69%	9%
USA	17%	24%	59%
Canada	26%	55%	19%
France	10%	80%	10%
Germany	4%	83%	13%

Evaluation prior to access surgery

History

Note any history of:

- previous proximal catheters
- previous peripheral IV catheters (subclavian or femoral)
- surgical procedures
- cardiac pacemaker
- IV drug use
- peripheral vascular disease
- smoking
- cardiac failure
- diabetes
- anticipated renal transplant from living donor
- clotting disorders.

Relevant examination findings

Including:

- pulses and bruits
- asymmetry of BP or pulses in limbs
- Allen test (for patent ulnar artery: compress both radial and ulnar artery at the wrist, wait for the hand to become pale, then release ulnar artery alone and watch for return of blood into the entire hand. If hand does not re-perfuse, ulnar artery not patent)
- presence of oedema.

Patients with previous central venous cannulation may require pre-operative imaging of central veins to exclude silent stenosis. Some units perform Doppler studies or angiography prior to surgery in patients with oedema, previous surgery, or, occasionally, routinely, to document location and size of all vessels from wrist to axilla. Vein mapping by tourniquet venous palpation and ultrasound (US) may be useful to select the best vein for anastomosis. Some data suggest veins need to be >2.5mm (by US) without stenosis, and arteries >2mm diameter without inflow stenosis.

All patients with CKD, and staff dealing with them, should be educated to preserve arm veins. Forearm cephalic veins should not be used for IV lines or venepuncture, and subclavian catheterization should be avoided in all patients with renal disease (including those on PD or transplanted).

Permanent vascular access

Choice is between AVF and a synthetic bridging graft. An AVF consists of a subcutaneous anastomosis between an artery and vein, usually in the forearm, which matures over several months by venous dilatation and thickening of the vein's wall (arterialization). A graft is an artificial connection between an artery and vein, usually made of PTFE (polytetrafluoroethylene, Teflon®) or, increasingly, biological material such as bovine veins. A tunnelled central line can be permanent vascular access, especially in patients with small vessels, but should not be first-line access of choice. (See Fig. 2.6.)

Fistulae

Good evidence for long-term patency, lower complication rates, lower morbidity, and improved performance (flow) with time in fistulae rather than grafts. Choice of location for AVF (in order of preference):

• radiocephalic (wrist)
• radiobasilic (wrist)
• brachiocephalic (elbow)
• brachiobasilic transposition (involves freeing and transposition of basilic vein at time of AVF formation)
• then forearm prosthetic grafts, thigh fistulae and thigh grafts, and axillo-axillary grafts.

An AVF can be created after the failure of a bridge graft when the proximal veins have dilated. AVFs should be constructed well in advance of need (at least 3–4 months). Up to 40% of AVFs may fail to mature.

Synthetic grafts

Should not be first choice for permanent access.

Usually made from PTFE. The material is porous, allowing ingrowth of fibroblasts and incorporation of the graft into the subcutaneous tissues. Can also be native transposed veins, bovine umbilical or mesenteric veins (ProCol®), or other synthetic or natural materials. The most common approach uses a forearm loop between the brachial artery and cephalic vein, extending 10cm down the forearm. Linear radiocephalic forearm grafts, upper arm loop grafts, and upper thigh femoral loops are also placed. Short grafts can deteriorate from repeated puncture at a limited number of sites. Long grafts have increased pressure, reduced flow, and increased thrombosis risk. Grafts are technically easy to cannulate, can be used soon after insertion (14 days ideally, but can be earlier), and can be easier to insert and repair.

Flows

Average flow through a forearm graft is 800–1200mL/min. Fistulae flows are more variable, but should always be >600mL/min.

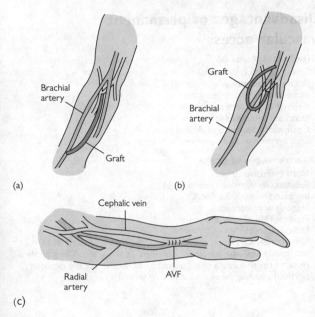

Fig. 2.6 Permanent vascular access for haemodialysis.
(a) Forearm straight PTFE graft. (b) Forearm loop PTFE graft. (c) Radial arteriovenous fistula.

Disadvantages of permanent vascular access

Disadvantages of AVF

- Slow maturation.
- Failure of maturation.
- More difficult to needle.
- Increase in size with age.
- Increased aneurysm formation.
- Cosmetic appearance of dilated veins.
- Steal syndromes and peripheral ischaemia

Disadvantages of grafts

- More extensive surgery.
- Substantially increased infection risk.
- Increased thrombosis risk (6×).
- Stenosis at anastomosis.
- Expected life of only 3–5 years.
- Difficult to remove.
- Skin erosion. Once skin erosion occurs, the graft is infected and does not usually heal with antibiotics, skin flaps, or skin grafts. The graft then requires revision into a new site (often with excision of the exposed portion) allowing the wound to heal by secondary repair.

Formation of permanent access

Formation of a fistula

- *Radial*: anastomosis of radial artery to cephalic vein at the wrist either end (vein) to side (artery), or, if the vessels overlie each other, side to side (increased risk of prominent hand veins, but potentially better fistula development).
- *Brachial*: increased risk of steal and oedema because of increased blood flow from brachial artery. Cephalic vein mobilized for anastomosis on to the brachial artery or a deep connecting vein from the median antecubital is used. Deeper brachial or basilic veins can also be transposed.

Patients should be well hydrated prior to surgery. BP should not be low or too high. Pre-operative dialysis should leave the patient above their dry weight. Patients with renal function should be given IV fluids to avoid dehydration when 'nil by mouth'. Local or regional anaesthesia usually used for distal surgery. Antihypertensive drugs should be avoided post-operatively. Dialysis should be delayed at least 24h post-operatively if possible, and care taken not to induce hypotension. Dry weight should probably be increased for the next week to avoid fistula thrombosis. There is no evidence for the benefit of aspirin, other antiplatelet agents, or anticoagulants for improving AVF survival after surgery.

Procedures to enhance fistula maturation

- Fistula hand and arm exercises may promote maturation, or at least increase patient awareness of their access.
- AVF with haematomas or oedema should be rested until swelling has resolved.
- Infiltrated or swollen fistulae or grafts should not be subjected to repeated cannulations. Single-needle use may be appropriate.

Formation of bridge graft

Appropriate vessels are isolated, and then the graft tunnelled subcutaneously. Kinking must be avoided. Standard vascular anastomoses are created. Systemic anticoagulation is rarely needed. Conflicting evidence for benefit of aspirin or low-dose warfarin in preventing graft thrombosis. Hydration state pre- and post-operatively should be carefully maintained, and hypotension avoided.

Stenosis of fistulae and grafts

Venous stenosis

- Less common with AVF than with grafts, but can be more severe.
- Usually occurs adjacent or just distal to the anast-mosis, or in the draining vein, and is caused by intimal and fibrous hyperplasia. Grafts can also develop intragraft stenoses.
- Screen by increase in venous pressure (insensitive), reduced blood flow (measure repeatedly by ultrasound dilution or Doppler US), or increased recirculation (more sensitive). Intragraft stenoses do not cause changes in pressure or recirculation.
- There is no evidence that repair of haemodynamically insignificant stenoses (of <50% vessel diameter) improves outcome or reduces thrombosis rate.
- Repair of stenoses in patent vessels is more effective than in thrombosed vessels: only 50% of grafts are patent 4 weeks after angioplasty for stenosis in a thrombosed graft, vs 80% patency at 28 weeks for angioplasty in non-thrombosed vessels.
- Surgical repair or angioplasty is less effective for AVF than for grafts. Angioplasty is often difficult in longstanding grafts with pronounced intimal hyperplasia.
- Stents have been used but can subsequently fibrose, make further thrombectomy difficult, and re-stenose inoperably.
- There are no controlled trials comparing different access interventions.

Good imaging prior to repair is important. Standard venography will often not visualize the anastomosis of an AVF or any proximal stenosis. Formal angiography (via femoral artery puncture and catheter insertion up to the axillary artery) provides better imaging of the feeding artery and anastomosis, but is more invasive. Venography combined with careful needle placement for contrast injection and with tourniquet compression can be used to visualize the arterial anastomosis properly. Magnetic resonance imaging (MRI) (or magnetic resonance venography) is increasingly being used to visualize the arterial and venous components of the AVF.

Thrombosis of fistulae and grafts

- Thrombosis is 6 times more common in grafts compared with AVF, but more severe in AVF.
- Usually secondary to stenosis or low arterial blood flow.
- Thrombus can be removed by thrombectomy using a balloon-tipped embolectomy catheter (Fogarty), but the underlying structural cause (in 80–90%) must also be treated.
- Angioplasty is often the preferred method for treating access stenosis or thrombosis.
- Salvage is often unsuccessful (surgical or angioplasty).
- Thrombus can also be removed using thrombolytic agents (tissue plasminogen activator (tPA), alteplase, or streptokinase, usually combined with heparin) instilled locally. tPA is used at 0.5–2mg, and subsequent 0.5mg aliquots. Standard or pulse spray catheters can be used. Infusion often continued for several hours.
- Alternatives include mechanical disruption via catheter.
- Treatment is rarely successful beyond 48h of thrombosis.
- Clopidogrel, combined aspirin and dipyridamole, or formal anticoagulation of grafts with warfarin to an international normalized ratio (INR) of 2 have not been shown to reduce the risk of thrombosis, and may increase bleeding risk.
- Omega-3 polyunsaturated fish oils have been shown to reduce thrombosis rates in grafts in small trials.

Screening for arteriovenous fistula/graft stenosis and thrombosis

Prospective monitoring of grafts and fistulae for haemodynamically significant stenoses has not been shown in prospective studies to improve access survival, although cohort studies have suggested reduced morbidity, hospitalization, need for surgical interventions, and thrombosis, and improved long-term patency with formal monitoring. Approximately 20% of patients with AVF require intervention each year, and more with grafts. Access failure is the most common cause for hospital admission in patients on HD. Grafts and fistulae can be monitored by:

- intra-access blood flow (Qa)
- static venous pressure
- dynamic venous pressure
- measurement of access recirculation using dilution techniques or urea concentration
- reduced delivered dialysis
- increased negative arterial pressures
- Doppler US.

Clinical features of inflow stenosis include flat access, excessive collapse of venous segment on arm elevation, abnormal thrill, or bruit (weak or discontinuous or high pitched) and for outflow stenosis, arm swelling and abnormal thrill or bruit. A blinded prospective study has shown a combination of bedside physical examination and routine Qa measurement by US dilution can detect >80% of stenoses in AVFs.

Access flow rates

Prospective monitoring is more beneficial for grafts than fistulae. Presence of a palpable thrill is associated with blood flow >450mL/min. Flow can be measured by Doppler US or dilution techniques (saline bolus or temperature). 'Normal' flow within an AVF is 500–800mL/min, and 600–1000mL/min in grafts (or even 3L/min). For grafts, thrombosis risk (over the following 6 months) increases when graft blood flow falls to <6–700mL/min, or has reduced by >25% over 4 months and is <1000mL/min. Serial measures are more useful than single measurements, and a trend to reduced blood flow is the most significantly predictive factor.

Flow can be measured using US measurement of the dilution of saline (e.g. Transonic® device); the blood lines are reversed, a bolus injected into the A line, and the effective dilution measured at the V line by US. This can be directly related to the access flow rate. Doppler US can be used to measure flow directly but can be confounded, especially by turbulence. Measurement of the brachial artery flow rate can be more reliable and is essentially the same as the access flow rate.

Dynamic venous pressure monitoring

Venous pressure arbitrarily recorded from the dialysis machine is a poor marker of venous stenosis. A more reliable method ensures measurements are made under controlled conditions on repeated occasions, e.g. measuring venous pressure from the HD machine at a blood flow rate (Qb) of 200mL/min during the first 5min of dialysis at every dialysis sessio. It is important that the same needles (length and gauge) and circuits are used. Patients with increasing pressures on consecutive occasions require venography, as do those with pressures above a given threshold (which needs to be determined locally). Dynamic venous pressure >125mmHg at Qb 200mL/min with a 15-gauge needle and a Cobe Centrysystem® 3 machine require investigation. With a Gambro AK10® and 15-gauge needle the cut-off is 150mmHg. Increasing pressure on sequential dialysis sessions is more significant than a single high value. It is less reliable or predictive than US dilution techniques, but simple to perform, repeatable, and requires no specialized equipment.

Doppler ultrasound

Can be predictive of graft stenosis and failure but requires experienced operator and expensive equipment. Marked interobserver variability in measurement of Doppler flow (see earlier in topic).

Magnetic resonance flow measurement

Accurate, very expensive, difficult to perform.

Ultrasound dilution techniques

Online measurement of dilution by US velocity changes is simple, reliable, repeatable, and valid. Will probably become the preferred method for prospective monitoring of access blood flow (see earlier in topic).

Measurement of recirculation

Predictive but very late sign of access stenosis since implies access blood flow rate already 350–500mL/min. Must be performed in standardized manner. Figures of >15% recirculation may imply stenosis, but the measure has a high false-negative rate. Can be done by US dilution techniques (saline or temperature) or serum urea measurement.

Decreased urea reduction ratio (URR) or Kt/V

Multiple factors can affect delivered dialysis dose, hence not very specific for access stenosis.

Venography or arteriography

Patients with suspected venous or arterial stenosis require formal imaging. Arterial stenosis manifests as low blood flows or 'sucking'. Venography often fails to demonstrate the fistula anastomosis and may therefore miss anatomic stenosis. Formal arteriography provides better imaging of the entire fistula or graft, including arterial inflow and draining vein, and may be used for suspected arterial problems. If venography is used then tourniquet compression of the arterial inflow may help ensure proper visualization of the anastomosis itself.

Other complications of fistulae and grafts

Inadequate flow

Low access blood flow prevents delivery of adequate dialysis, and increases risk of access thrombosis. Usually requires formal angiogram, and management of any arterial stenosis (angioplasty or surgical correction).

Ischaemia

Ischaemia of the hand and fingers can cause permanent loss of digits, small regions of infarction, or ischaemia on exercise. More common in the elderly and diabetics, or in patients with multiple failed fistulae. Patients should be told to report changes in sensation, temperature, or weakness. Minor degrees of ischaemia are common and manifest simply as reduced temperature or paraesthesiae; they do not require any intervention, and generally improve with time. More severe ischaemia may require urgent treatment by closing the fistula. Alternatively, some success has been reported using the DRIL procedure (distal revascularization interval ligation). The artery is ligated immediately distal to the AVF, and a saphenous vein used to bypass the ligation from artery proximal to the AVF to a more distal portion of the artery.

Oedema

This is common, especially if a side-of-vein anastomosis is used. In this case it can be converted to an end-of-vein anastomosis. Sometimes so severe requires closure of the AVF.

Aneurysm formation

Usually caused by repeated needling of a single (or few) site(s). Only requires repair if overlying skin becomes thinned, aneurysm becomes very large, there is spontaneous bleeding or limitation to needling sites, nerve compression, or for cosmetic reasons. Low flow in aneurysms predisposes to thrombosis.

Pseudoaneurysm

This is due to communication between the graft or fistula and a confined space of surrounding tissue. It can lead to ischaemia of the skin overlying the graft or fistula, poor haemostasis after needle withdrawal, and prolonged bleeding; it can also prevent full use of the graft or fistula. Should be repaired when skin is compromised, there is a risk of rupture, nerve compression, or lack of sites for needling.

Steal syndrome

Occurs when flow through the fistula or graft has lower resistance than other distal vascular beds and arterial inflow is limited (e.g. by arterial calcification or stenosis). Under these conditions, distal blood flow is reduced (see ➋ Ischaemia, this topic). When severe, it can lead to digital gangrene. Access requires revision or banding to increase the resistance, moving the arterial inflow more proximally, or sometimes closure.

Infection
Mostly a problem with grafts and catheters. Particularly common in patients with (temporary) central catheters who develop a Gram-positive bacterae-mia. It is difficult to eradicate bacteria once a graft is colonized, and very prolonged courses of antibiotics or removal of the graft may be required. AVF infections are rare and should be treated as for endocarditis (6 weeks of antibiotics). Patients with grafts should receive prophylactic antibiotics during dental work, catheterization, etc.

Extravasation injury
Usually occurs when the venous needle transfixes either the graft (more commonly) or AVF, or becomes dislodged during dialysis, or by blood leak-age from inadequate haemostasis after dialysis. It can cause rapid swelling of the limb before the dialysis machine blood pump stops, access thrombo-sis, compartment syndrome, neuropathy, critical ischaemia, or can become infected. Drainage may be required.

Superior vena cava (SVC) or central vein obstruction syndrome
Presents usually as grossly swollen arm with dilated veins across the chest, or with neck and facial swelling too. Occurs with stenosed subclavian veins (most common), SVC, or internal jugular veins secondary to previous cen-tral catheters, or more rarely just to very large venous return. Management initially may be simply expectant. Some benefit from anticoagulation, venoplasty (only 20–40% patent at 6 months), venoplasty and stent inser-tion (but stents may come loose or drift proximally in central veins) or open surgery.

Tunnelled cuffed catheters

These should be used in patients requiring temporary venous access for >3 weeks. Often inserted while awaiting permanent access formation or maturation, but also increasingly used for long-term access in patients who have exhausted all other access options, or sometimes (mostly inappropriately) as first-line, long-term access. However, some centres report extremely low infection rates and excellent long-term success of tunnelled catheters, but this is rare. Preferred site is the right internal jugular vein. Can also be inserted into external jugular veins, subclavian veins, femoral veins, or translumbar into the inferior vena cava. Should not be inserted into the same side as a maturing fistula if possible, and subclavian route should only be used if no jugular access available. Insertion should be performed under fluoroscopy to confirm the position of the tip in the right atrium, and US should be used to aid localization of the vein. (See Table 2.8.)

Many different lines are available with little objective evidence for major differences (Permcath®, Vascath®, Tesio®, Ash Split Cath®). They can either be dual lumen with round or oval cross-sections, or two single-lumen lines inserted in the same vein. Should be able to provide flow rates of at least 300mL/min (often 400mL/min). Ingrowth of fibrous tissue into the cuff lowers the rate of infection in the short and long term and provides subcutaneous tethering.

Insertion similar to temporary lines using a modified Seldinger approach, with tunnelling performed either prior to venous insertion or after, depending on the nature of the catheter and its distal connectors. Adequate anaesthetic must be used for the tunnelling.

Table 2.8 Tunnelled cuffed catheters

Advantages	Disadvantages
Universally applicable	High morbidity especially from infections, thrombosis, and venous stenosis
Can be inserted into multiple sites	Risk of stenosis affecting permanent access
Can be used immediately	Low blood flow rates
No venepuncture required when using the catheter	Cosmetic appearance
Easy to place and relatively inexpensive	Discomfort
Thrombotic complications to treat	Relatively short life expectancy easier Complications at time of insertion.

Complications

Same as for temporary IV access (but all less common) including immediate complications at time of insertion, infections, thrombosis, and venous stenosis. Left internal jugular and subclavian sites have higher rates of venous stenosis and thrombosis. Femoral site has increased rates of infection. Infections are not trivial, and staphylococcal sepsis especially is associated with mortality. Rates of complications much lower for tunnelled than temporary catheters.

Temporary vascular access

Temporary percutaneous access should be used when access is required for <3 weeks. Usually made of polyurethane, which is stiff at room temperature and softens at body temperature. (See Table 2.9.)

- Can be tunnelled or non-tunnelled.
- Non-tunnelled access can be inserted at the bedside under US control, should be placed immediately before use, and should have its position confirmed by radiography.
- Right internal jugular vein is the preferred site (good evidence), but can be placed in subclavian or femoral veins.
- The subclavian approach should be avoided in all patients who may require permanent access at a later stage because of the risk of subclavian stenosis, which might compromise future fistulae, although infection risk slightly lower with subclavian than internal jugular lines.
- Femoral route should only be used in bed-bound or immobile patients, but also useful in patients who cannot lie flat for line insertion (e.g. severe pulmonary oedema, kyphosis). Highest infection risk.
- US should be used to aid insertion, especially for internal jugular lines.
- Non-cuffed catheters have increased complication rates (especially infection) if left in place for >5 days.
- Femoral catheters are generally changed after 1–3 days, and internal jugular catheters after 5–14 days.
- Infection rates increase substantially after 14 days for neck lines.
- Non-infected catheters can be changed over a guidewire.
- Temporary catheters should provide flow rates of up to 250mL/min.

Table 2.9 Temporary vascular access

Advantages	Disadvantages
Easy to insert	Infection
Low cost	Venous stenosis or thrombosis
Can be used immediately	Local complications during insertion
Easy to change	Short life
	Easily dislodged

Insertion of vascular access catheters

Insertion of vascular access catheters

A modified Seldinger approach is used. Should be done under US guidance to visualize the internal jugular vein and carotid artery (or femoral vessels), with an assistant, under full sterile conditions. US guidance certainly reduces complications for internal jugular lines. Each patient must be individually assessed for factors that might make any one location better or worse (e.g. obesity, groin infections, COPD).

- Localize the appropriate vein using cutaneous markers. For the internal jugular, a high approach is half way between the mastoid process and the sternoclavicular joint, just lateral to the carotid artery pulsation. A low jugular approach can be used immediately superolateral to the sternal end of the clavicle. The femoral vein lies immediately medial to the femoral artery just distal to the groin crease.
- Place the patient in a Trendelenburg position (head down) for all neck lines.
- Scrupulous sterility to avoid immediate line infections and bacteraemia—the operator should wear gloves, gown, and mask.
- Surround the puncture site with sterile towels after skin preparation with iodine solution.
- Before beginning, ensure all the necessary equipment is available, unpacked, and laid out within easy reach of the operator. Do not begin until everything is ready.
- Infiltrate local anaesthetic initially with a 23- or 25-gauge needle to minimize discomfort, and subsequently infiltrating right down to the vein. Avoid excess volume that will distort the anatomy.
- Advance a large insertion needle (sufficient diameter to accommodate the guidewire) carefully into the vein, at a 45° angle to the skin. For the internal jugular vein it is easy to aim in too medial a direction—the ipsilateral nipple is the correct target. It is helpful if the needle is placed on a 10mL syringe containing 2–3mL of saline, through which continuous suction is applied.
- One hand should remain gently palpating the adjacent artery at all times, while the other guides the introducer needle forward while applying suction.
- The needle must only be moved forwards once in the subcutaneous tissues, and never swung from side to side (the cutting edge may lacerate a blood vessel and cause a large haematoma).
- If the vein is not located within 2–3cm of the skin surface, the needle should be withdrawn almost completely, and then reinserted in a slightly more medial or lateral direction.
- Most inexperienced operators start too laterally when trying to localize the internal jugular vein.
- Once a flush of venous blood is seen in the syringe, the introducer needle must not be moved.
- The free hand should gently hold the hub of the needle, while the syringe is removed.
- Insert the guidewire into the needle and advance carefully. There should be no resistance to the wire.

- Remove the needle over the wire while holding the wire in place, and make a small incision through the skin over the wire at the entry point.
- Pass a dilator over the wire (do not push the wire into the vein—very embarrassing) into the vein briefly, and then remove.
- Advance the catheter over the wire into the vein, and then remove the wire.
- Withdraw blood through each lumen of the catheter to ensure ease of flow.
- Flush each lumen with 5–10mL saline.
- Insert heparin into each lumen to prevent thrombosis. Only insert the required volume (usually 0.9–1.7mL) to avoid systemic heparinization. Use 1000units/mL heparin.
- Stitch the line in place (but do not puncture the catheter with the needle) and cover with an adherent dressing (try to avoid stitches with permacaths as they may be a focus for infection). Mupirocin ointment applied to exit may reduce infection rates.

In general, 15cm lines should be used for right internal jugular vein, 20cm for left internal jugular, and 20–25cm lines for femoral access.

Catheter locks

Heparin locks have been used for many years and are relatively safe but lines continue to fail from thrombosis and bleeding risks exist. Evidence suggests low-concentration heparin (100units/mL) locks are most cost-effective with lowest overall risks. Risks include systemic anticoagulation from heparin leakage and heparin-induced thrombocytopenia.

Alternatives include *trisodium citrate* (4%, 30%, or 46.7%), most evidence supporting use of 4%, with lower bleeding events. Risks include metallic taste and peri-oral/digital paraesthesiae.

Thrombolytics (tPA) have also been used as locking solutions but are not currently recommended for routine use.

Antimicrobial line locks have been shown to reduce infection episodes in units with higher line infection rates (see ➔ Box 2.1, p. 133).

Systemic *warfarinization* aiming for INR 1.5–2.5 should be reserved for high-risk patients with recurrent CVC malfunction, and antiplatelet drugs alone are not sufficient to prevent thrombosis.

Complications of temporary access insertion

These include:

- *arterial puncture* (increased with internal jugular lines)—managed by direct pressure for 5–15min (except the inaccessible subclavian artery); if possible heparin should be avoided during dialysis (if this is to be performed immediately)
- *haemothorax* (especially subclavian lines)—may require chest drain insertion
- *pneumothorax* (especially subclavian lines)—may require chest drain insertion
- *haematoma*—avoid heparin if immediate dialysis needed
- *cardiac arrhythmia*—usually self-terminating after withdrawal of the wire
- *air embolism*—rare during catheter insertion; the patient should be placed head down on their left side and given cardiorespiratory and oxygen support as necessary; it is rarely necessary to aspirate air directly from the right ventricle
- *loss of insertion guidewire* into the right atrium/vena cava; can usually be rescued by an interventional radiologist.

Other complications of vascular catheters

Infection

A very common and important problem. (See → Management of access (catheter) infections, p. 132.)

Positional malfunction

Commonest cause of early failure (<7 days) and includes poor position or kinking.

Fibrin sheath formation

Commonly forms if the tip is abutting the vessel wall, causing a reduction in blood flow. It can be lysed with urokinase (but large volumes needed (200,000–250,000units over 2–6h) or by mechanical stripping using intraluminal brushes or snare loops via the femoral vein. If catheter is removed it is important not to reinsert new catheter down existing fibrin sheath. Fibrin tails or flaps can cause partial occlusion and act as one-way valves (often preventing blood withdrawal). Can form as early as 5–7 days after placement.

Catheter thrombosis

Can be mural thrombosis from vessel wall injury or intraluminal within the catheter. Most common with femoral lines when it often leads to venous thrombosis. Can be minimized with heparin instilled into the lumens between uses. Initial management should be a forceful flush of saline in a 10mL syringe (little risk). Most commonly treated using intraluminal urokinase or other thrombolytic agent, usually tPA. Urokinase usually instilled into the catheter, using 5000 units/mL to fill the volume of the catheter itself. If the catheter is fully clotted this is difficult. Urokinase should be used as soon as reduced flows are noted. Urokinase can be left in place for 5–15min, or between dialysis sessions. Some units make up the urokinase in a solution of heparin (2000–5000 units). Alternatively 1.25–2mg of tPA can be used in place of 5000 units of urokinase. May need to be repeated and left for 30–60min. Some centres use systemic thrombolysis with 250,000units urokinase (or 30mg tPA) into the venous port over 3h throughout a dialysis session when reduced flows are noted. This is more expensive and has an increased risk of bleeding complications.

Mechanical disruption using a wire or brush can be tried, but is less successful, or catheter exchange over a guidewire.

Thrombosis not prevented by low-dose warfarin, but full anticoagulation (INR >1.5) may reduce risk. If thrombosis is extrinsic to the catheter (within vessel itself) full anticoagulation should be instituted (INR 2–3) and continued for 1 month, and the catheter removed.

Use of lytic therapies such a tPA as locking solutions between dialysis sessions (in place of heparin) may reduce incidence of thrombosis, line occlusion, and need for line changes.

Venous stenosis

Venous stenosis (especially subclavian) or thrombosis may present acutely or be silent. May occur in up to 50% of subclavian lines. Diagnosed by clinical features (limb/facial swelling, poor flows, recirculation) and venography. Venoplasty may be needed but stent insertion not very successful in major veins. Veins difficult to plasty as walls very labile. Anticoagulation usually necessary to prevent thrombosis. Intraluminal brachytherapy may help if available. Thrombosis can be treated with intraluminal thrombolytic agents.

Recirculation

Not a major problem unless short femoral lines used, in which case can reach almost 20%. Usually only 3–10%.

Monitoring for access dysfunction

Should be undertaken by close monitoring of blood flow (Qb) and pre-pump negative arterial pressure. Since Qb will vary with pressure, measuring Qb at a preset pre-pump pressure at each session 5min after the start of dialysis can be a useful strategy. A decline of >10% may indicate an impending problem.

Management of access (catheter) infections

Very common. Occur during 15–60% of catheter insertions, increasing with duration of use. Incidence rates range from 0.6 to 7 episodes per 1000 catheter days. Usually caused by *Staphylococcus aureus* or *S. epidermidis* (up to 70%), and increasingly by MRSA (meticillin-resistant *S. aureus*); occasionally by enterococci or Gram-negative rods. Significant cause of morbidity (and mortality). Serious metastatic infections occur in 3–44% of episodes (heart, bones, veins, spine, lungs, brain, etc.). Infection may be reduced by elimination of nasal carriage of staphylococci with regular nasal mupirocin, scrupulous insertion technique, dressing, and exit care, and use of mupirin creams to exit site. Antibiotic-/silver-impregnated lines are expensive but do reduce infection rates and are especially useful in units with high infection rates. Chlorhexidine 2% exit site cleansing provides superior antisepsis to povidone-iodine 10% solution. Medical grade honey has been shown to be as effective as mupirocin.

Temporary catheters should be removed immediately if infection is suspected.

Physicians are sometimes more resistant to removing tunnelled catheters since some form of access is needed for patients on HD. Infection may be more common with internal jugular than subclavian lines (but much more common still with femoral lines). Presence of a fever without another focus, positive blood cultures with an appropriate organism, or purulent exit site should lead to removal of the catheter. Blood cultures should be performed from peripheral veins as well as through the catheter to ensure correct interpretation of a positive culture result. If possible, patients should remain free of further percutaneous catheters for 24–48h to minimize risk of recolonization of the new catheter. Some data suggest permacaths can be safely exchanged over a guidewire (after initiation of antibiotic treatment) even after an episode of line sepsis.

Blind treatment is often necessary in patients with fevers prior to culture results. Knowledge of local organisms and their antibiotic sensitivities is crucial for the correct choice of antibiotic, but IV vancomycin (20–30mg/kg weekly) and gentamicin (1–2mg/kg after each dialysis session) are commonly used to cover likely organisms, especially if MRSA is a possible infectious cause. First-generation cephalosporins have been used as an alternative, but most are no longer being manufactured. Alternatives to gentamicin for Gram-negative cover include 3rd-generation cephalosporins or meropenem. Antibiotics should be continued for at least 2 and possibly 3 weeks if uncomplicated infection, but 6 weeks for *S. aureus* infection and any complications, e.g. distal infective emboli. Some units always change the line if the infecting bacteria is *S. aureus*.

Catheter exchange over a guidewire can be successful as bacteria adherent to the line are a particular cause of maintaining bacteraemia and resistance to antibiotic penetration.

Patients with persistent fevers or elevated CRP should be examined carefully for metastatic staphylococcal infections (endocarditis, osteomyelitis, spinal abscess, disc infection, intracerebral abscesses).

The formation of biofilm within the catheter also predisposes to infection and prevents antibiotic penetration. Thrombolytics are useful in improving antibiotic access to bacteria in biofilm.

Antibiotic line locks or citrate can be used to ensure full eradication of infection in biofilm, and have been demonstrated to reduce infection. (See Box 2.1.)

> **Box 2.1 Antibiotic and citrate line locks reported to reduce infection rates**
> - Citrate (4–46.7%; use precise volume of line: caution with highest strengths)
> - Gentamicin (20mg/mL) plus heparin (5000IU/mL) to volume of line
> - Gentamicin (5mg/mL) plus heparin (5000IU/mL)
> - Gentamicin (20mg/mL) plus citrate (4.67%)
> - Ceftazidime (0.5mL of 10mg/mL solution) plus vancomycin (1mL of 5mg/mL solution) plus heparin (0.5mL of 10,000 units/mL solution)
> - Cefotaxime (10mg/mL) plus heparin (5000IU/mL)
> - Vancomycin (100mcg/mL) plus gentamicin (20mcg/mL) plus heparin
> - Taurolidine (1.35%) plus citrate (4%)
> - Minocycline (3mg/mL) plus EDTA (30mg/mL).

Prevention of infection of dialysis access

Infection rates are linked with personal hygiene of the patient, experience of staff, and nature of the access. Education of patients and staff is crucial to minimize infection risks.

- Hand washing minimizes nosocomial spread of infection.
- Skin preparation—cleaning skin with 70% alcohol or 10% povidone-iodine after washing reduces infection. Alcohol only bacteriostatic for 1min. Iodine only fully bacteriostatic after 2–3min. One caution is the potential for alcohol to dissolve polyurethane, and for povidone-iodine to dissolve silicon.
- Careful nursing of percutaneous catheters including use of bacteriostatic dressings (especially povidone-iodine) and careful examination for early exit-site infections. The lumens should not be exposed to the air, but should have syringes inserted once the caps have been removed. Catheter caps should be soaked in povidone-iodine before removal.
- Dry dressings rather than transparent films reduce infection at exit sites.
- Regular application of topical mupirocin 2% to the exit site reduces S. aureus infections. There are concerns over a potential for resistance and increased fungal infections, but these have not emerged as clinically significant.
- Eradication of nasal staphylococcal carriage with intranasal mupirocin, often needed long term—affects up to 60% of HD patients—reduces infection rates.
- Percutaneous lines impregnated with antibiotics (minocycline and rifampicin; chlorhexidine and silver sulfadiazine), silver, or other antimicrobial agents are increasingly available and reduce infection rates significantly. Cost-effective by US$200 per catheter if institution rate of catheter-related bacteraemia is >2%.
- Antibiotic or citrate (3–46.7%, with or without taurolidine) line locks can also reduce infection rates in units with high infection rates, or used at time of systemic infection to help clear biofilm infection.

Arteriovenous shunt (Scribner shunt)

Very rarely used now. Usually placed between radial artery and cephalic vein (at the wrist) or posterior tibial artery and long saphenous vein (at the ankle). A rigid plastic tip is inserted into a distal artery and vein, and each is connected to a silicone tube, which emerges through the skin. The two external tubes are joined via a small rigid connector, allowing continuous flow of blood through the shunt. Shunts can be used immediately. The exit site requires careful nursing as infections are common. For dialysis the silicone tubes are clamped, the connector opened, and the end of each tube attached to the venous and arterial lines of the dialysis machine. At the end of dialysis the silicone tubes are rejoined through a new sterile rigid connector.

Complications

As the artery is tied distal to the shunt insertion, the hand or foot requires an intact second arterial supply (ulnar or dorsalis pedis artery). This should be confirmed prior to formation of a shunt (Doppler or Allen test).

- Proximal venous stenosis causes early clotting of a shunt.
- Infection with *Staphylococcus* spp. common, and may cause septic pulmonary emboli, endocarditis, mycotic aneurysms.
- Clotting is common—especially in the face of hypotension or dehydration. Patient or nurse should palpate the shunt for a pulsation at least every 12h. Manual declotting can be performed using suction (with a syringe), or a balloon-tipped catheter (Fogarty). Urokinase or tPA can be infused. An angiogram should be performed to exclude venous stenosis if a shunt clots.
- Bleeding is a major risk if the two silicone tubes become disconnected. Patients must be educated to carry clamps at all times, and to apply direct pressure to the tubes if bleeding occurs.

Cardiopulmonary recirculation

There are two types of recirculation: cardiopulmonary and access. Both reduce the efficiency of dialysis by reducing the concentration of urea (and other solutes) at the dialyser inlet.

Cardiopulmonary recirculation

During dialysis via an AVF or arteriovenous graft (AVG), dialysed blood is returned to the venous circulation to be mixed with undialysed venous blood returning from peripheral tissues. The mixed blood becomes the arterial supply to the dialyser after being pumped through the pulmonary circulation. Thus the urea concentration at the dialyser inlet will be slightly less than the true arterial urea concentration were no dialysis to be occurring. This reduction in inlet urea is usually ~3–7%, but can be much higher in patients with poor cardiac output or high access flow rates.

Cardiopulmonary recirculation can be calculated approximately by:

$$\frac{Dialyser\ Clearance\ (K)}{Cardiac\ Output\ -\ Access\ Blood\ Flow}$$

Access recirculation

This occurs when blood that has just been dialysed returns directly to the dialyser inlet. It is usually caused by retrograde blood flow within a fistula or graft, when flow through AVF or AVG falls below 350–500mL/min, or when venous blood is drawn up as arterial blood through a dual-lumen catheter.

Measured using a two-needle urea-based technique (i.e. using the dialysis needles only) but non-urea-based dilution methods increasingly common. The three-needle peripheral vein method overestimates recirculation unpredictably, and requires additional venepuncture (for arterial, venous, and peripheral venous samples).

Recirculation >10% (urea method) or >5% (dilution method) requires further investigation (by venography).

Recirculation does not occur unless access flow rate is less than the dialyser blood pump flow rate, and is a marker of venous stenosis.

Two-needle measurement of recirculation

- Perform test after 30min of dialysis with UF switched off.
- Take arterial (A) and venous (V) blood samples from the access lines.
- Reduce blood flow rate to 120mL/min for 10s then switch off pump.
- Clamp arterial line above sampling port and take systemic arterial sample (S) from arterial line.
- Resume dialysis.
- Measure urea in arterial, venous, and systemic sample (A, V, and S).

$$Recirculation = \frac{S-A}{S-V} \times 100$$

This method is less accurate than dilution techniques, but easy to perform and reliable. Dilution methods are increasingly used though as more dialysis machines come equipped with appropriate technology.

US dilution techniques for measurement of recirculation

Recirculation can be easily measured using US measurement of the dilution of saline (e.g. Transonic® device) or by temperature change, as for measuring flow but with blood lines not reversed. A bolus of saline injected into the V line will be detected at the A line if there is significant recirculation.

The first dialysis session in chronic and acute kidney disease

Planned dialysis for ESKD is very different from dialysis for an acute uraemic emergency. In ESKD, access may have been planned and formed several months previously, the patient is aware of the procedure, and in general the metabolic derangement of CKD will have been progressing slowly. A first chronic dialysis session may be performed as an outpatient. However, correction of metabolic abnormalities in ESKD can still have similar effects to that seen in HD for acute uraemia.

In AKI, access will usually be a temporary catheter, the patient may be confused, catabolic, sick, or just frightened. There is some evidence that episodes of hypotension during dialysis may delay recovery from AKI (especially ATN) and should be avoided.

Factors to be considered include:
- length of session
- blood flow rate
- choice of dialyser
- anticoagulation
- dialysate composition
- fluid removal (UF)
- skill of nursing staff and presence of medical staff.

Anticoagulation

Heparin-free dialysis is preferred for a first dialysis session, to minimize the risk of pericardial bleeding, bleeding from access sites, or intracerebral bleeding in the setting of hypertension. Anticoagulation (heparin or other) can be introduced subsequently.

Nursing and medical staff

A first dialysis session requires skilled staffing, for monitoring both the patient and equipment, and for patient reassurance. Complications may be severe or unexpected.

Length of session

Together with blood flow, this is the major determinant of the quantity of dialysis administered. Major concern is the dialysis disequilibrium syndrome, which occurs from overcorrection of uraemia. Can occur in either AKI or CKD if blood urea levels are reduced too quickly, or the initial blood urea is particularly high. *A first dialysis should only reduce blood urea by 30%.* For most patients, an optimum first session is ~2h. Many patients will require daily dialysis for a few days before instituting a standard dialysis regimen. A second session is typically 3h, and the third 3.5–4h. Reduced hours are only necessary if the blood urea remains very high on the second or third day (but beware very catabolic patients who do need increased dialysis times after the first session). Marked urea rebound is common in acute dialysis.

Blood flow

Usually ~150–200mL/min for the first session. Larger patients may require a slightly longer session (2.5h) or slightly higher blood flows (250mL/min).

Dialyser

High-efficiency dialysers (KoA >400) are not needed for the first few dialysis sessions. If they are used, the length of session or blood flow should be reduced. There is conflicting evidence as to the benefit of biocompatible membranes on morbidity, length of time to recovery of renal function, or infection rates in AKI, but no studies document a detrimental effect, and hence they are increasingly used in AKI. Atopic patients may be more at risk of reaction to ethylene oxide sterilant. Patients on ACEIs can in rare cases develop anaphylactic reactions when dialysed with AN69® membranes.

Ultrafiltration

No more than 2L should be removed during a first dialysis session. For patients with severe fluid overload or pulmonary oedema, isolated (or additional) UF can be used first to remove fluid. Some patients are 'dry' and require additional fluid.

Dialysate for use in first session

Bicarbonate

Preferred to acetate to minimize risks of hypotension. Patients at severe risk of alkalaemia may need reduced bicarbonate concentrations (<35mmol/L). Patients with metabolic alkalosis can easily have their systemic pH worsened (raised) by hyperventilation. Patients with severe acidosis should aim to have their serum bicarbonate raised to 15–20mmol/L, and may also need a relatively low dialysate bicarbonate to avoid overcorrection.

Sodium

Avoid correction of hyponatraemia too rapidly by altering the dialysate sodium. In general, 140–145mmol/L is satisfactory. For patients with serum sodium <130mmol/L keep dialysate sodium no more than 15–20mmol/L higher than the pre-dialysis serum sodium. For hypernatraemic patients, the dialysate sodium should be equal to or slightly higher (1–3mmol/L) than the plasma sodium. Hyponatraemic dialysate (relative to blood) may cause hyponatraemia in venous blood returning to the patient and lead to acute hypotension as water moves into the interstitial compartment.

Potassium

Serum potassium will be reduced with correction of acidosis. Use 4–4.5mmol/L dialysate potassium if serum level ≤4.5 mmol/L, and 2–3mmol/L if serum level >5.5mmol/L. For severe hyperkalaemia, dialysate potassium of 2mmol/L is usually satisfactory, but some physicians use 0mmol/L dialysate potassium. Serum potassium must be carefully monitored after dialysis in this case.

Calcium

Avoid low calcium dialysate as it may contribute to hypotension.

Dialysate flow

Rate does not need altering (500mL/min).

Complications during dialysis

Common complications during dialysis

See Table 2.10.

Other complications are less common, including:
- air embolism
- seizures
- haemolysis
- severe dialysis disequilibrium
- first-use syndromes
- acute urticaria
- cardiac tamponade.

Dialysis disequilibrium syndrome

This can occur in either AKI or CKD if blood urea levels are reduced too quickly, or in those with very marked uraemia or pre-existing alterations in mental state. Manifests as headache, nausea, disorientation, restlessness, blurred vision, asterixis, fits, coma, and even death, occurring during or after dialysis. Milder symptoms may include cramps, nausea, and dizziness. Probably caused by cerebral oedema due to osmotic influx of water into the brain after removal of urea by dialysis, before equilibration across cell membranes occurs. Cerebral acidosis may play a role. It is rare in patients initially dialysed for 2h at low blood flows. Slow removal of urea minimizes risk. Initial blood urea reduction during a first dialysis should be <30%. In patients at highest risk (severe uraemia, abnormal mental state) some physicians use prophylactic phenytoin (1000mg loading dose, then 300mg/day). Symptoms are self-limiting over a few hours. Patients with severe fitting can be treated with IV mannitol (10–15g) or hypertonic saline (5mL of 23%).

Table 2.10 Common complications during dialysis

Hypotension	25–60% of treatment sessions
Cardiac arrhythmias	5–60% (usually asymptomatic)
Cramps	5–25%
Nausea and vomiting	5–15%
Headache	5–10%
Back pain	2–5%
Chest pain	2–5%
Itching	1–5%
Fever	1%

Hypotension

This occurs in 6–30% of dialysis sessions and can be episodic or, less commonly, persistent. Can be classified as hypovolaemic, distributive shock or from pump failure. More frequent in patients with lower body mass and cardiac disease. IDH forms part of a vicious cycle maintaining hypertension and fluid overload: the response to a drop in BP is frequently to infuse normal or hypertonic saline, leaving the patient hypertensive, necessitating further use of antihypertensive agents, which in turn worsen IDH by inhibiting appropriate reflexes (tachycardia, vasoconstriction). Hypotension is usually multifactorial. Often manifest by nausea, vomiting, cramps, and yawning, in addition to a fall in BP. IDH has been associated with myocardial and cerebral ischaemia, mesenteric ischaemia, and frontal lobe cerebral atrophy, but whether this is as a marker for co-morbidity or as a causative factor is not clear. (See Table 2.11.)

Patients most at risk are older patients, females, with diabetes, raised serum phosphate, coronary artery disease and those with autonomic neuropathy.

The major factor in preventing IDH is correct assessment of dry weight.

Table 2.11 Common causes of hypotension

Patient-specific causes	Treatment-specific causes
Diabetes	Rapid fluid removal (high UF rate)
Autonomic neuropathy	Antihypertensive agent use
Reduced cardiac reserve (especially LVH and diastolic dysfunction)	Rapid reduction in plasma osmolality (leading to water movement from the vascular into interstitial compartment)
Arrhythmias	Warm dialysate
Poor nutritional state	Low sodium dialysate
High weight gain	Low dialysate osmolarity
Ingestion of food during dialysis (increased splanchnic venous pooling)	Use of acetate as buffer (a vasodilator)
Antihypertensive agents impairing cardiac stability and reflexes	Bioincompatibility
Septicaemia	
Release of adenosine during organ ischaemia (e.g. induced by hypotension; adenosine is a vasodilator and inhibits norepinephrine release)	
Subclinical myocardial ischaemia	

Less common causes of hypotension
- Pericardial effusion or tamponade.
- Reactions to dialysis membranes.
- Increased dialysate magnesium.
- GI bleeding.
- Disconnection of blood lines.
- MI.
- Haemolysis.
- Air embolism.
- Chronic persistent hypotension occurs in ~5% patients, usually those on dialysis >5 years, and systolic BP is often <90mmHg before starting dialysis. Such patients may have depressed LV function, valve disease, etc. but often an underlying cause is not found. Increased circulating vasodilators such as nitric oxide and adrenomedullin may contribute, together with adrenergic unresponsiveness.

Hypotension from excessive ultrafiltration

Hypotension from excessive ultrafiltration

During UF, as water is removed from the vascular compartment, blood volume is maintained by movement of water from tissues (refilling). This can only occur until the true dry weight is achieved. Hypotension will be induced if UF is too rapid or excessive, as adequate refilling will not occur under these circumstances. Most patients with ESKD also have diastolic dysfunction, which impacts on cardiac output especially under conditions of reduced vascular filling. Cardiac 'stunning' during dialysis may also contribute.

Factors making uncontrolled UF more likely

- Dialysis machines without volumetric control of UF can lead to rapid fluctuations in UF rates.
- Patients who drink too much between dialysis sessions have excessive (and unachievable) UF requirements during the dialysis session. This is usually driven by salt consumption (often hidden in foods). Salt intake of 0.5g/day will lead to a 1.5kg weight gain on average in a 70kg anuric patient. Weight gain should be 1kg/day.
- Excess blood flow is a rare cause of hypotension.
- Incorrect target dry weight (too low) will lead to hypotension. This occurs especially during recovery from an acute illness when lost muscle weight is being recovered.

Management of hypotension

Episodes of hypotension are uncomfortable and very distressing for patients, lead to significantly impaired quality of life, morbidity, and contribute to cardiovascular mortality. Repeated and careful assessment of dry weight is crucial to minimize hypotension.

Immediate management requires volume resuscitation:

- Place patient head-down.
- Administer 100mL bolus of normal saline (some units use 10mL of 23% saline, 30mL of 7.5% saline, 50mL of 20% mannitol, or albumin solutions).
- Reduce UF rate to zero.
- If BP does not normalize rapidly, further saline may be given.

Hypertonic saline may increase thirst, prevent achievement of dry weight, and worsen fluid overload. Albumin is very expensive.

In most cases, hypotension is due to excess UF, and is rapidly corrected. Other explanations should be sought if BP does not respond to reasonable saline replenishment, especially cardiac causes, GI bleeding, and sepsis.

If hypotension occurs repeatedly, review:

- dry weight (too low?)
- use of short-acting antihypertensive agents before dialysis (give drugs after dialysis; does not apply to most modern long-acting agents)
- UF rate
- weight gains between sessions (carefully counsel patient especially about salt, limit weight gain to 1kg/day, look for hidden fluids such as soups, and salt intake)
- dialysate sodium (keep above plasma sodium)
- use bicarbonate not acetate dialysate
- lower dialysate temperature to 34–36°C (but makes some patients feel uncomfortable)
- increase Hb
- avoid food intake during dialysis (but balanced against nutritional intake—for some patients this can be the only time of encouraged food intake).

If all else fails, the following drug treatments can sometimes help:

- Levocarnitine 20mg/kg/treatment IV at the end of dialysis may improve IDH. Overall evidence limited or poor.
- Midodrine (an oral α_1 agonist) 2.5–10mg 30min before dialysis; increases peripheral vascular resistance, increases venous return and cardiac output; can give second dose in middle of session.
- Sertraline 50–100mg/day PO.

First-line management

Careful clinical reassessment of dry weight.

Dietary sodium restriction reinforcement.

Refrain from food intake during dialysis (unless malnourished).

Use of a dialysate temperature of 36.5°C.

Check dosing and timing of antihypertensive agents

Second-line management

Try objective methods to assess dry weight.

Perform cardiac evaluation (echocardiography).

Gradual reduction of dialysate temperature from 36.5°C (lowest 35°C).

Switch to haemodiafiltration.

Consider individualized blood volume monitoring and controlled feedback.

Prolong dialysis time and/or increase dialysis frequency (daily short dialysis or nocturnal).

Use dialysate calcium concentration of 1.50mmol/L.

Third-line management

Consider midodrine (PO 2.5–10mg) before dialysis.

Consider levocarnitine (IV 20mg/kg/treatment) supplementation after dialysis.

Consider PD.

(Information from European Best Practice guidelines.)

Prevention of hypotension

Prevention is crucial. Hypotension is unpleasant for patients, makes achievement of euvolaemia difficult, and leads to persistent fluid overload and hypertension. As cardiovascular disease is the major cause of mortality in ESKD, controlling hypertension is of paramount importance. Episodic IDH prevents this happening.

Time on dialysis

Slower, longer dialysis often cures episodic hypotension but is not favoured by patients. Patients need educating.

Sodium ramping or profiling

This can be used to minimize symptoms of hypotension and cramping by optimizing vascular refilling—dialysate sodium is set at a high level (e.g. 144–155mmol/L) during the first hour (or 2h) of dialysis, and then either stepped downwards in intervals or reduced gradually over the next 3h. Controlled trials have shown reduced hypotensive episodes, but also a tendency to increased thirst in patients, and subsequent increased fluid intake (counterproductive) because of salt loading. May be beneficial for some patients but must be prescribed very carefully. Overall the mean delivered sodium dialysate concentration must be lower than that of plasma, not just the sodium concentration at the end-point. Trials suggesting benefit have usually combined it with UF profiling.

Sequential UF and isovolaemic dialysis

Helps some patients achieve dry weight without hypotension, but tends to be less effective than sodium profiling. UF is performed initially without dialysis during the first hour or 2h of a session, ensuring fluid loss occurs while plasma urea and sodium concentrations may be highest, and allowing most rapid refilling of the vascular compartment. Subsequent dialysis is performed with minimal further UF. Tends to increase dialysis session time. Pulsed profiles may result in increased IDH.

Temperature modelling

The patient's temperature is kept 0.5°C below normal by reducing the dialysate temperature (36.5–35°C). This essentially leads to cutaneous vasoconstriction, which helps maintain BP during dialysis. Can be very effective in preventing hypotension.

Carnitine

There is some evidence that carnitine deficiency may contribute to hypotension on dialysis (and to muscle fatigue, cardiomyopathy, and anaemia), and may be helped in some patients by regular IV levocarnitine therapy (see ➜ Carnitine and ESKD, p. 410) after dialysis or daily oral levocarnitine (500mg/day) alone or in combination with daily oral vitamin E (200IU/day).

Dialysate calcium

Low calcium dialysate is associated with impaired myocardial contractility, and prospective studies have shown improved IDH with higher dialysate calcium (1.5mmol/L or 1.75mmol/L vs 1.25mmol/L). Use of higher dialysate calcium, however, may contribute to a positive calcium balance.

Haemodiafiltration

Convective therapies may offer greater cardiovascular stability than routine HD. Incidence of IDH is generally reduced in patients receiving HDF, but studies are conflicting. Conflicting reports of benefit on patient reported symptoms after switching from HD to HDF.

Peritoneal dialysis

Some patients may need to switch to PD if IDH is persistent and uncontrollable.

Blood volume monitoring

May be helpful in individual patients. Sometimes referred to as crit-line monitoring. Continuous optical measurement of Hct or plasma protein concentration will allow assessment of blood volume (by change in concentration of Hb or plasma proteins). Expert software systems can 'learn' to identify changes in blood volume preceding symptomatic hypotension, and intervene to prevent hypotension occurring (e.g. by slowing the UF rate). This remains controversial. In general, a decrease in blood volume >8–10%/h indicates hypovolaemia is imminent. However, an individual patient usually has an RBV limit below which hypotension occurs. This is particularly useful when performed repeatedly, but there are large interpatient variations in responses. Despite this potential benefit, prospective RCTs have shown no benefit or even a detrimental effect overall, possibly because patients do not achieve dry weight, and remain fluid overloaded.

Examples of real-time blood volume record are shown in Figs 2.7, 2.8, and 2.9.

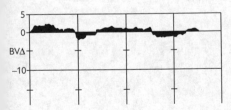

Fig. 2.7 This trace shows no reduction in RBV over 4h of dialysis, indicating that the patient remains overhydrated.

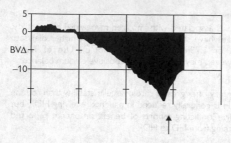

Fig. 2.8 This trace shows a sharp drop in blood volume (leading to cramping and hypotension) and need for a clinical intervention at arrow (turning UF to zero and a bolus of saline).

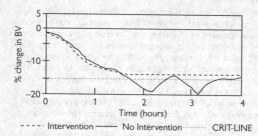

Fig. 2.9 In this example during one HD (no intervention) the patient has two hypotensive episodes requiring saline boluses. During the second dialysis, an intervention threshold has been set at −15% (the crit-line), and the UFR rate was automatically adjusted to keep the blood volume profile trace above this line. The patient remained symptom free.

Other complications during dialysis

Cramps

Occur in up to 90% of dialysis treatments, mainly towards the end of dialysis. A significant cause for early termination and underdialysis. Cause not entirely clear, but associated with hyponatraemia, hypotension, hypovolaemia, hypoxia, and carnitine deficiency. Cramps are increased in patients using low-sodium dialysate and requiring increased UF.

Management

Minimize interdialytic weight gain and need for excessive UF, prevent dialysis hypotension, higher sodium dialysate, or sodium profiling. Acutely, IV saline (normal or hypertonic) and IV 50% glucose are very effective (but saline will contribute to hypertension and volume overload). Local massage offers some relief.

Carnitine supplementation and quinine sulfate may help some patients. Quinine is best used 2h before dialysis. Vitamin E (200–400IU) was as effective as quinine in an RCT. Some patients respond to diazepam, carbamazepine, amitriptyline, phenytoin, or alcohol. Carnitine replacement therapy helps some patients (20mg/kg IV after each session—see ➜ Carnitine and ESKD, p. 410). A single study of daily oral vitamin E (200 IU/day) or daily oral levocarnitine (500 mg/day) for cramps and hypotension suggested significant benefit of both but especially combined treatment.

Nausea, vomiting, and headache

Common, and usually associated with hypotension. May be a minor manifestation of disequilibrium syndrome due to excess urea removal, or in patients with persistent marked uraemia. Rarely precipitated by caffeine or alcohol withdrawal during dialysis.

Management

Treat and prevent hypotension. Antiemetics and paracetamol may help if not precipitated by hypotension. Reduction of blood flow rate (by 25–30%) during first hour of dialysis sometimes useful (but overall dialysis time must be lengthened to maintain dose of dialysis). Use bicarbonate rather than acetate dialysis.

Chest pain

Commonly caused by angina, but also by hypotension, dialysis disequilibrium syndrome, haemolysis, and air embolism. Recurrent angina during dialysis should be investigated cardiologically, and can be treated with nitrates or β-blockers. Both agents may cause hypotension.

Air embolism

Rare, as air detectors will clamp venous blood lines if air is detected in the return circuit. May occur while manipulating CVCs. Introduction of 1mL/kg air may be fatal.

In sitting patients, air tends to move upwards into cerebral venous circulation and cause fitting and coma. In recumbent patients, it causes chest pain, dyspnoea, chest tightness, and cough, and may pass through the pulmonary vascular bed and embolize into arterioles causing acute neurological signs.

Foam is usually seen in the venous blood line. Churning sound may be heard on cardiac auscultation.

Management

Clamp venous line and stop blood pump. Place patient in left lateral position, with head and chest down. Administer 100% O_2 (enhances nitrogen diffusion out of air bubbles), and cardiopulmonary support as necessary. Rarely, percutaneous aspiration of air from the ventricle is necessary.

Haemolysis

Severe haemolysis is rare, but can cause chest pain, abdominal or back pain, chest tightness, headache, nausea, and malaise. Life-threatening hyperkalaemia can occur if unrecognized. Should especially be considered if several patients complain of similar symptoms simultaneously. Venous blood may develop a darker appearance, and plasma will appear pink in clotted or spun blood samples. Hb falls. Causes include:
• overheating of dialysate
• contamination with bleach, formaldehyde, or peroxide from water purification or reprocessing
• chloramine, nitrates, or copper from water supply
• hypotonic dialysate
• kinks in blood tubing
• malfunctioning blood pump.

Management

Stop blood pump immediately and clamp lines. Risk of severe hyperkalaemia. Check potassium and Hb. Haemolysis may continue for several hours after removal of precipitant. Seek cause urgently, as multiple patients may be affected if it is due to water or a central dialysate problem.

Complications during dialysis: dialyser reactions

Also called first-use syndromes, but can occur with re-used dialysers. Can be severe anaphylactic reactions (type A) typically occurring within the first few minutes of dialysis (but can occur up to 30min), or milder reactions (type B; often back and chest pain) occurring minutes to hours after starting dialysis. (See Table 2.12.)

Table 2.12 Dialyser reactions

	Type A: anaphylactic	Type B: mild
Prevention	Seek cause	Change from cellulose to modified cellulose or synthetic membrane
	Avoid ethylene oxide-sterilized dialysers and rinse all dialysers well, with increased volumes. Stop ACEIs, especially if using AN69® or PAN membrane. Change membrane type. If occurs with different dialysers on several occasions, try heparin-free dialysis	Re-using dialysers may help

Blood clotting during haemodialysis

Contact between blood and the various plastic surfaces within the extra-corporeal circuit initiates platelet adherence, activation of the intrinsic clotting pathway, and thrombosis. Clotting is promoted by slow blood flows, high Hb, high UF rate, intradialytic blood transfusion, or parenteral nutrition containing lipid. Most dialysis sessions require anticoagulation, usually with heparin. Low-MW heparin (LMWH), epoprostenol, and regional anticoagulation with citrate or heparin–protamine are also used. Heparin-free dialysis is possible. Heparin-bonded plastics may allow true regional anticoagulation, but are not yet available. Heparin-binding dialyser membranes (e.g. AN69ST®) reduce the need for systemic heparinization after an initial rinse with heparinized saline.

Clotting during dialysis

Not trivial. Can contribute to anaemia and necessitate blood transfusion (with risk of HLA sensitization). Leads to underdialysis. Features:

- blood becomes very dark in circuit
- streaking in dialyser
- visible clots in bubble trap
- visible clots in venous lines
- clots in arterial end of dialyser (not just small strands)
- venous pressure will drop if clot forming in dialyser, or rise if clot distal to monitor
- arterial pressure may rise.

Anticoagulation for haemodialysis: heparin

Heparin

A highly charged anionic glycosaminoglycan extracted from bovine or porcine tissues, binds antithrombin III to inactivate factors II, IX, X, XI, and XII. Comprises a heterogeneous mixture of molecules with varying MWs. Half-life 30–120min. Side effects include pruritus, thrombocytopenia (rare in HD), hyperlipidaemia (especially hypertriglyceridaemia), osteoporosis, hair loss, and allergy (rare). Major complication is bleeding (in up to 50% of high risk patients).

Heparin-induced thrombocytopenia (HIT) is a potentially serious although rare problem (overall incidence 2.6% of patients exposed to heparin for more than 4 days). Risk of HIT from LMWH 30 times lower. Type I HIT is non-immune, mild, and resolves despite continues use of heparin. Platelet count is rarely <100. Type II HIT is antibody mediated, causes thrombocytopenia usually 5–10 days after use of heparin and thromboembolism. Median nadir platelet count is 55×10^9/L, and severe thrombocytopenia (<15) is rare. It does not resolve spontaneously and recurs on challenge. The antibody induced in HIT II binds the heparin–platelet factor 4 complex on platelets and induces both thrombocytopenia and clumping, activation, and thrombosis. It resolves 1–2 weeks after stopping heparin. LMWHs are *not* safe in patients with HIT type II (50% cross-reactivity). Diagnosis is by the 4T scoring system (thrombocytopenia degree, timing of onset, thrombosis and excluding other causes) and then immunological assays of antibody to PF4 or heparin. Alternative anticoagulants that can be used on dialysis are danaparoid, lepirudin, fondaparinux, and argatroban. Catheter locks should avoid heparin: alternatives include tPA (1–2mg/mL), urokinase (1250–2500IU/mL), and lepirudin (1–5mg/mL). Trisodium citrate and taurolidine have been used but cases of catheter thrombosis reported.

Monitoring heparin

Activated clotting time (ACT) is most commonly used. A number of automated methods are available. Cheap, rapid, repeatable, and easy to perform. An activator is added to the blood sample, and the time for clotting to occur is recorded (normal 90–140s). Target ACT usually baseline +80% (200–250s) during dialysis, reducing to baseline +40% at the end of the session. Patients with high baseline ACT should have a reduced target ACT.

Whole-blood activated partial thromboplastin time (aPTT) sometimes used (target 120–160s).

Anticoagulation for haemodialysis: heparin administration

Routine heparin administration

Bolus injection followed by infusion or repeated bolus injections, after priming circuit with heparinized saline. Some degree of heparin adsorption to the dialyser and circuit occurs. There are no good studies demonstrating the best method, and there are a wide range of methods in use in practice.

Infusion method
- Reliable and easier for nursing staff.
- Initial bolus usually ~2000U (~50U/kg).
- Continuous heparin infusion into arterial line at ~500–2000U/h, monitored hourly, more frequently in new patients (to achieve target of ACT baseline +80%).
- Adjust infusion rate to clotting time.
- Stop heparin 60min before end of dialysis.

Bolus method
- Initial bolus usually ~4000U but sometimes lower at 1000–2000U.
- Give second bolus of 1000–2000U when ACT reaches baseline +50% (~2 h). Some units never give a second bolus.
- Repeat ACT in 30min. Two or three doses of heparin usually required.
- Increase initial bolus if ACT not increased to baseline +80% (can check ACT 3min after initial administration). Increase dose proportionately to increase in ACT required.
- Avoid or reduce initial bolus in uraemic patients or those with prolonged baseline ACT.
- Time to stop heparin can be determined from the ACT and the half-life of heparin for a given patient. Usually 1h before the end of dialysis.

Tight (or minimal) heparin

For patients at moderate risk of bleeding. Target ACT is baseline +40% (~150–200s; reduced if initial ACT prolonged). Achieved by 30min bolus injections of 500U, or, preferably, constant infusion of 250–2000U/h (usually ~600U/h), after reduced (or no) initial bolus (~750U; check ACT after 3min). Monitor ACT every 30min. Heparin continued until the end of dialysis.

Anticoagulation for haemodialysis: heparin-free dialysis

Heparin-free dialysis should be used for actively bleeding patients, those with pericarditis, coagulopathy, thrombocytopenia, intracerebral haemorrhage, recent surgery, and recent renal transplant. With careful nursing can usually sustain a full 4h dialysis session. Only 5% risk of complete circuit clotting. Requires well-functioning vascular access. New dialysis membranes (e.g. AN69ST®) bind heparin avidly and can avoid the need for systemic heparinization. Patients with HIT type II cannot be exposed to any heparin, even in initial rinse.

Common protocol

- Rinse circuit with heparinized saline (3000–5000U/L saline).
- Flush the rinse to drain and do not return it to the patient.
- Use high blood flows (>400mL/min).
- Rinse circuit every 15–30min with 25–200mL saline, while occluding arterial line (but little evidence for benefit).
- Increase UF rate to remove extra saline.
- Careful inspection of dialyser and monitoring of venous pressure for early signs of clotting.
- Avoid blood transfusion (unless into venous return through a large-bore tube).
- Requires more intensive nursing.

Regional anticoagulation for haemodialysis

Regional heparin with protamine reversal

Rarely used now and probably should be avoided. Largely replaced by heparin-free techniques. Protamine binds heparin and prevents its anticoagulant activity. Heparin is infused constantly into the dialyser inlet while protamine is infused into the venous line. ACT is maintained in the circuit at ~200–250s, and also monitored in the blood returning to the patient (should be back to baseline). 1mg protamine reverses ~100U of heparin.

- This is difficult to monitor correctly and provide the correct dose of protamine.
- More importantly, rebound bleeding can occur after 2–4h (and up to 10h) when heparin dissociates from the protamine. Can be severe.
- Protamine can cause flushing, hypotension, and bradycardia.

Regional citrate anticoagulation

Where routinely used it is a reliable and effective means of anticoagulation. Requires careful nursing, increased patient monitoring, and can have significant adverse effects if not well managed. Citrate complexes calcium, which is necessary for activation of all coagulation pathways. Calcium must be absent from the dialysate and replaced in the venous return.

Requires calcium-free dialysate, trisodium citrate solution (132mmol/L— stock solutions usually 46.7%), calcium chloride (50mL of 10% calcium chloride diluted into 100mL normal saline, or a 5% solution), and two IV infusion pumps.

Various regimens have been validated, for example:

- baseline ACT is measured
- trisodium citrate solution (132mmol/L) is infused into the arterial line at ~270mL/h
- start blood flow
- start calcium chloride infusion into venous line at ~30mL/h
- ACT should be measured in the arterial line distal to the citrate infusion and kept at ~100% above baseline (~200s)
- titrate citrate infusion to ACT
- check arterial calcium every 30min and keep in normal range
- titrate calcium infusion to plasma calcium level
- ensure neither citrate nor calcium pumps stop working during the procedure
- if dialysate bypasses, reduce citrate and calcium infusions by half
- at the end of dialysis stop both calcium and citrate infusions.

Complications

- Hypocalcaemia or hypercalcaemia.
- Hypernatraemia (from sodium citrate).
- Metabolic alkalosis (citrate is metabolized to bicarbonate by the liver).

Other methods of anticoagulation for haemodialysis

Low-molecular-weight heparin

Recommended (preferred) by European guidelines for ease of use, efficacy, fewer side effects (especially lipids, potassium, and bleeding), and has become first-line anticoagulant in Europe. Obtained by fractionation of heparin. Causes greater inhibition of factor Xa, less thrombocytopenia (but can still occur), less bleeding, less dyslipidaemia, less hyperkalaemia, less hair loss, and may require less monitoring than heparin. Activity expressed as anti-Xa activity units. PTT and thrombin time not usually prolonged. Expensive, and overall benefit over heparin debated. Should not be used in patients with HIT type II as antibodies can be cross-reactive.

Given as single bolus at beginning of dialysis. For example: enoxaparin 0.7–1mg/kg, or 40mg stat dose (0.25mg/kg if very high risk bleeding). Can be monitored if necessary to maintain anti-Xa activity at 0.5–1.0 units/mL (but not commonly needed).

Epoprostenol

Induces inhibition of platelet aggregation and vasodilatation. Usually infused IV at 5ng/kg/min (range 4–8ng/kg/min). Causes little bleeding at this dose, but more clotting than full heparinization. Hypotension common. Other side effects include headache, flushing, nausea, vomiting, and chest and abdominal pain. Very expensive.

Danaparoid

A low-MW glycosaminoglycan conjugate of heparin sulphate. Expensive. Usual dose 3750units as IV bolus (2500 units if <55kg) or 40 units/kg before first two dialysis sessions (then reduce to 3000 or 2000). Monitor antifactor Xa levels (aim for 0.5–0.8 units/mL). 100–400 units/hour in CRRT.

Recombinant hirudin (lepirudin)

Originally derived from leeches. Forms complex with thrombin and inhibits platelet aggregation. Administered as a single bolus at the start of dialysis (0.08–0.15mg/kg). Effective, expensive, and has a prolonged half-life, which may cause bleeding after repeated use. Patients develop non-neutralizing antihirudin antibodies, which enhance its potency. May only need repeat dosing after 6–12 days. Can be monitored by aPTT (aiming 1.5–2.5).

Argatroban

A thrombin inhibitor similar to hirudin. Particularly useful in patients with HIT type II. Care in patients with liver disease (reduce dose). Give 10mg initial dose into dialysis circuit (or 250mcg/kg) and then 25mg/h (or 0.5–2mcg/kg/min). Aim for activated aPTT 1.5–2.0 or anti-Xa activity 0.2–0.4 units/mL.

Nafamostat mesilate

A thrombin inhibitor. Use at 20–40mg/h and keep aPTT at 2.0. Can cause hyperkalaemia.

Fondaparinux

A synthetic pentasaccharide which binds antithrombin 3 and has high anti-Xa activity. Half-life prolonged in renal failure and longer than LMWHs. Can be used in patients with HIT. Dose usually 2mg IV pre-dialysis.

Aspirin and ticlopidine

These are not effective anticoagulants for HD.

Dialysis adequacy

Outcomes of haemodialysis

Mortality is easily measured, but morbidity and quality of life are equally important outcomes (but difficult to quantitate). Survival on dialysis has increased for all patient groups over the last decades, and is now predominantly determined by co-morbidity. Older patients with significant co-morbid illnesses, late presentation for dialysis, and poor overall functional capacity have a <25% 1-year survival after starting dialysis. Patients without other significant diseases and preserved social functioning have almost 100% 1-year survival, and 80% 5-year survival. Age is a less significant predictor of poor outcome than co-morbidity. Cardiovascular disease remains the most common cause of death, the origins of which pre-date initiation of dialysis.

There is little value therefore in concentrating solely on small solute removal by dialysis, although it is a useful marker for quantitating dialysis dose delivered. It is possible to remove urea quickly using high flux dialysers and high blood flows, but patients treated in this way do not have the lowest morbidity or mortality.

Adequacy of dialysis

- Adequate dialysis maximizes well-being, minimizes morbidity, and helps a patient retain social independence.
- Adequate dialysis is not simply a dose of dialysis exceeding a given number, and should not be defined by solute clearance alone.
- Optimum dialysis is a method of delivering dialysis, producing results that cannot be further improved.
- Dialysis prescription should be individualized, monitored, and reassessed regularly.

Assessment of adequacy should include:
- patient well-being (physically, mentally, socially)
- nutrition (lack of malnutrition)
- small solute clearance (urea kinetic modelling (UKM))
- adequacy of UF
- control of BP
- protein catabolic rate (PCR)
- control of anaemia, acidosis, and bone disease.

Clearance of medium and large molecules (e.g. $\beta_2 m$) is not routinely measured, but may be a better marker of dialysis adequacy, and may be approximately assessed by surrogates such as control of extracellular volume and BP (controversial).

Measurement of solute clearance

- Measurement of pre-dialysis serum urea and creatinine concentrations is not useful. Low levels may reflect good dialysis, but more commonly reflect malnutrition, reduced protein intake, and loss of muscle mass. Increasing the dose of dialysis may lead to an increase in serum urea and creatinine as nutrition and well-being improve.

- Clinical assessment of uraemia is difficult as signs and symptoms occur late, and are confounded by anaemia (or its successful treatment), and other complications of ESKD (cardiac disease, especially heart failure, bone disease, depression).
- Do not forget residual renal function (assessed from urine collections), which may well be significant in the first few months after the start of HD, but subsequently declines.
- More sophisticated measures of solute clearance are determined from urea reduction post-dialysis, UF rate, body size, and urea generation rates. Urea clearance is uniformly used as a marker of small solute removal and can be measured by:
  - URR
  - formal UKM
  - calculation of Kt/V from urea reduction during dialysis.

The National Cooperative Dialysis Study (NCDS) first showed that an average urea concentration and PCR were important determinants of short-term morbidity and mortality. Subsequent studies have attempted to determine the best way of calculating urea clearance, and the effect of different clearances on various outcomes. The Kt/V (fractional urea removal rate) was identified as a dimensionless numeric construct, which could best model urea clearance, and relates K (urea clearance), t (time on dialysis), and V (volume of distribution of urea, roughly the same as total body water). Since the NCDS, targets for urea clearance have been established (often with little good evidence) based on the Kt/V. This has created a need to measure Kt/V reproducibly, which is a major cause of problems. Small variations in blood sampling, dialysis time, and measures of patients' weight can cause large errors in calculated Kt/V and subsequent alterations to prescribed dialysis dose. A Kt/V of 1.3 in a small white woman is not the same as in a large Afro-Caribbean man. Excessive emphasis on Kt/V does not necessarily improve patient well-being.

Dialysis adequacy: urea kinetic modelling

UKM is simply a method for describing and modelling the combined effects of urea removal and urea generation, while taking into account the total distribution of urea within the body, and hence providing a measure of both solute clearance and nutrition. UKM calculates the Kt/V, but also includes assessment of residual renal function and the urea generation rate. It also allows prediction of the effect of changes in various factors (e.g. size or type of dialyser, time of dialysis) on solute removal. Many dialysis machines now come with software for calculation of Kt/V already installed, and increasingly collect the appropriate data as necessary (blood flows, time, UF rates, and pre- and post-dialysis urea levels).

Kt/V in principle is easy to calculate: t represents time on dialysis (directly measurable), V the volume of distribution of urea (calculated from body weight and height/surface area), and K is the dialyser urea clearance (known for each dialyser from *in vitro* studies). If a given Kt/V is to be achieved, the time of dialysis necessary can be calculated for a given patient. This analysis provides a measure of prescribed dialysis dose (Kt/V) and not the actual delivered Kt/V. Problems arise because of calculated V may not reflect the true V, and K measured *in vitro* may not be the same as occurs *in vivo*. There has been debate whether V or body surface area should be used as the denominator.

Formal UKM uses data collected from the patient over two dialysis sessions to determine the rate of clearance of urea during the dialysis session, and the rate of generation of urea between dialysis sessions. Samples collected are a pre-dialysis and post-dialysis urea for the first dialysis treatment during a given week, pre-dialysis urea for the second session, pre- and post-dialysis weight for the first dialysis session, and actual dialysis time in minutes. Correct blood sampling is crucial.

Post-dialysis blood must not be contaminated with saline washback or with recirculated blood (a spuriously low post-dialysis urea level will overestimate dialysis delivered). Blood sample should be taken within 1–2min of pump slowing to ensure the initial urea rebound due to access recirculation has occurred, and arterial and venous urea concentrations have equilibrated. The true post-dialysis serum urea level after subsequent redistribution (rebound) can be modelled mathematically and included in the UKM calculation. If patients still make urine, a 24 or 48h urine collection should be included for measurement of residual renal urea clearance to be added to the Kt/V.

The rate of decline in urea during the dialysis session is a function of both K and V (as redistribution of urea from body compartments occurs during dialysis), while the increase in urea between sessions is a function of V and urea generation rate. UKM uses computer modelling to suggest what parameters to change in order to alter the dose of dialysis delivered. Most conventional UKM takes the post-dialysis urea as a true measure of post-dialysis urea (so-called single-pool model). In reality the serum urea rebounds quite considerably for 45–60min after the end of dialysis as redistribution from tissues occurs. Some UKM techniques use double-pool models, with modelling of the rebound included, but the clinical significance of this is unclear.

Residual renal function should be included in any assessment of delivered dialysis dose, and may contribute significantly during the first few months on HD. (See Table 2.13.)

Table 2.13 Blood sampling for UKM

Pre-dialysis sample	Post-dialysis sample
For dialysis using AVF or AVG	
Take before *any* dialysis has begun from fistula needle	Set the UF rate to zero. Slow blood pump to 50mL/min for at least 10s
	Stop blood pump
	Take sample within the next 20s (alternatively slow pump to 100mL/min, over-ride alarm to keep blood flowing, wait 15–30s then take sample from A line) Second alternative: stop dialysate flow but keep blood pump running; wait 5min then take blood sample from anywhere in circuit
	For single-needle dialysis, clamp blood lines and discard 1st (dead volume) blood aspirated
For dialysis using percutaneous catheter	
Discard 1st 10mL blood from catheter	Take blood 30s after slowing pump

Calculation of Kt/V

Single pool (sp) Kt/V can be calculated from the pre- and post-dialysis urea in a single treatment, the time of the session, and the UF volume. This can be a useful measure of delivered dialysis.

One validated formula accurate over a range of Kt/V from 0.7 to 2.0 is (Daugirdas):

$$Kt/V = -\ln[Upost/Upre - 0.008t] + [4 - 3.5Upost/Upre] \\ \times (Wpost - Wpre)/Wpost$$

Where Upost = post-dialysis urea; Upre = pre-dialysis urea; Wpost = post-dialysis weight; Wpre = pre-dialysis weight; t = time of dialysis in h; Wpost − Wpre is the UF volume. (Sometimes 0.03 is used in place of ($0.008 \times t$) for simplicity.)

Less accurate approximations for the Kt/V from URR include:

$$Kt/V = 2.2 - 3.3 \times (Upost/Upre - 0.03 - (Wpre - Wpost)/Wpost)$$

accurate over a range of URR between 55% and 75%, but which otherwise underestimates Kt/V) and:

$$Kt/V = (0.026 \times PRU) - 0.46$$

or

$$Kt/V = 0.024 \times PRU - 0.276$$

Where PRU is the percentage reduction in urea during dialysis.

A URR of 50% corresponds approximately to a Kt/V of 0.8, 58% to 1.0, and 65% to 1.2.

Equilibrated Kt/V

This is increasingly used rather than simple Kt/V and can be calculated by:

$$eKt/V = art\ Kt/V_{sp} - (0.6 \times art\ Kt/V_{sp}/t) \\ + 0.03 \text{ (when using arteriovenous access)}$$

or

$$eKt/V = ven\ Kt/V_{sp} - (0.47 \times ven\ Kt/V_{sp}/t) \\ + 0.02 \text{ (when using veno-venous access, i.e. catheter)}$$

It remains unclear whether spKt/V or eKt/V is more useful.

There are also concerns that in women using Kt/V may lead to under-dosing of dialysis: if a formula using surface area as a denominator is used, women require significantly more dialysis.

Dialysis adequacy: other measures of solute clearance

Kt

It has been proposed that V (effectively a measure of body size) may directly alter patient outcome, independently of the effect on urea clearance. This suggestion has arisen partly because black patients have a better survival on dialysis than white patients (at least in the USA) and smaller patients, despite a lower relative URR. Also patients with the highest Kt/V have increased mortality, probably due to increased malnutrition, an effect not noted when comparing Kt alone with outcome. Increasing use is therefore being made of the uncorrected Kt, but as yet correlations with outcome are lacking. This measure also emphasises the critical importance of time itself in determining adequate dialysis: increasing evidence suggests increased mortality with even slightly shorter dialysis sessions regardless of formal small solute clearance achieved, although this may be confounded by a number of factors.

Urea reduction ratio

This is the simplest measure of delivered dialysis. It does not include the time of dialysis, effects of UF, or body size, but is correlated with Kt/V and still provides useful information.

$$URR = (1 - Upost/Upre) \times 100$$

[alternatively described as $(Upre - Upost)/Upre \times 100$]

Solute removal index

The total quantity of urea removed during a dialysis session is measured from the concentration and volume of the spent dialysate. The method does not require blood sampling, but has yet to be validated against appropriate outcome measures, and necessitates collection of the entire spent dialysate volume.

Quantification of clearance in HDF

This needs to take account of both diffusion and convection (ultrafiltration). In general, small solute removal is measured by Kt/V as with conventional HD, and additionally the effective convection volume (total volume of undiluted fluid ultrafiltered during treatment). In pre- or mid-dilution HDF the UF volume must take account of the degree of dilution using a dilution factor.

Dialysis adequacy: online measures of clearance

Online clearance monitors can provide automatic measures of delivered Kt/V and urea clearance. This can be done in a number of ways:

- Online urea sensors may allow the direct measurement of urea removed during a dialysis session. Dialysate is passed through a disposable urease column and the amount of urea quantified. URR and Kt/V are calculated in real time using conventional formulae. The normalized PCR (nPCR) can also be calculated.

- Online measurement of ionic dialysance (which correlates with urea clearance) using a biosensor in the dialysate flow path (the Diascan™) produces a continuous measure of Kt/V (based on predicted V). Essentially, the dialysate conductivity is measured at the inlet and outlet, which produces a measure of the ion flux during dialysis, which correlates with urea clearance. Dialysis machines are increasingly coming equipped with such monitors.

- Continuous measurement of ultraviolet absorbance of the spent dialysate allows estimation of toxin removal over time and can provide a measure of Kt/V.

Residual renal function

Residual renal urea clearance (Kru)

When HD is first begun, residual renal function may contribute greatly to the total amount of solute clearance. For all patients passing urine, Kru should be calculated from 24h or preferably 44h (interdialytic) urine collection and measurement of urea clearance. Patients must be instructed to collect all the urine passed between two dialysis sessions (for a 44h collection), and note the exact time of the collection:

Kru (mL/min)

$$= \frac{\text{Urine urea} \times \text{Urine volume (mL)} \quad \text{Urine urea} \times \text{Urine volume (mL)}}{(\text{Plasma urea}_1 \times 0.25) + (\text{Plasma urea}_2 \times 0.75) \times \text{Time (min)}}$$

for thrice-weekly HD, urea_1 being the urea at the beginning of the urine collection (end of 1st HD) and urea_2 the urea at the end of the urine collection. It is possible to add the Kru to the calculated Kt/V to produce a summary value often labelled as KT (or KtV), although there are mathematical problems with this. KT = Kt/V when there is no residual function:

For 3× weekly dialysis:

$$KT = Kt/V + (5.5 \times Kru/V)$$

Or alternatively:

$$KtV = Kt/V + 5.9 \times Kt/V \cdot Kru$$

Whether this value can be equated to the Kt/V for determining inadequate dialysis is unclear. It may be that residual function provides a more 'important' function than HD, but this has not been proven. Many studies, however, have shown that the presence of residual renal function is strongly associated with improved survival on dialysis (both HD and PD). Residual renal function declines rapidly in HD patients after initiation of dialysis.

Other markers of adequacy

- *Acidosis* should be controlled so patients have a normal pre-dialysis serum bicarbonate level. Bicarbonate transfer during dialysis is proportional to URR (and Kt/V). Dialysate bicarbonate can be varied according to individual needs.
- *UF* should be sufficient to keep the patient euvolaemic. Compliance with salt and fluid restriction is important. Increased oedema or ascites increases V, and hence reduces Kt/V if K and t are not increased. Increased dialysis time is also necessary to allow redistribution of fluid from interstitial compartments into the vascular compartment during dialysis.
- *Malnutrition* is a key marker of dialysis inadequacy and is easily missed. Early weight loss is often accompanied by fluid retention as the dry weight is not reduced in line with loss in muscle mass.
- Some dialysis units in the USA use an overall score generated from multiple factors to compare 'adequacy' between units. For example, the Davita quality index is based on a combination of mean Kt/V, Hb, PTH, PO_4, albumin, standardized mortality ratio, and presence of CVC line for the dialysis population.
- The *HD product* has also been suggested as a good marker for adequacy of dialysis:

$$HDP = \text{no. of hours per dialysis session} \times (\text{no. session per week})^2$$

And where the minimum acceptable should be 72 (i.e. 8h × 3/week or 2h × 6/week).

This score emphasizes the importance of time spent on dialysis and frequency rather than small solute clearance, in order to take into account middle and large molecule clearance, BP control, etc. This formula and its minimum target would suggest that 4h × 3/week is always *inadequate* dialysis.

Protein catabolic rate

PCR (usually normalized for weight: nPCR; g/kg/day) is derived from the urea generation rate and is usually calculated during UKM.

- nPCR can also be derived from nomograms relating plasma urea, nPCR and total urea clearance (KT).
- Urea generation is not a pure marker of protein intake (though it is often misconstrued as such), as increased muscle catabolism will also increase nPCR, although protein intake is often reduced in this circumstance.
- Patients with nPCR <0.8g/kg/day have increased morbidity and mortality, and generally patients need an nPCR <1.0g/kg/day to maintain positive nitrogen balance.
- Patients with a low nPCR need a careful assessment for protein malnutrition.

PCR can be calculated approximately from:

$$PCR = (\text{pre–post blood urea nitrogen}) \times (0.045/T)$$

Where T = number of days between blood samples.

Targets for adequate dialysis

- Adequate for the patient or a health economy?
- Adequate or optimum?
- A healthy patient, in a good frame of mind, without admissions to hospital for intercurrent illnesses.
- There is no universally accepted method for calculating Kt/V nor a clearly defined target.
- Kt/V should not be the sole criterion for adequate dialysis.
- The HEMO study has answered some questions but has generated much debate (see ➜ The HEMO study, p. 174).

Kt/V

The NCDS (a prospective randomized, but short-term study) identified a Kt/V <0.8 as a marker of increased morbidity and mortality.

There is increasing evidence that more dialysis is better; however, whether there are limits to an improvement in outcome with increasing dialysis, or the precise thresholds for underdialysis remain unclear. Furthermore, it may well be that beyond a certain level of urea clearance other factors become significantly more important in determining outcome, such as BP control. (See Table 2.14.)

The UK Renal Association and the US K/DOQI have recommended a minimum (not target) spKt/V of 1.2. Mean or median values for a dialysis unit should therefore be substantially higher for most patients to attain this goal. Prescribed spKt/V may also need to be higher (1.3) to achieve a delivered spKt/V of 1.2. Whether solute clearance targets should be higher remains contentious. Bear in mind that an spKt/V of 1.2 still represents only 15% of native renal clearance, and is equivalent to eKt/V = 1.05 or URR ~70%. European guidelines are currently recommending a target spKt/V of ≥1.4 (eKt/V ≥1.2) with thrice-weekly HD. Targets should almost certainly be higher for women.

The HEMO study has NOT shown any benefit of increasing spKt/V above 1.3 when dialysing 3×/week.

URR

The minimum target, as recommended by the UK Renal Association, is >65%, which in reality requires a target of 70%.

Table 2.14 Recommended targets for urea clearance spKt/V (eKt/V)

	Minimum	Suggested
K/DOQI	1.2	1.3
UK Renal Association	1.3 (>1.2)	1.4–1.45 (>1.3)
European Best Practice guidelines	1.3-4 (>1.2)	

nPCR

The nPCR target is 1.0g/kg/day.

- Smaller patients and women probably need higher target Kt/V.
- High-flux dialysis is likely to lead to greater urea rebound and overestimation of delivered Kt/V. Patients receiving high-flux dialysis probably need higher targets for Kt/V (especially when using standard single-pool calculations).
- Increasing Kt/V usually is associated with an increase in nPCR.
- High weekly Kt/V values are more common in countries using longer dialysis (Europe vs the USA), and overall mortality rates are lower in this setting. One centre in France (Tassin) has used low-flux cellulose dialysers for many years, and dialyses all patients for 8h three times per week. Average weekly Kt/V is 1.67. Probably more importantly, almost all patients have normal BPs, and do not require antihypertensive medication. Mortality and morbidity are significantly lower than almost all other units in the world.
- Daily dialysis (either long overnight or short hours) giving the same overall weekly Kt/V as 3×/week HD has been reported to provide significantly better BP control, fewer symptoms, and better quality of life.

Frequency of measurement

Dialysis dose should be assessed every 3 months in stable patients, and at least monthly in unstable patients. Formal UKM should be routinely used, although URR and Kt/V can be used in addition. An individual URR can be associated with Kt/V, which vary enormously. One study found a median URR of 0.6 associated with median Kt/V of 1.12, but ranging from 1.0 to 1.3.

The HEMO study

The HEMO study[1] attempted to determine whether a higher dose of dialysis, as judged by urea clearance (spKt/V 1.7 vs 1.3), or high-flux dialysers provided lower mortality and morbidity.

- A prospective RCT of 1846 patients established on 3×/week HD in 72 dialysis units in the USA. 72% patients were black. Re-use was common.
- Patients enrolled 1995–2000, having been on HD for ≥3 months. Many patients had their dialysis dose decreased from previous levels once they entered into the trial.
- Excluded if residual urea clearance >1.5mL/min, albumin <26g/L, unable to achieve the high Kt/V target in <4.5h on two of three occasions, or serious co-morbidities.
- Patients randomized to either standard or high-dose dialysis and to either low- or high-flux dialyser (3 or 34mL/min β$_2$m clearance).
- Targets were well achieved: mean URR was 66% vs 75%, mean spKt/V 1.3 vs 1.7.
- Survival was identical in patients achieving lower or higher solute clearances.
- Mortality was 17.1% in the standard group and 16.2% in the high-dose group (lower than in the USA in general).
- Survival was identical in those using low- or high-flux dialysers.
- Mortality was 17.1% vs 16.2%.
- Patients achieving a Kt/V of 1.3 were no better off if using a low- or high-flux dialyser (morbidity or mortality).
- Patients on dialysis for longer (>3.7 years) had some morbidity and mortality benefit when using high-flux dialysers.

Overall, therefore, the study suggested that dialysis delivered 3 times per week is currently being driven as hard as possible using current targets, and there is no advantage in attempting to increase the amount of small solute clearance. The study did exclude sick, older, unwell patients with co-morbidities, had a relatively young mean age, and most patients started with a relatively high Kt/V (1.4).

The more recent MPO study[2] also attempted to examine the benefits of high flux dialysis and also showed no major benefit overall compared with the use of low flux dialysers on overall mortality.

References

1. Eknoyan G et al. Effect of dialysis dose and membrane flux in maintenance hemodialysis. N Engl J Med 2002; 347: 2010–19.
2. Locatelli F et al. Effect of membrane permeability on survival in hemodialysis patients. JASN 2009; 20: 645–54.

Increasing dialysis dose delivered

The most common reasons for a lower than expected Kt/V are:
- lower blood flow actually used or provided than prescribed
- reduced time on dialysis, due to patient's late arrival, late initiation of dialysis, early termination at patient request or clinical indication, needle difficulties, recurrent machine alarms
- access recirculation
- dialyser clotting
- technical errors in collection of blood samples
- increased sequestration of urea in peripheral tissues, especially muscles, partially dependent on cardiac output.

Increasing the dose

Dialyser surface area, blood flow rates, and time on dialysis can all be increased.
- Increases in blood flow are often limited by the quality of the access. However, patients and nurses often underestimate what blood flow access can achieve before attempting to increase flow rates. Increasing blood flow beyond the capability of the access will lead to partial collapse of the arterial blood lines, increased machine alarms, and stoppages during dialysis. Using a larger diameter needle can improve blood flow, and ensure maximum flow through the access.
- Increasing dialyser size has a relatively modest effect on dialysis dose delivered.
- Increasing dialysate flow from 500 to 800mL/min can increase KoA by 15%; however, this rarely translates to increased Kt/V in practice with newer dialysers, for unexplained reasons.
- Changing the dialyser may increase dialysis dose, but there is little value in using high-efficiency dialysers if access is poor (for example). Dialysers with higher KoA will provide increased solute clearance.
- Increasing time is the major factor that will increase dose of dialysis. Increasing time increases urea and large molecule clearance, and also allows more extensive equilibration between body compartments, maximizing total body urea reduction. Patients do not like increasing time on dialysis, and increasing time increases the cost of dialysis. Patients, staff, and healthcare providers need education.
- Changing from conventional HD to haemofiltration can increase the clearance of large-MW molecules (by convection).

Prescribing chronic haemodialysis

If more dialysis is better (which is probably true although never proven; but see ⊃ The HEMO study, p. 174) then patients should receive the maximum amount of dialysis they will accept. In practice, the dose of dialysis delivered is the minimum acceptable to the patient and the provider, and is limited by the cost of dialysis and the time constraints. Dose of dialysis is rationed by cost in almost all countries.

Urea clearance

Used as a target for the amount of dialysis prescribed, but should not be the sole criterion for adequate dialysis. For 3 sessions per week a Kt/V of 1.2 is suggested as an absolute minimum. Kt/V can be increased by increasing the number of sessions per week, time on dialysis (length of sessions), size of dialyser, KoA (urea clearance) of dialyser, or blood flow. Computer modelling can allow an estimation of Kt/V using various combinations of dialyser, time in dialysis, and blood flow. Predicted Kt/V must always be checked, as delivered dose is almost always less than expected. Higher than expected Kt/V should not generally lead to a reduction in the amount of dialysis provided, unless for very good reasons.

Causes of unexpectedly low delivered dialysis include:
- blood flow delivered less than pump speed (with high venous pressures, high negative arterial pressures, poor access, poor needle placement)
- access recirculation
- dialyser clotting
- inaccuracy in the dialyser clearance figure used
- reduced treatment time (interruptions causing shortening of dialysis time, non-compliance)
- error in blood sampling (pre-dialysis urea too low or post-dialysis urea too high, taken before the end of dialysis or >5min after the end).

Patient factors

Number of sessions

It is impossible to achieve adequate solute clearance or UF control by twice-weekly dialysis. Small patients with significant residual function (at the start of dialysis) may just receive sufficient extra clearance. However, with loss of residual function they will rapidly need thrice-weekly sessions. A target Kt/V of 1.8–2 has been suggested for each session for twice-weekly dialysis, if this is unavoidable.

Time

The initial time required for dialysis can be estimated from the target Kt/V, the patient's V (from published nomograms based on sex, weight, and height), and the dialyser clearance (based on published KoA and blood flow).

Increasing time of dialysis is the single best way if increasing the amount of dialysis delivered, but is often resisted by patients (and staff). Whether patients have the same outcome from dialysis sessions delivering the same Kt/V but of differing lengths (e.g. 2.5h vs 4h) is not clear. However, there is evidence that long sessions provide significantly better control of BP, dry weight, and higher MW clearance, and dialysis units using long dialysis often achieve lower morbidity and mortality (e.g. Tassin, France, uses 8h 3× per week with low morbidity and mortality). Most units cannot provide 8h dialysis sessions because of the overall number of patients needing dialysis, and the resistance of patients themselves to such long hours. Nocturnal dialysis may change this, and more frequent short dialysis (see ➔ Home haemodialysis, p. 238).

Blood flow

Can have a major impact on solute clearance. All patients should have flows of >250mL/min, and preferably >400mL/min. When using high KoA dialysers even higher blood flows should be used to maximize the benefit of increased solute clearance (350–450mL/min). Patients can have increased intradialytic symptoms and hypotension if acetate dialysis is used with high blood flows, but not with bicarbonate.

- High blood flows require larger needles (14-gauge rather than 16-gauge) and shorter blood lines.
- If access is inadequate or needles too small, the pump will generate increased negative pressure and delivered blood flow will be less than the pump speed.
- High venous pressures can also lead to reduced blood flow at high pump speeds.
- Increased access recirculation occurs at high blood flows if the access flow rate is inadequate (poor arterial inflow).

Antihypertensive medications

Short-acting drugs may need to be omitted pre-dialysis to avoid hypotension during UF.

Patient monitoring during dialysis

Weight pre- and post-dialysis, BP, temperature, access site, development or changes in AVF or AVG, blood testing (usually monthly).

Dialyser factors

Dialyser KoA

The larger the KoA, the greater the clearance of urea achievable in a given time, and the more expensive the dialyser. High KoA dialysers may be associated with more acetate-related side effects in units still using acetate buffers. Large patients almost always need high KoA dialysers (>700) to achieve even minimum targets of urea clearance.

Dialyser size

Increasing size has relatively little impact on dose of delivered dialysis.

Dialyser membrane

The importance of the biocompatibility of the membrane remains contentious. Synthetic membranes are more biocompatible. Membranes can have low or high permeability (flux), which will affect larger MW solute clearances particularly. More permeable membranes will also allow increased backfiltration of dialysate during UF (important if water quality not sufficient). Membranes with higher water permeability need careful control of UF.

UF rate

The amount of fluid to be removed during each session must be prescribed. This requires knowledge of a patient's dry weight, and accurate weighing prior to each dialysis session. The weight difference is the excess water intake over water loss during the interdialytic period. A maximum of 4kg can be removed during a single dialysis session, and increased UF is associated with hypotension, reduced time of dialysis, inability to reach dry weight, hypertension, and probably with increased morbidity and mortality. Patients should aim for a maximum weight gain of 2–3kg between dialyses. Patients require careful and repeated education about the importance of minimizing fluid gain. Dry weight should be constantly reassessed as patients lose or gain muscle mass. UF rate can be constant throughout dialysis or varied (often made higher for the first 2h, and then reduced or stopped) to try and minimize intradialytic symptoms. Blood volume monitoring (BVM) may help maximize UF without problems for individual patients.

Dialysate

Flow rarely varies from 500mL/min, though can be increased to 800mL/min for patients using high KoA dialysers. Bicarbonate is preferred to acetate under all circumstances. Calcium, potassium, and sodium concentrations can all be varied. Sodium can be varied continuously by monitoring the dialysate conductivity. Sodium profiling or ramping is used to help maximize UF without inducing symptoms of hypotension, cramps, etc.

Anticoagulation

LMW or unfractionated heparin regimen (or alternative anticoagulant) needs prescribing (initial bolus and infusion or subsequent boluses).

Laboratory tests for patients on regular haemodialysis

The tests in Table 2.15 should be performed, usually monthly (unless clinically indicated more frequently). Blood tests should be taken pre-dialysis.

Table 2.15 Laboratory tests for patients on regular haemodialysis

Test	Comments
Urea	Absolute measure difficult to interpret (diet, catabolism, GI bleeding, residual function, liver disease, alcoholism). URR and formal UKM need measuring rather than blood urea in isolation
Creatinine	Absolute value difficult to interpret (muscle mass, nutrition). Higher values associated with lower mortality overall because of association with better nutrition.
Albumin	Strongly associated with outcome. Mortality increases at all levels <40g/L. May be marker of nutrition or else reflection of inflammatory response (opposite of CRP)
Calcium and phosphate	Renal bone disease not cured by dialysis. Calcium may be high, low, or normal, and varies with treatment with vitamin D analogues, phosphate binders, etc. Calcium in dialysate may need reducing in patients with hypercalcaemia. Patients with high phosphates need dietary advice, modification of phosphate binder use. Difficult to increase clearance with dialysis unless using haemofiltration
Bicarbonate	Should be maintained in normal range. Can increase dialysate bicarbonate in persistently acidaemic patients
PTH	Increased secretion controlled with vitamin D analogues or calcimimetics. Measure 2–6-monthly depending on need
Vitamin D	Measure if PTH raised; vitamin D deficiency common in dialysis populations and may need separate supplementation
Cholesterol	Cardiovascular disease remains major cause of death. Hypertriglyceridaemia more common than hypercholesterolaemia. Patients should be managed as for secondary prevention of cardiovascular disease
CRP	Increased levels significantly associated with mortality, regardless of cause. High levels indicate that a raised ferritin not necessarily a marker of replete iron stores
Glucose	Especially in patients from high-risk groups for developing diabetes (e.g. Asians, Maoris)
Hb	Aim for 11–12.5g/dL. Higher values may not be helpful (increased mortality in high-risk patients) but anaemia associated with cardiac disease, IDH, bleeding

Table 2.15 (*Contd.*)

Test	Comments
Ferritin, iron, transferrin saturation	For iron stores. Maintain ferritin levels 400–800ng/mL (assuming CRP normal)
Platelets	Thrombocytopenia may be induced by heparin
Liver function tests (AST, ALT, bilirubin)	Marker of hepatitis (especially viral). Especially if patients have dialysed in high-risk units (e.g. while on holiday)
Virology (HBV, HCV)	Often only measured 3-monthly. Patients should be immunized against HBV to minimize risk
Cytotoxic antibodies	For all patients on a transplant waiting list, especially after blood transfusions (usually 3-monthly)
UKM, URR, Kru, nPCR	Certainly 3-monthly, preferably monthly

Dry weight

The dry weight is used in HD as the target for fluid removal. It should be the weight of the patient who is in normal fluid balance, without oedema, or excess interstitial or intravascular water. It is clinically defined as the lowest weight a patient can tolerate without intradialytic symptoms and hypotension. However, intradialytic symptoms are also affected by the distribution of body water, the balance between UF rate and the rate of plasma refilling from interstitial compartments, lean body mass, nutritional status, and cardiac dysfunction. It is usually estimated by trial and error, and assessed by episodes of hypotension, overt volume overload, or hypertension.

Clinical assessment

Clinical assessment of dry weight is difficult, as it depends on solute and water content of various tissue compartments, accurate appraisal of the causes of intradialytic symptoms, and a patient's weight gain or loss.

- History of salt intake is crucial, and examination of jugular venous pressure (JVP), oedema.
- Weight gain may represent good nutrition and increasing muscle mass, or increasing volume overload due to overestimate of dry weight in the face of malnutrition and true weight loss. Measuring weight accurately is vital, using the same scales for a patient which are regularly calibrated.
- Hypotension on dialysis may be due to excessive UF because of an incorrect assessment of dry weight (too low), or because the rate of UF is too high to allow plasma refilling from volume-overloaded interstitial compartments.
- The greatest problems can arise early in dialysis when patients may be malnourished, but salt and water overloaded without oedema. Improvement in the patients' nutritional status can then lead to incorrect assessment of dry weight.

Long-term inaccurate assessment of dry weight can lead to persistent volume overload, hypertension, LVH, and increased risk of cardiovascular mortality. At least 80% of hypertension in dialysis patients is due to chronic hypervolaemia. It is sometimes claimed that hypertension is dialysis or UF resistant, implying a patient is truly at their dry weight. This is very rare. In the Tassin dialysis unit using 8h HD thrice-weekly, <2% of patients require antihypertensive medication. Long slow dialysis can achieve much better volume control than short fast dialysis. Mortality in Tassin is also reduced (75% 10-year survival). Similar results can be achieved by daily dialysis.

There is no gold standard for dry weight assessment.

Novel measures of dry weight

A number of techniques have been developed to try and improve the identification of true dry weight. None has yet been successfully imported into routine clinical practice although some units are now using bioimpedance, and several devices can produce real time measures of excess fluid during dialysis. One study of bioimpedance-guided adjustment of fluid status has shown significant benefits on BP, antihypertensive drug use, and dialytic hypotension. (See Table 2.16.)

Table 2.16 Novel measures of dry weight

Technique	Mechanism	Advantages	Disadvantages
Serum atrial natriuretic peptide	Released from atrial tissue with increased pressure; levels increase with overhydration	Ease of use. Sensitive for volume overload	No use in patients with heart failure Cannot detect underhydration Normal range?
Vena cava diameter	Measured by echocardiography or US. Increased diameter with overhydration	Reflects intravascular volume. Sensitive for overhydration	Difficult in heart failure Interoperator variation Large interpatient variation
BioImpedance	Electrical impedance in the body is proportional to total body water. Spectral analysis can distinguish intra- from extracellular water	Ease of use. Reproducible. Detects underhydration. Can be used continuously during dialysis. Measures interstitial and intracellular water as well as intravascular	Confounded by temperature and ion effects. Insensitive at detecting volume removal from trunk (main source)
BVM	Change in Hct or protein concentration (detected optically) is inversely proportional to change in blood volume	Ease of use. Continuous (real time) measure. Allows for prevention of hypotension	Plasma volume not only dependent on hydration state. Interpatient variability

Re-use of dialysers

This is the repeated use of a dialyser marketed for single use, for the same patient for multiple dialysis sessions. Extremely common in the USA (in ~40% of HD units, but falling, and rare in Europe and Australasia (0–20% of dialysis units), and prohibited in Japan. More commonly used for high-flux dialysers to reduce the unit cost. Safe when properly instituted and managed, although one study has suggested reduced mortality on switching patients from re-use to single-use dialysers. Number of re-uses for a single dialyser varies widely, with a median of 14. (See Table 2.17.)

Contraindications

Patients with sepsis or HBV antigenaemia. HIV and HCV infections are not absolute contraindications if strict precautions preventing cross-infection are in place.

Potential problems

- Atypical mycobacteria commonly found in tap water can be resistant to lower concentrations of disinfectants.
- Formaldehyde is an atmospheric pollutant and irritant, can cause contact dermatitis, and is associated (rarely) with the formation of anti-N-form antibodies (formaldehyde exposure leading to the development of antibodies to the N antigen on red blood cells, causing cold agglutination and haemolysis).
- Requires staff training and monitoring.
- Accurate record keeping mandatory, especially if automated.
- Patients need regular monitoring to ensure continued *in vivo* dialysis efficiency.

Table 2.17 Re-use of dialysers

Advantages	Disadvantages
Economic—more widespread use of costlier high-flux dialysers	Possible exposure of patients and staff to chemicals
Reduction in treatment cost	Possible infection risk
Possible reduction in intradialytic symptoms	Loss of dialyser efficiency with time
Reduced exposure to residual chemicals used in manufacture of new dialysers	Risk of endotoxin exposure
Enhanced biocompatibility for unmodified cellulose membranes	Labour intensive
Reduced environmental burden of discarded (used) dialysers	Anti-N-form antibodies in patients using formaldehyde-reprocessed dialysers

Medico-legal issues

Strict regulations cover the re-use of dialysers labelled by manufacturers as 'for single use'—regulated by the FDA (Food and Drug Administration) and HCFA (Health Care Financing Administration) in the USA, and the Medical Devices Authority in the UK. The responsibility for multiple use of dialysers falls on the dialysis unit and medical practitioner. Informed consent from patients may be appropriate.

Technique

Can be manual or automated. Involves four key steps: rinsing, cleaning, performance testing and disinfection.
- Label dialyser.
- Rinse with heparinized saline and dialysis grade water under pressure.
- Inspect for clots, cracks, etc.
- Rinse blood compartment repeatedly with dialysis grade water at 4L/min.
- Instil cleansing agent into blood compartment for 1min (sodium hypochlorite 1%, periacetic acid/hydrogen peroxide/acetic acid mixture, or hydrogen peroxide).
- Performance testing:
  - measure *dialyser total cell volume (or fibre bundle volume)* for degree of fibre occlusion (volume of fluid necessary to prime blood compartment fully) and compare with baseline figure; dialysers no longer used if cell volume reduced by >20%
  - *pressure-leak test* using pressurized air or nitrogen through blood compartment, or negative pressure applied to dialysate compartment; damaged fibres will rupture and leak air
  - *in vitro clearance studies* are performed intermittently using sodium chloride and cyanocobalamin, and UF coefficient determined by water transfer under pressure.
- Disinfect blood and dialysate compartments with periacetic acid/hydrogen peroxide/acetic acid mixture (Renalin®), formaldehyde, or glutaraldehyde. Store for up to 24h. Presence of disinfectant must be confirmed, usually by coloured indicator added to the disinfectant. Heat sterilization can be used with some polysulfone dialysers (105°C for 20h).

At next use:
- verify label (ideally with patient)
- remove disinfectant with saline and warmed dialysate flushes
- ensure removal of trapped air
- verify lack of residual disinfectant by colorimetric testing.

Haemodialysis and surgery: pre-operative

Morbidity and mortality are increased in patients with ESKD having almost any surgery (overall mortality of 4% and morbidity of 50%). Causes include coronary artery disease and MI, problems with electrolyte (especially potassium) and fluid balance, increased bleeding, drug interactions, drug (analgesics and anaesthetic agents) accumulation, and hypotension.

Biochemistry

Baseline assessment should include Hb, electrolytes, albumin, calcium and phosphate, glucose, and coagulation screen.

- Hyperkalaemia is the major electrolyte abnormality provoking anxiety in anaesthetists, although patients with CKD tolerate hyperkalaemia better than normal individuals.
- In an emergency, surgery can be performed in a patient with potassium of 6–6.5mmol/L and without ECG abnormalities. Otherwise medical measures (especially insulin and dextrose, and salbutamol) or dialysis (2h sufficient) should be instituted.
- Blood transfusions will increase serum potassium.
- A mild degree of acidosis is safer than alkalosis, which may worsen during induced hyperventilation and predispose to arrhythmias.
- Acidosis will worsen if normally compensated by increased ventilation, which becomes reduced during anaesthesia.
- Anaemia should be corrected (to improve bleeding time, cardiac state, and tissue oxygenation, and reduce risk from intra-operative blood loss) preferably by EPO rather than blood transfusion (in patients awaiting renal transplant).
- Transfusion may necessitate dialysis to control the volume and potassium load.
- There no defined safe Hb level for surgery.

Cardiac assessment

Baseline ECG and CXR needed in all. Many patients will require more extensive cardiac assessment prior to routine (non-emergency) surgery, e.g. echocardiography, stress testing (dipyridamole thallium or stress echo techniques), or even coronary angiography for high-risk patients.

Dialysis

Patients should be well dialysed (Kt/V >1.3) and in a good nutritional state (nPCR >1.0g/kg/day) prior to surgery, to minimize risks of infection, poor wound healing, and bleeding. Intensive (daily) dialysis prior to surgery has not been shown to improve mortality; it reduces the need for dialysis in the first post-operative day, but may induce electrolyte disturbances.

Fluid balance

Patients should be at their dry weight—fluid overload is associated with increased risk of pulmonary oedema peri-operatively and poor wound healing. Dehydration can be associated with hypotension. Intravenous fluid management can be difficult and needs careful assessment.

Hypertension

Should be optimized by volume control prior to surgery. If patient remains hypertensive, short-acting or parenteral agents should be used to control BP (labetalol, hydralazine, nitrates, very rarely nitroprusside).

Intravenous access

All unnecessary lines should be avoided, especially subclavian. Fistula or graft should be labelled and shown to the anaesthetist, and BP cuffs or external constraints should not be used on this limb.

Haemodialysis and surgery: bleeding risks

Bleeding times are prolonged in patients with ESKD, due especially to endothelial and platelet dysfunction. Risk can be minimized by:

- ensuring good dialysis prior to surgery
- correction of anaemia
- administration of desmopressin (0.3–0.5mcg/kg IV or 3mcg/kg intranasally); desmopressin can, however, cause rarely coronary artery vasoconstriction (and angina or MI) or flushing reactions and should therefore be avoided in any patient with known coronary artery disease; the effect of desmopressin begins after 1h and lasts for up to 24h
- rarely cryoprecipitate or fresh frozen plasma (FFP) are needed, but the volume of both of these may be a problem
- oestrogens are also effective but need to be given several days in advance (0.6mg/kg/day IV for 5 days or 2.5–25mg conjugated oestrogens orally: best evidence available for intravenous treatment)
- heparin should be avoided during dialysis itself if dialysis is necessary prior to surgery, or surgery delayed for 4h (protamine is rarely needed to reverse the effect of heparin)
- aspirin, NSAIDs, or clopidogrel should be stopped for several days (preferably 2 weeks) if possible.

Heparin used during dialysis and in CVC line locks can significantly prolong the aPTT in some patients even many hours after dialysis is completed and despite careful control of anticoagulation during dialysis. In patients at high risk of bleeding, minimal or heparin-free dialysis should be used and citrate for CVC line locks.

Haemodialysis and surgery: peri-operative

Renal failure has varying effects on anaesthetic and sedating agents:
• thiopental dose needs reducing
• propofol is well tolerated and is hepatically metabolized
• halothane and nitrous oxide are safe
• enflurane is metabolized to fluoride, and methoxyfluorane to oxalate, both of which may reduce residual renal function
• ketamine can cause exaggerated hypertensive episodes
• suxamethonium has been associated with severe hyperkalaemia (it increases serum potassium by at least 0.5mmol/L)
• atracurium has a shorter half-life than pancuronium (renally excreted) and is therefore the preferred paralysing agent
• the free fraction of benzodiazepines is increased in ESKD, and the sedating metabolites are often renally excreted.

Analgesics

Pethidine (meperidine) should be avoided as its hepatic metabolites nor-meperidine and norpropoxyphene have extremely long half-lives in ESKD, and can be sedating, cardiotoxic, neurotoxic, and cause central nervous system (CNS) irritability and respiratory depression. Morphine (and codeine) is metabolized to morphine glucuronides, which have prolonged action in ESKD. Fentanyl is a safe opioid (no active metabolites). Paracetamol can be used at normal doses.

Fluid and electrolyte balance

Requires careful monitoring, almost always with CVPs. Fluid overload must be avoided. Potassium should not be included in IV fluids. Serum potassium requires monitoring if blood transfusions are required. During cardiac surgery patients can be filtered while on bypass.

Vascular access thrombosis

Surgery is associated with episodic hypotension and hypertension, and AVF or grafts may thrombose during surgery.

Haemodialysis and surgery: post-operative

- Patients need careful assessment immediately after surgery, and daily thereafter, particularly for *fluid balance*, *electrolyte disturbances*, and the dialysis access viability. Fluid overload and pulmonary oedema are common complications of generous hydration peri- and post-operatively. Hyperkalaemia is also common (blood transfusion, potassium-containing fluids, tissue damage, muscle compression, depolarizing muscle relaxants).
- *Hypertension* is common—pain, anxiety, lack of usual antihypertensives pre-operatively, fluid overload—and should be treated with oral agents if at all possible.
- *Hypotension* needs careful assessment (bleeding, volume depletion, cardiac dysfunction, sepsis).
- *Fever*—infections are very common in ESKD patients after surgery, and include wound infections, pneumonia, sepsis, and line-related bacteraemia.
- *Nutrition* must be carefully assessed—patients should have early institution of nutritional support (enteral if possible). Hypophosphataemia is common in patients not eating after restarting dialysis (or CRRT), and should be supplemented.

Dialysis peri-operatively

- Patients should preferably be dialysed within 1 day prior to surgery—electrolyte disorders and fluid balance thereby corrected and reduces need for urgent dialysis in immediate post-operative period.
- Post-operatively, *heparin-free* or regional citrate dialysis should be used, if possible.
- Patients may need daily dialysis or CRRT for post-operative volume overload, especially if oxygenation impaired.
- Dry weight can reduce rapidly after surgery in immobilized patients who are not eating adequately, leading to volume overload (peripheral and pulmonary oedema) if not recognized.

Haemodialysis in transplant recipients

Up to 50% of patients have delayed graft function after a transplant, and require dialysis in the post-operative period. Patients should be warned of this prior to transplantation. Dialysis should be avoided if possible for the first 24h post-transplantation to minimize the risk of hypotension causing further insult to the transplanted kidney. Recurrent post-operative hypotension may be associated with prolonged graft non-function. Heparin should be minimized or avoided. The influence of the biocompatibility of the dialyser membrane on delayed graft function is controversial and unresolved. Special care should be taken to avoid line-related infection in patients with percutaneous IV catheters. They should be removed once renal function is properly established. HD does not alter the dose of most immunosuppressive drugs used routinely for transplantation, but they should be given after dialysis if possible.

Haemodialysis in terminal care

Patients should not be denied dialysis simply because they have a terminal illness. Patients with extensive malignancies or severe heart failure (for example) who develop renal failure should be properly assessed. AKI caused by volume depletion may only require a few days of dialysis before recovering. If the aetiology (or recoverability) of the renal failure is unclear, dialysis can be introduced explicitly as a trial for a short period of time. Dialysis may also allow patients extra time in which to make final arrangements. Under these circumstances it is best for the duration of the trial period to be explicitly discussed, so that dialysis can be withdrawn later (if appropriate). In some patients, conservative management may be more appropriate (of potassium, acidosis, anaemia, etc.).

Conversely, patients who develop a terminal illness while on dialysis should continue to be dialysed. Withdrawal of dialysis may be raised by the patient, their family, or the care team, and requires careful and repeated discussion (see ➲ Withdrawal of dialysis, p. 605), and may of course be appropriate and can be planned carefully.

Specialist palliative care teams are usually available in the community and hospitals, and can provide expert skills in the management of specific problems. Good pain relief is important, and renal failure should not stop prescription of adequate analgesia. Pain is poorly managed by nephrologists, and is common. Opioid metabolites can accumulate (especially norpropoxyphene and norpethidine), so pethidine- and dextropropoxyphene-containing analgesics should generally be avoided. Fentanyl and alfentanil are effective and safe (hepatically metabolized), and can be used as transcutaneous patches. NSAIDs may cause increased GI bleeding in patients with renal failure and a gastric protectant should probably be used. SC midazolam (often combined with diamorphine) can be useful in controlling discomfort and agitation (and uraemic twitching if dialysis has been withdrawn).

Haemodialysis for non-renal disease

Congestive heart failure

Conventional therapy includes diuretics, ACEIs, spironolactone, β-blockers, digoxin, and nitrates, and can control symptoms, reduce mortality, and delay progressive ventricular dysfunction in patients with mild to moderate heart failure. Patients with severe heart failure are more resistant to these therapies, have avid salt and water retention to maintain systemic BP, and have a 30–50% 1-year mortality.

PD and haemofiltration have both been used to remove excess water and salt gradually without compromising BP, and to reverse sympathetic and renin–angiotensin overactivity. UF over a few weeks can also restore the sensitivity of kidneys to β-diuretics. Mortality can be reduced in patients with severe heart failure offered dialysis, and quality of life improved.

Patients should be fully investigated to exclude other potentially treatable causes for pulmonary oedema (renal artery stenosis) or signs of heart failure (e.g. constrictive pericarditis).

Psoriasis

Both HD and PD have been used to treat extensive psoriasis even in patients without renal failure. A number of small controlled studies, including sham HD, have been conducted, with mixed results. In patients with renal failure, psoriasis can hinder the delivery of RRT of any modality because of the degree of skin involvement, the risk of secondary infection leading to either line sepsis or peritonitis, and the difficulties in performing surgical procedures through involved skin.

Psychiatric illnesses

Haemofiltration, HD, and plasma exchange (PE) have been used to treat schizophrenia, obsessive–compulsive disorders, and a number of other psychoses both in adults and in children, with no convincing evidence for benefit overall.

Nursing a patient on haemodialysis

Approaching patients on haemodialysis

Established renal failure

HD is the most common RRT used for patients with ESKD. Prior to starting a chosen RRT, patients should be given information and counselling about the different treatment modalities, namely HD, PD, transplantation, and conservative treatment. RRT will generally be considered when GFR falls below 15mL/min, and patients become symptomatic with signs of early uraemia, weight loss, volume overload, hypertension, or electrolyte imbalance. HD requires patients to come to a dialysis unit usually 3 times a week for at least 4h. However, the duration and frequency can vary, and dialysis treatment can also be done at home. Increasing use is being made of frequent (often daily) dialysis, nocturnal dialysis, and home dialysis.

Considerations for the renal nurse when performing HD treatment include:

- patient assessment clinically including dry weight and fluid assessment and vital signs
- review HD therapy: dialysis access, prescription, blood results, dialyser, connection, blood flow rate, anticoagulation, dialysate fluid, fluid removal, time
- review blood test results, need for blood products or medications, general health and well-being of patient
- patient and relative support.

More widely, when caring for patients with ESKD nurses should pay attention to:

- fluid balance
- vital signs: temperature, pulse, respiration, BP, oxygen saturation
- weight
- nutritional support and dietary advice
- medication
- care of vascular access
- availability of and access to transplantation
- patient education: disease process and its treatment needs
  psychosocial aspects of ESKD: concerns regarding employment, potential loss of earnings, health, sexual functioning, loss of self-esteem, depression.

It is the responsibility of the renal nurse to perform HD treatment safely and effectively with minimal complications whilst maintaining patient comfort at all times. Patients should be encouraged to be involved in their care to promote self-care and independence. Any changes to a patient's HD treatment must be documented, and individualized care plans written for any problems identified.

Nursing care of vascular access

Vascular access is the HD patient's lifeline; access failure and access complications are a significant cause of morbidity and even mortality. Two kinds of permanent accesses are used for patients who need long-term dialysis: AVFs and synthetic AVGs. Tunnelled central lines have significantly increased risks especially of infection, and in general should not be considered permanent access for HD; however, there may be circumstances where they are the ideal form of permanent access, e.g. older people with short life expectancy on dialysis, but only if infectious complications can be minimized. The AVF is considered the best long-term vascular access for HD because it provides optimum blood flow for dialysis, long life, and is less prone to infection and clotting. It is ideally formed in the non-dominant arm, either the forearm or upper arm. Grafts have higher infection and thrombosis risks and are more expensive.

Permanent vascular access (ideally an AVF) should be established several months before the patient requires dialysis to ensure that it is mature and ready for cannulation once treatment begins. The latest clinical practice guidelines from the UK Renal Association (2011) state that 'at least 65% of patients should commence dialysis with an arteriovenous fistula' and '85% of all prevalent patients on HD should receive dialysis via a functioning arteriovenous fistula'. Maintaining access patency requires clinical skill expertise, regular monitoring for continuing of care, ongoing education, and commitment from nursing staff for improved quality patient care. An access that is functioning well should deliver blood pump flow rates above 300mL/min.

Considerations before formation of fistula/graft

- General well-being of the patient: ensure patient is fit for surgery.
- Type of renal failure: AKI or established ERF. Forming permanent access in patients with AKI is inappropriate.
- Blood pressure and hydration status of patient: patients need to avoid dehydration, hypotension, and hypertension at the time of formation of AVF, and dehydration especially can cause access thrombosis.
- Infection: to ensure patient is free from any infection at time of formation of access and prevent infections subsequently.
- How quickly the patient needs to commence dialysis.
- Any underlying disease: such as diabetes, peripheral vascular disease, or thrombotic tendencies.
- Investigations/imaging of the patient's blood vessels may be needed, e.g. by Doppler US.

Pre- and post-operative care of access

Pre-operative care of AVF or AVGs

This begins as soon as vascular assessment has been completed and the site for access decided. The patient should be well informed of the surgical procedure and full explanation given of the aftercare of access. The patient is told that the arm should not be used for venepuncture or BP monitoring. Care prior to surgery:

- Baseline observations of temperature, pulse, respiration, BP, oxygen saturation, weight, blood glucose if patient is diabetic including any virology screening such as MRSA.
- Obtain haematology, biochemistry and clotting blood sampling
- Ensure consent form has been signed by patient.
- Ensure all necessary investigations and results have been reviewed prior to procedure.
- Administer any pre-medication, prophylactic antibiotics and all other relevant medication as prescribed prior to procedure.
- Patient is adequately hydrated and above their target weight if recently dialysed, and may need omission of antihypertensive medication.

Surgery can be performed under local, regional, or general anaesthetic.

Post-operative care of AVF or AVGs

Immediately following surgery, post-operative observations must be carried out (half-hourly at first) and the site should be checked for the following:

- Excessive bleeding, haematoma, swelling, pain, signs of infection such as raised temperature.
- Check warmth to ensure peripheral circulation.
- Assess access patency: palpate fistula gently for thrill ('buzzing sensation' of blood through the fistula) or listen for bruit ('whoosh' of blood through the fistula heard through a stethoscope).
- Check radial pulse, colour, movement, warmth, and sensitivity of affected limb to ensure blood flow reaches extremities.
- Monitor BP and hydration status: keep BP up and avoid dehydration to prevent access clotting.
- Elevate/support the access arm to help minimize oedema and swelling.
- Assess patient for pain, administer post-operative analgesia as prescribed.
- Report any abnormal findings to medical team ASAP.

Patient education

Good fistula or graft care will help maintain the patency of the vascular access. The nurse should discuss the care of the AVF or AVGs and answer any concerns the patient may have. Prior to discharge leaflets on AVF or AVG care should be given for further reference. Patient education is vital in the survival of their access. It is the responsibility of the nurse to advice patients to:

- check at least once daily for thrill or bruit
- avoid jewellery, tight straps, or constrictive clothing which will restrict the limb
- avoid carrying heavy loads with the affected arm
- the limb should not be exposed to extremes of heat/cold
- never to allow anyone to perform BP, venepuncture, or administer IV drugs into access arm
- avoid sleeping on the access arm
- gentle arm/hand exercises should be performed on the access arm to aid maturation of the AVF and increase awareness of the fistula
- use the access site only for dialysis
- wash skin over access with soap and water daily before dialysis
- keep the access clean at all times; the fistula/graft must be observed for signs of infection, including pain, swelling, redness, tenderness, or pus.

Any signs and symptoms of infection or absence of bruit/thrill must be reported to the renal unit immediately. Delay of even a couple of hours may render the AVF non-repairable. The fistula may need a minimum of 6–8 weeks to mature—ideally ≥12 weeks.

Cannulation of fistulae

Also called needling.

Pre-cannulation assessment of a fistula/graft
- Type and location of access.
- Visual inspection (anastomosis, discoloration, redness-infection, oedema, bruising, aneurysm, haematoma, prior needle marks).
- Manual palpation of access and palpation using tourniquet (thrill-patency, tenderness, temperature).
- Auscultation/ listening with stethoscope (listen for bruit; bruit should be continuous).
- First cannulation should always be undertaken by an experienced nurse.

Skin preparation

Following pre-cannulation assessment, preparation of the needle sites is crucial. Cannulation is an invasive procedure; therefore the limb should be washed with soap and water, and cleaned with an alcohol-based solution according to local renal unit policy to minimize the risk of infection.

Once the skin has been cleaned, the vessel should not be palpated. A tourniquet may be used to cause distension of the vessel to help visualize potential cannulation sites. Local anaesthetic is needed in some patients, most commonly intradermal lidocaine 1–2% (max 0.5mL) or lidocaine spray on the site of cannulation. The site should be left for one minute. Topical anaesthetics that contain lidocaine can also be used, but usually need to be applied by the patient 30–60min prior to cannulation.

Cannulating the fistula/graft

Needle site placement should always take into account needle site rotation. Proper needle site rotation will extend the lifespan of the fistula, preventing pseudoaneurysm formation. Fistulae that are cannulated throughout their length mature more evenly and last longer.

Needle gauge selection is dependent on the size of the vessel. Initially a smaller needle (16 to 17 gauge) may be used. Larger needles will be required if high blood flows are to be achieved (14 to 15 gauge) especially for high-flux or high-efficiency dialysis. A small increase in needle diameter can lead to a large increase in blood flows, and large needles minimize stress-related haemolysis.

The needles should be placed in the vein proximal to the fistula itself. The arterial needle is placed in the distal aspect of the vessel and can be pointing either away or to the heart. Placing the arterial needle near the anastomosis will achieve the best blood flow (but keep needles at least 1.5–2cm away from anastomosis). The venous needle is placed at least 5cm from the arterial needle, pointing towards the heart to minimize the risk of blood recirculation. If there are insufficient sites for two needles, single-needle dialysis can be performed.

Documenting the care delivered at each dialysis session and a written care plan are important in order to preserve the patient's access and to detect any complications at an early stage. Both are also important as a tool for communication among staff and a quality measure that patients are receiving high standards of care. The care plan and documentation should include:
• needle size and cannulation technique
• blood flow achieved throughout treatment
• arterial and venous pressures
• any problems with cannulation
• any signs of infection.

Cannulation technique

This is vital for the preservation of access. Repeated cannulation of the vessel in the same area causes weakening of the vessel wall and can lead to formation of aneurysms and pseudoaneurysms.
• The 'rope ladder' technique uses the entire length of the fistula with equal distribution of the puncture sites, developing the complete vessel. May also though lead to small dilatations over the whole fistula.
• The 'area puncture' technique, usually known as site rotation, is the repeated puncturing of 1 or 2 sites. This technique has an increased risk of aneurysm formation due to repeated punctures of the same sites, with stenosis in adjacent regions.
• The 'button hole' technique requires the needle to be inserted into exactly the same needle tract in the same direction, same depth, and same angle for every cannulation. This technique is especially beneficial for patients who self-cannulate, and for patients with limited cannulation sites due to construction, location, or condition of fistula, and may have a reduced aneurysm rate. It may take 2–6 weeks to develop the track, after which relatively blunt needles can be used for cannulation.

If cannulation is unsuccessful, repeated attempts should be avoided. Damage to the fistula may occur. The nurse should not exceed 3 cannulation attempts. If the site becomes swollen, the area should be avoided until the swelling/bruising has gone.

Complications of fistulae and their management

Nurses play an important role in managing vascular access-related complications through assessment and detection of possible complications.

Thrombosis

This is one of the most common complications of AVF. In AVF it is often caused by venous stenosis resulting in reduced blood flow, infection, or severe episodes of hypotension. The formation of stenosis can lead to recirculation, damage to the vessel wall, and eventually clotting of the fistula. The AVF/AVG loses its thrill and bruit and may feel firm. No blood or blood clots can be aspirated after cannulation. Urgent treatment is required to prevent the failure of the access (surgery or thrombolysis).

Poor arterial flow and increased venous pressure

Lead to reduction in blood flow and require investigation before access thrombosis or significant recirculation occurs. Poor flows can lead to clotting of the AVF/AVG. An angiogram or Doppler US should be performed to detect stenosis or thrombosis. Recirculation tests can also be used to determine the significance of venous stenosis. Recirculation >10–15% suggests access malfunction. Patients with low blood flow or low arterial pressures need an arteriogram (via the femoral artery) to examine the arterial inflow into the fistula (in addition to the venous limb) or a venogram with use of tourniquets to allow retrograde flow of contrast to visualize the arterial inflow. Patients with high venous pressures or thrombosis need a fistula venogram using a needle placed proximally within the AVF. For grafts, angioplasty may be required, or surgery to replace the narrow segment of the loop.

Infection

Infection and low blood flow are much less common in AVFs than in AVGs and venous catheters. Clinical practice guidelines from the UK Renal Association (2011) state that 'infection of an AVG has a worse prognosis than infection of AVF. Infection can be caused by:

- inadequate disinfection of the skin
- contamination of the needle
- manipulation of the needle during dialysis
- scratching of the puncture site
- poor personal hygiene
- contamination due to bathing.

Infected access must be managed urgently as it can lead to thrombosis or sepsis if left untreated. The vascular access must be observed for signs and symptoms of infection such as redness, swelling, pain, and a raised temperature. Bloods cultures must be obtained and the access site swabbed to confirm diagnosis. Antibiotics may be necessary. Nurses must adhere to strict aseptic technique procedure during cannulation and when dealing with access at initiation and discontinuation of dialysis.

Aneurysm formation

This is seen in patients on long-term dialysis. It is associated with stenosis and repeated needle puncture of the same or nearby sites. Surgery is indicated when the aneurysmal dilatation is >2cm, pulsatile pain is present in the aneurysm, and the overlying skin appears glossy and discoloured. Surgery is also necessary if there is a risk of rupture.

Steal syndrome

The name is derived from the stealing of (arterial) blood which would normally flow to the palmar arch. Patient can complain of:

- cold sensation and pale colour of the fingers
- ischaemic pain
- diminished or absent pulses
- necrosis of the finger tips may occur—in severe cases this may be associated with infection.

Investigations such as pulses, BP, pulse oximetry, Doppler, duplex US should be carried out. Patient needs to be strictly monitored for any signs of ischaemia which will require surgical intervention.

Grafts

Arteriovenous grafts

- Created surgically, using synthetic materials such as PTFE to connect vein and artery.
- Should only be created when AVF formation is not possible.
- Usually placed in the forearm, either straight or looped.
- Pre- and post-operative care is the same as for AVF formation.
- Bruising and pain are more extensive after surgery because of the SC tunnelling required for insertion of the graft.
- Advantage of a graft is that it can be cannulated after 3 weeks, if the surgical procedure is without complication, and sometimes immediately if absolutely necessary.
- Infection is said to occur in 5–15% of patients.
- Clotting and stenosis at the site of the anastomosis are more common.
- Care of the graft is the same as for AVF.

Scribner shunts

Quinton and Scribner invented the shunt in 1960. It is very rarely used now. The Scribner shunt was a U-shaped Teflon® tube permanently installed between an artery and a vein in a patient's forearm. The tubing is connected externally to make a loop.

Disadvantages

- High risk of infection.
- Cumbersome and difficult to use.
- High incidence of clotting in the blood vessels or shunt.
- Risk of blood loss if disconnection occurs.
- Short life of the shunt, risk of falling out, and accidentally being pulled out by patients.

Advantages

- Good blood flow.
- Possibility for dialysis several times each week without blood vessel damage.
- No new incisions need to be made.

Percutaneous tunnelled vascular catheters

Cuffed tunnelled percutaneous catheters

Used generally for patients who have immature or failed permanent access, or are awaiting access formation, or needing short-term dialysis. Increasingly used as longer-term access in patients with short life expectancy, and in patients who have no other access available (multiple failed AVF/AVGs or inadequate veins). It is performed using ultrasonographic and fluoroscopic guidance. They are placed in the internal jugular (preferable) or subclavian vein, and tunnelled subcutaneously over the anterior chest wall. They can also be inserted into the femoral vein or inferior vena cava (rarely). The catheter can be used immediately. They can be a form of permanent access in some circumstances, but should not generally be first choice access. X-ray must be done to confirm position prior to initiation of dialysis. Some patients will require anticoagulation therapy to improve access survival.

Advantages
- Catheter can be used immediately for dialysis.
- Can be readily inserted as day case procedure.
- Easy removal and replacement.
- Needle-free connection to dialysis machine.
- No risk of developing aneurysmal AVF.

Disadvantages
- Very significantly increased infection rates over AVFs/AVGs.
- Complications of insertion, e.g. pneumothorax.
- Lower blood flow rates usually.
- Increased risk of venous stenosis.
- Thrombosis within the catheter.
- Development of fibrin sheath resulting in poor/no flow.
- High risk for sepsis, haemorrhage, or air embolism.

Infection risks can be minimized using expert line insertion, careful nursing, and scrupulous line care. Under these circumstances infection rates can approach those of AV fistulae.

Catheter handling

Should always be performed aseptically, especially when uncapping or recapping before and after use. Sterile syringes should be placed into the open end if not immediately connected to dialysis lines. Alcohol solutions used for skin cleansing may dissolve polyurethane catheters, and betadine may dissolve silicon catheters. Hypochlorite 0.1% is safe for all catheters.

Percutaneous temporary vascular catheters

Temporary vascular catheters

Placed in the internal jugular, subclavian, or femoral vein under full sterile conditions by a trained operator. Those placed in the femoral vein can be used immediately after insertion. Internal jugular and subclavian catheters will require a CXR to confirm their position. Femoral lines must be removed prior to discharge. Internal jugular and subclavian lines can be left for 7–10 days, but the infection risk increases rapidly with longer periods. The use of temporary vascular access is known to be associated with serious complications such as infection, venous stenosis, and venous thrombosis. Femoral lines are associated with a high risk of femoral vein thrombosis and infection rates tend to be higher with femoral line. The date of insertion should be documented and lines should be removed as soon as possible.

Pre- and post-operative care of vascular catheter insertion

Pre-operative care of vascular catheter insertion

Explain pre-operative procedure and expected outcome following insertion of vascular catheter and allow time for patient to express concerns. Care prior to insertion:

- Baseline observations of temperature, pulse, respiration, BP, oxygen saturation, weight, blood glucose if patient is diabetic.
- Obtain haematology, biochemistry and clotting blood sampling, and virology (e.g. hepatitis B screening) and swabs for MRSA.
- Ensure consent form has been signed by patient.
- Ensure all necessary investigations and results have been reviewed prior to procedure.
- Administer any pre-medication, prophylactic antibiotics, and all other relevant medication as prescribed prior to procedure.

Surgery can be performed under local, regional, or general anaesthetic.

Post-operative care of vascular catheter insertion

Post-operative observations must be carried out (half-hourly at first):

- Check catheter site for excessive bleeding, haematoma, swelling, pain, signs of infection such as raised temperature.
- Assess patient for pain, administer post-operative analgesia as prescribed.
- Ensure patient has CXR following insertion and image has been checked to confirm correct positioning prior to use.
- Ensure the catheter dressing is performed using an aseptic non-touch technique and use clear semi-permeable dressing for clear visibility.
- Administer any medication, prophylactic antibiotics, and all other relevant medication as prescribed.
- Report any abnormal findings to medical team urgently.

Ensure permanent access has been planned especially for patients with CKD stage 5 (GFR < 15) prior to removal of vascath. If temporary catheter is no longer required or if presence of any underlying infection, remove vascath and tip should be sent off for microbiology.

Patient education

The nurse should discuss the care of the vascular catheter and answer any concerns the patient may have. Prior to discharge, leaflets on catheter care should be given for further reference. Patient education is vital in the care and management of their access. It is the responsibility of the nurse to advice patients to:

- keep catheter exit site clean and dry at all times
- avoid soaking exit site through swimming, shower, or bath
- apply waterproof dressing over exit site before taking a bath
- ensure the catheter clamps are clamped and the caps in place at the ends of the catheter at all times when not in use

- the dialysis catheter must only be used by the dialysis staff unless authorized by the nephrologist
- inform the dialysis staff of any pain, swelling, or bleeding around the exit site
- prevent any pulling or use of excessive force as catheter could become dislodged
- if any part of catheter develops a hole or leak, the catheter must be clamped off above the problem area and reported to the renal unit immediately.

Complications of vascular catheters and their management

Catheter exit site infection

The exit site should be observed at each dialysis session for signs of infection, including redness, swelling, pain, fever, or drainage from exit site. If a semi-permeable transparent dressing is used, the dressing can be changed when required. Strict aseptic technique should be used when changing the dressing and infections promptly treated. Record the patient's temperature; obtain an exit site and nasal swab and venous blood cultures if the patient has pyrexia. Consider using mupirocin 2% on the exit site at each dressing change if high incidence of staphylococcal exit site infections in the unit.

Blocked catheters

A common problem. Adequate flushing of catheters with a minimum of 10mL of normal saline, and correct instillation of heparin post-dialysis should prevent this.

Management

- An intraluminal catheter brush can be inserted to withdraw the clot with caution; the length of the catheter must be known to ensure the wire does not protrude into the vein.
- Urokinase thrombolysis has become common practice in the treatment of blocked catheters. Various doses are used, e.g. 5000 units given as an infusion or to fill the dead space of the catheter. Can be left in the catheter either for a short time (10–30min) or between dialysis sessions (2 days) or applied as an infusion.
- If the problem persists, a new catheter will be necessary.
- In patients with limited access sites, urokinase may need to be used at each dialysis session.
- Alternatives include tPA (1.25–2mg).

See also sections on catheter infections (→ Management of access (catheter) infections, p. 132; → Exit site infections, p. 318).

Strategy for improving vascular access

Nurses play an important role in improving vascular access through preventing unnecessary venepunctures to promote vein preservation. Written care plans and documenting care delivered at each dialysis session are important in order to preserve patients' access and to detect complications at an early stage. Documentation at each session should include:
• needle size and needling technique
• blood flow achieved throughout treatment
• arterial and venous pressures
• any problems with cannulation
• any signs of infection (pain, swelling, redness or bleeding around the catheter site)
• any presence of clots or obstruction in catheter.

If evidence of any problem, immediate actions such as radiological investigations, blood investigations, observations, strict monitoring, and appropriate referral for early detection, prevention, and management of access. Patients should be continually educated about the importance of looking after their vascular access and early reporting of any complications.

Local policies and standards

Each renal unit should develop written policies and procedures that are evidence based on ways of improving access for their patients:
• early referral and pre-surgery assessment
• cannulation
• recirculation studies.

Monitoring and rescuing access at risk through weekly access meetings where individual patient's access problems and complications can be discussed.

A multidisciplinary team approach is paramount in the management of long-term survival of fistula/graft and to promote favourable outcome for the patient. Good vascular access is the key to the overall management of a HD patient.

Preparation for haemodialysis

Dialysis equipment preparation

Ensure that all consumables are available according to the dialysis prescription. Alarm testing or function test (according to the manufacturer's instructions) should be performed prior to the initiation of treatment to minimize the risk of machine-related complications. The machine should be free from all alarms before the patient is connected. Priming of the dialyser should be thorough and should occur immediately prior to the start of treatment. The nurse initiating the treatment should check the machine and circuit carefully before connecting the patient. Checking should ensure that all air is expelled from the dialyser to prevent foam in the circuit once treatment has begun. Most dialysers are steam sterilized; however, if the dialyser has been chemically sterilized extra priming should be performed. Once primed, the machine may be placed in recirculation mode until the patient is ready. The machine should then be programmed according to the dialysis prescription and in line with the needs of the patient. This should include the desired fluid loss, the hours of treatment, heparin dose, if required, dialysate flow rate, temperature adjustment, and any additional modifications to treatment. See ➔ Chapter 2 for details on dialysis adequacy and prescribing dialysis.

Patient assessment

This is the key to preventing complications during treatment and should be accurately performed before each dialysis session. Pre-dialysis assessment includes performing observations of temperature, pulse, respiration, BP, oxygen saturation, and weight of patient. These observations are vital as baseline information as well as establishing the dialysis prescription, particularly for weight loss/UF requirements. A review of the patient's last dialysis records should be carried out and any recent interdialytic complications discussed with the patient. The general well-being of the patient should be considered. It is vital to assess the current fluid status of patient to decide on the most appropriate fluid removal technique best suited for each patient.

Dry weight assessment

Accurate assessment of dry weight is vital to the management of patients on dialysis. It must be ongoing and should be performed prior to the initiation of each dialysis session. Dry weight is the weight at which there are:
• no obvious signs of fluid overload
• no elevated JVP/CVP
• no peripheral oedema
• no signs of dehydration
• patient is normotensive.

Performing dry weight and fluid assessment of a patient

The nurse should consider the following:

Patient history
- Breathlessness at rest or on exertion
- Disturbed sleeping pattern: nocturnal dyspnoea
- Productive cough
- Excessive salt intake
- Recent appetite: anorexia may have led to loss of flesh weight
- Headache (BP related)
- Medical diagnoses (e.g. heart failure, cancer, etc.)
- Dialysis history: review of previous UF
- Urine output: residual renal function
- Fluid allowance: usually 500mL (any measurable fluids) plus previous day's urinary output.

Clinical signs and symptoms
- Oedema (e.g. lower extremities, periorbital)
- Breathlessness at rest or on exertion
- Hypertension (usually volume related); lying, sitting, and standing; BP >130/80 is almost always indicative of volume overload
- Hypotension: if severely overloaded or cardiac compromised
- Weight gain since last dialysis: more accurate if the same scale is used on all occasions
- JVP: raised and distended in fluid overload
- Chest auscultation: any crackles indicating pulmonary oedema.

Diagnostic procedures
- CXR: it is the responsibility of the nurse to prepare patient and liaise with medical team to ensure result is known. May show pulmonary oedema.
- Bioimpedance: increasingly used in some units to assess dry weight.
- Serum albumin: if albumin levels low then can lead to low UF capacity, which precipitates volume overload.
- Hb: if Hb levels low can lead to low UF capacity, which precipitates volume overload.
- Serum sodium: low levels can lead to low UF capacity as above.

Patient education

It is the responsibility of the nurse to advise patients on:
- fluid allowance: residual renal function
- intra-dialytic weight gain
- signs and symptoms of fluid overload
- importance of record keeping
- positive aspects of controlling fluid.

Nursing staff should liaise with the medical team if necessary to ensure accurate fluid assessment and dry weight of patient.

The haemodialysis prescription

Fluid removal on haemodialysis

When deciding on the total volume of fluid to be removed, the nurse must consider the UF rate and the physical condition of the patient, including cardiovascular compliance. Recent blood results and current medication should also be taken into consideration. Removal of fluid during dialysis is dependent upon the movement of fluid into the vascular space. Refilling depends on the volume of excess fluid for removal from the ECF. This will continue throughout the dialysis session and for a period of time after, until homeostasis is achieved.

A UF rate that remains high (>0.8–1.0L/h) throughout treatment is poorly tolerated by many patients. Patients with large interdialytic fluid gains, and those with poor plasma refill capability, are particularly at risk of developing fluid-related complications, with symptoms including headache, nausea, dizziness, hence the need to adapt a suitable fluid removal technique. Dry weight and fluid removal techniques must be reviewed frequently to minimize the risk of fluid overload or volume depletion.

Different fluid removal techniques include the following:

• Fluid profiling: fluid removed in stages or at a constant rate. Larger volumes removed at the start with UF rate at a maximum when blood osmolality is at its highest (when patient less likely to become hypotensive). Rest periods may be incorporated for patients with poor plasma refill, e.g. patients with diabetes and older people or the option of removing equal amount of fluid throughout the dialysis session.

• Isolated UF: large volume of fluid removed without HD especially for patients who are fluid overloaded. The time for adequate dialysis must be considered when using this method.

• Sodium profiling: dialysate sodium manipulation to increase osmotic pressure to prevent dialysis induced hypotension. By using higher dialysate sodium at the start of dialysis, more fluid can be removed, but can lead to sodium overload and excess thirst and fluid gains between dialysis sessions.

• Low dialysate temperature: dialysate temperature reduced to enable vasoconstriction, which increases cardiac output and BP. Core temperature is used as baseline. Aim to maintain dialysate temperature at patient's baseline of 0.5°C below baseline.

• Blood volume monitoring: determines circulating blood volume usually relative to start point in various ways, either by US or by measuring the photo-absorbency of blood, both as a marker of the relative concentration of blood or protein. Can indicate when rate of fluid removal too high. Whether this tool overall improves fluid management is not clear.

For details on the rest of the HD prescription see ➔ Chapter 2.

Dialysate options

Should be made following an assessment of blood results. The main considerations are:

• hypercalcaemia (Ca >2.8mmol/L) → low calcium dialysate (1.00–1.25mmol/L)
• hypocalcaemia (Ca <2.0mmol/L) → high calcium dialysate (1.50–1.75mmol/L)
• hyperkalaemia (K+ >6.0mmol/L) → low K+ dialysate (0–2.0mmol/L)
• hypokalaemia (K+ <3.5mmol/L) → high K+ dialysate (3.0–3.5mmol/L)
• patients with diabetes should use a dialysate containing glucose ranging from 1.0 to 2.0g/L to minimize the risk of hypoglycaemia.

Dialyser selection

This is dependent upon the individual patient's need for small and large solute clearance, UF, dialysis treatment time, use of haemofiltration, biocompatibility of membrane, and size of the patient. In practice, individual units often keep a small range of dialysers (with two or three different sizes and membranes).

There are cost implications of various dialysers, hence re-use of dialysers in some countries and dialysis programmes, which has its limitations such as possible infection risk, loss of dialyser efficiency over time, and staff/patient exposure to chemicals. The clinical benefit of biocompatible membranes is controversial; however, there is evidence to suggest that they are associated with fewer dialyser reactions and better clearance of middle molecules.

Education and technical services offered by a supplying company may also be important.

In AKI, dialyser selection will be made following assessment of the patient's biochemistry and fluid balance and for CRRT most units will have access only to 1 or 2 dialysers often varying by size.

A good dialyser is integral to dialysis adequacy. The renal nurse need to be aware of the importance of selecting the right dialyser dependent on patient requirements such as:

• needs of the patient: surface area, clearance required and KuF
• access: achievable blood flows
• cardiac status of patient
• dialysis time
• desirable extras: middle molecule clearance, biocompatibility and cost.

Anticoagulation for haemodialysis

The regimen should be individualized and reviewed on a regular basis. The aim is to administer the minimum amount required to achieve therapeutic effects. The prescription should be based on:

- measured ACT
- patient's diagnosis and general well-being
- type of access
- clarity of dialyser and circuit after dialysis
- any coagulation complications post-dialysis.

Heparin is the usual form of anticoagulation used for HD, although LMWHs are increasingly used and recommended first line in Europe. Due to its frequent use, many dialysis units develop ways of prescribing heparin to meet the demands of the patient. These include the use of patient group directions, which provides a framework for the prescription and administration of medicine without the need for an individualized prescription.

Heparin may be administered by:

- initial bolus dose
- initial bolus + maintenance dose
- maintenance dose only
- intermittent doses.

There are 3 main regimens used in the administration of heparin:

- *Routine*: patients with low bleeding risks or an established regimen.
- *Tight*: patients with slight bleeding risks, e.g. patients on additional anticoagulants or those who do not yet have an established regimen.
- *Heparin free*: patients with high risks for bleeding, e.g. immediately pre- or post-surgery, first HD with associated uraemia.

Alternatives are usually prescribed on an individual patient basis and include LMWH, e.g. enoxaparin sodium, regional citrate, epoprostenol, argatroban, and danaparoid.

Points to consider

- In AKI, the heparin prescription should be reviewed at each dialysis session.
- Uraemic patients may have platelet dysfunction and active bleeding.
- Patients having invasive procedures performed should be dialysed on a tight or heparin-free regimen after the procedure.
- During heparin-free dialysis, high blood flow and saline flushes every 15–30min are used to prevent clotting of the circuit. The saline flushes should be incorporated into the total fluid loss required. Heparin-free dialysis can rarely result in the loss of the whole blood circuit due to clotting.
- Heparin locks in CVCs can cause significant systemic anticoagulation (by slow leak of heparin from the line), and must be removed before dialysis.

Initiation of treatment

The nurse should check the machine before initiating dialysis to ensure it is free from alarms and that the extracorporeal circuit is air free to minimize the risk of air embolism. The nurse must ensure the patient's pre-dialysis observations and fluid assessment are carried out taking into account the individual patient prescription prior to initiation of dialysis.

Initiating dialysis with an AVF/AVG

- Ask patient to wash their arm with handwash or soap and water if able. Clean arm with 2% chlorhexidine gluconate in 70% isopropyl alcohol.
- Place waterproof towel beneath fistula limb of patient.
- Apply tourniquet if required to palpate and identify appropriate cannulation sites.
- Administer intradermal lidocaine anaesthetic (1–2%) or Xylocaine® spray to cannulation site, leave for 1 min.
- Release tourniquet if applied.
- Attach a 10mL syringe primed with saline 0.9% to each fistula needle (use dry needle for blood sampling).
- Reapply tourniquet and insert fistula needles using appropriate needling techniques. Release tourniquet.
- Check blood flow from each needle site by flushing with 5mL of saline 0.9%. Tape fistula needles securely to skin.
- Begin treatment by connecting needles to arterial and venous lines with blood pump at 150mL/min.
- Once desired pump speed achieved, initiate dialysis and document all care delivered.

Initiating dialysis with vascular catheter

- Remove dressing using non-sterile gloves. Assess exit site and catheter for signs of infection, displacement or holes.
- Remove gloves, apply alcohol hand gel, position sterile field and put on sterile gloves.
- Clean the catheter exit with 2% chlorhexidine gluconate in 70% isopropyl alcohol solution using strict non-touch technique.
- Apply clear semi-permeable dressing to cover the exit site.
- Another sterile glove should be worn and non-touch technique used to clean catheter limbs, clamps, and hubs.
- Remove Luer locks, connect 2.5mL syringe and withdraw 2.5mL of blood from each catheter limb or according to catheter dead space volume.
- Attach 5–10mL syringe primed with saline 0.9% to catheter. Withdraw slightly first, then infuse saline 0.9% into catheter.
- Leave syringes attached to catheter limbs.
- Begin treatment by connecting lumens to arterial and venous lines with blood pump at 150mL/min.
- Once desired pump speed achieved, initiate dialysis and document care delivered.

On connection, the nurse should pay keen attention to the extracorporeal circuit and the patient to ensure that that there are no obstructions to blood flow, no air is visible, and all connections are secure.

Before leaving the patient, the nurse should ensure that:

• the arterial and venous lines are secure
• the patient is comfortable
• the patient's observations have been rechecked and are stable
• blood glucose levels have been assessed for diabetic patients
• the machine is in dialysis mode and free from all alarms
• anticoagulation has begun
• at least 500mL saline 0.9% is attached to the circuit for emergency use
• the correct fluid loss has been programmed into the machine
• fluid removal technique is in progress if necessary
• nursing documentation has been completed
• used dressing packs have been discarded
• the patient has access to a nurse call system if not visible to nursing staff.

Intradialytic monitoring

It is the nurse's responsibility to monitor patients during dialysis and respond to any unexpected outcomes with appropriate intervention to minimize the risk of dialysis-related complications. The frequency will depend on the stability of the patient. It is recommended that all patients have the following obtained and documented on at least one occasion during treatment:

• general condition
• BP
• pulse
• venous pressure
• arterial pressure
• volume of fluid removed
• UF rate
• heparin dose delivered.

Less stable patients or those with large fluid gains will need more frequent observations performed. Continuous monitoring is advised during a first dialysis or in an acute setting. During dialysis, the nurse should ensure that medications given during dialysis, e.g. anticoagulation therapy, iron therapy, Hb management, intravenous medication, and nutrition supplement are administered safely as prescribed. If blood or blood products are given, the volume should be accounted for in the total UF volume. Nursing documentation should be completed and should be accurate and up to date.

Universal precautions should be adhered to at all times and asepsis maintained within the dialysis unit for the protection of both nursing staff and patients. Each dialysis unit should have agreed local infection control policies which should consider national and international guidelines.

Each time a clinical procedure is performed ensure:

• hands have been washed
• clean gloves and clean plastic apron are worn
• face protection (visor) should be worn as there is a risk of blood/chemical splashes
• the availability of bacteriostatic substances for blood spillage or exposure.

Discontinuing haemodialysis

Once dialysis treatment is complete the machine will give either an audible or visual indication that the programmed hours of treatment have been achieved. Prior to this, it is important to ensure that the necessary consumables are prepared to avoid delay with the procedure. This will need ~5min in advance to minimize the risk of infection. Assess patient's general status and BP to ascertain washback volume. The nurse should check if the patient is prescribed any medications post dialysis. Administration time varies dependent on the drug to be given (determined by local drug administration protocols) but may occur just before, during or after wash back. The rinseback line should be attached to at least 500mL of saline 0.9%.

Post-dialysis blood sampling

Should be performed 0–2min after the blood pump is switched off, having been slowed previously. Rebound of some electrolytes will occur and needs to be taken into consideration. A substantial proportion of electrolyte rebound occurs late (2–30min after finishing dialysis).

Washing back

Blood in the extracorporeal circuit is returned to the patient using normal saline at a blood pump speed of 150–200mL/min. The aim is to use as little normal saline as possible to minimize the risk of fluid overload. 200–400mL is commonly needed and given. More saline 0.9% may, however, be given if the patient is hypotensive. When the venous line is light pink, the rinseback procedure should be stopped. The patient should be assessed again at this stage so that more saline 0.9% can be administered if required.

Terminating dialysis with an AVF/AVG

- Place a clean waterproof sheet and create a sterile field underneath the patient's access limb.
- Stop the blood pump.
- Clamp the arterial line and arterial fistula needle.
- With clean gloves, attach the arterial line to the rinseback line so the blood is returned via the venous needle.
- Flush the arterial needle with 5–10mL saline 0.9%
- Commence washback at blood flow rate of 150mL/min.
- Stop pump when blood has been returned to patient.
- Remove venous fistula needle first and then the arterial needle to minimize the risk of bleeding from the arterial site. Apply pressure to the venepuncture sites with sterile gauze.
- Once bleeding has stopped (usually a few minutes later), cover the site with gauze and tape or a dressing—this should stay on ovenight.
- Self-care should be promoted and the patient may assist where possible.
- Document all care delivered.

Terminating dialysis with a percutaneous vascular catheter

- Create an aseptic field under the catheter limbs using waterproof sheet.
- The use of sterile gloves and the aseptic non-touch technique is paramount.
- The catheter hubs should not be left exposed and should be cleaned prior to the replacement of sterile caps.
- Stop pump. Clamp arterial line and arterial lumen of catheter.
- Using sterile gloves remove the arterial line from the patient.
- Once the arterial line has been attached to the saline 0.9%, commence blood pump to a maximum flow of 150–180mL per minute.
- Flush arterial lumen of the catheter with at least 10mL of saline 0.9%.
- Stop blood pump once blood has been returned to patient.
- Flush venous lumen of catheter with at least 10mL of saline 0.9%.
- Instil individual patient prescription of heparin/citrate/urokinase into the dead space of each lumen (1000–5000 units/mL), using the correct volume indicated on each limb. Note that over filling the lumen can result in excess coagulation and bleeding risk to patients.
- Place hubs on end of each catheter limb to prevent blood loss and minimize infection and embolism risk to the patient.
- Document all care delivered.

Post-dialysis evaluation

The importance of patients completing their prescribed dialysis time in view of achieving dialysis adequacy is paramount. Post-dialysis clinical observations are crucial in ensuring safe discharge of patients.

- BP should be checked to assess any evidence of hypertension or hypotension. It is important that BP is normalized, particularly if patient is travelling back home.
- Post-dialysis weight should be compared with both pre-dialysis weight and dry weight, to ascertain if programmed weight loss has been achieved. The nurse should also assess how well the patient has been able to tolerate fluid removal.
- Assessing fluid status will ensure correct establishment of dry weight.

Discrepancies between desired and achieved weight loss can be caused by:
- incorrect weight recorded at start of dialysis
- incorrect calculation of weight loss
- faulty UF control
- patient consuming extra fluid during treatment
- IV fluid administered during treatment without accounting for this in total UF volume, e.g. blood, medications, and saline 0.9%.

In addition to the above clinical assessments, the patient's overall physical condition should be assessed and appropriate actions taken to ensure safe discharge. The nurse is responsible for reviewing post dialysis findings with accurate documentation, appropriate communication, within the healthcare team to ensure continuity for future dialysis sessions (blood results, any access problems, appearance of circuit) and discuss changes to individualize dialysis prescription in view of inadequate dialysis.

Dialysis machine alarms

Although dialysis machines vary, all have common alarm features:
- alarms directly related to patient safety which cause the blood pump to stop
- warning alarms related to patient safety if they are not corrected, but do not cause the blood pump to stop.

With both of these types of alarm, an audible and visual prompt will be present to alert the operator to the need for action. (See Table 3.1.)
Alarms should immediately be corrected.

Table 3.1 Dialysis machine alarms

Alarm	Cause
High venous pressure	Incorrect positioning of venous fistula needle
	Venous stenosis
	Clot within the vessel
	Clotted circuit or dialyser
	Occluded venous lines
Low venous pressure	Error at the venous pressure sensor
	Dislodgement of venous fistula needle
	Saline infusions
	Poor arterial flows
	Blood leak in return circuit
Low arterial pressure	Incorrect positioning of arterial fistula needle
	Arterial vessel stenosis
	Clot within the arterial vessel
	Occluded arterial blood lines
	Poorly developed fistula
	Poor flows from vascular catheter
	Hypovolaemia/dehydration
Air and foam detector *Do not reset or over-ride alarm if air is present*	Transfusions/drug administration
	Turbulence within the chamber caused by high blood flow
	Hole or tear in vascular catheter
	Dislodged needle
Blood leakage	Damaged dialyser fibres causing leakage of blood through the dialyser membrane and possible contamination of blood with dialysate
	Air in the dialysate causing a false alarm
Conductivity	Incorrect concentrate, kinks in the dialysate tubing, empty concentrate cans, or a machine fault

Venous pressure

Will vary according to type of vascular access, needle gauge, and the diameter of the dialysis blood lines. Venous pressures >120–150mmHg at a blood flow of 200mL/min need investigation, usually with a fistulagram. Such pressures though are common if blood flows of 400mL/min are achieved.

Arterial pressure

Can be measured by a pressure transducer giving a direct reading or by sensors that detect changes within an arterial pump insert. If the pressure falls below a set value, the arterial pressure alarm is triggered. An arterial pressure greater than −250mmHg can result in an inaccuracy of the delivered blood flow of >±10%. With a blood flow of 300mL/min the arterial pressure should not exceed −200mmHg.

Action
Remove or readjust needle to prevent extravasation and damage to the vessel
Avoid stenosed area. Investigate urgently
Arrange embolectomy, surgery, or thrombolysis. Refer for fistula angiogram
Change complete circuit and review anticoagulation
Remove occlusion
Refer to operator manual
Re-cannulate with new needle. Observe for bleeding or extravasation
Investigate for cause
Identify leak and correct
Remove or readjust needle
Avoid stenosed area. Investigate urgently
Avoid area. Arrange surgery or thrombolysis
Remove occlusion
Allow more time for maturation. May need fistula angiogram
Urokinase infusion into catheter or change
Ensure patient is not below dry weight
Stop infusion or review when complete
Reduce blood flow until turbulence ceases
Increase the level within the chamber. If fine air bubbles within the circuit, disconnect the patient and recirculate until circuit is clear. If patient may have received an air embolus, place in Trendelenberg position, disconnect lines; attempt to withdraw the air from the fistula needle or line, and alert emergency team.
Test the effluent dialysate for the presence of blood
If blood is present discard circuit and resume dialysis
Correct fault

Care of dialysis machines

Dialysis machines are expensive and must be utilized efficiently. In some renal units, 3–4 treatments will be performed daily on a single machine. Dialysis machines must be well maintained and correctly used, adhering to the operators' guidelines supplied by the manufacturer.

Educational support is usually available from the machine manufacturers to provide training for new staff, and to teach existing nurses the full range of treatment options available with each machine.

Technical staff are usually based within each renal unit to ensure machine faults are repaired promptly, and routine maintenance work is carried out. If technical staff are not based on site, an on-call service will be in operation. Efficient technical support is vital in minimizing delays caused by machine faults.

Machine faults should always be dealt with urgently. If a fault is noted before the commencement of treatment, the machine should be removed and replaced with an alternative machine. Spare machines are needed for this. If a fault is noted during treatment, the nurse will need to decide whether to discontinue treatment and prepare an alternative machine. If the fault is likely to affect the patient's treatment, dialysis must be discontinued. Alarm testing of the machine should be performed prior to each treatment. It is the responsibility of the nurse to ensure this has been safely completed. Only trained operators should use dialysis machines. If patients prepare their own machine or perform their own treatment, a detailed training programme must be completed.

In the event of a power failure, the dialysis machine will shut down and the operator must be able to return the blood to the patient. To do this, the nurse should remove the venous line from the venous clamp and hand crank the blood pump until all the blood has been returned using the rinseback procedure. It is, therefore, essential to ensure that all dialysis machines have a handle available for this purpose (some machines have a handle built into the blood pump).

Cleaning of dialysis machines

- External cleaning of the machine must take place after each dialysis treatment.
- Visible blood should be cleaned with a bleach solution and disposable cloth.
- The dialysis machine should then be cleaned with an evidence-based virucidal disinfectant. Even though local policies may vary, it is important to use a solution that is active against blood-borne viruses and is not harmful to the machine.
- Scrupulous attention should be paid to the cleaning of machines to prevent the spread of infection.
- After each treatment the machine should be either chemically cleaned or heat disinfected.
- It is advisable to disinfect the machine if it has not been used for 48h.
- Extra chemical cleans may be required with acid solutions to prevent precipitation within the machine.

Psychological care of haemodialysis patients

The psychological impact of ESKD can be huge as it affects every aspect of a person's life, and the prospect of dealing with this for nursing staff can be daunting. Patients experience complex physical, psychological, and social problems. For patients and their families, life with maintenance dialysis requires major changes for an indefinite period of time. Some or many of their daily activities and lifestyle need to be adapted to life on dialysis. These may include dietary and fluid allowance, taking regular medications, ability to continue working, potential loss of earnings, and loss of self-esteem and independence, especially if role changes within the family.

The nurse must be aware of the anxiety and distress that this can cause. During this period, the patient will need support and understanding, and must have complete confidence and trust in the nursing team. The nurse needs to be sensitive to the needs and stressors caused by ESKD and provide adequate discussion and explanations of the nature of the illness, treatment benefits, complications, risks, and alternative methods of treatment to the patient and family.

The relationship between the nurse and patient is a unique one to renal nursing and will continue through several treatment modalities. The most important aspect in maintaining the trust between the nurse and the patient is developing a partnership in care. It is essential that the nurse explains and discusses all aspects of HD treatment with the patient. The nurse must respect patients' rights, cultural differences, and preferences, in order to promote their autonomy and empower them to make choices about their health and healthcare. Being supportive to the patient and family in helping them adjust to their illness and treatment, and encouraging helpful attitudes and coping strategies is vital in order for them to be able to make informed decisions and set realistic goals. Without this involvement, patients can experience loss of control and increased dependence on the nursing staff.

Specific concerns experienced by patients on HD often centre on:

- fluid and dietary allowances
- life restricted by dependence on a machine
- cannulation problems
- body image issues
- complications during dialysis
- fluid removal during treatment resulting in hypovolaemia or fluid overload
- machine problems/alarms
- unexplained changes in treatment
- length of time spent waiting for machines
- transport to and from dialysis units
- holidays.

Effective patient education can enhance a patient's quality of life as well as help a patient cope with living with a chronic illness like ESKD.

The dialysis unit

Staffing

With the increase of dialysis-dependent patients who are elderly with complex medical needs, maintaining adequate staffing levels has become a pressing issue facing renal units. The nurse-to-patient ratio has fallen over recent years and will vary according to the dependency of patients and local policy. The UK National Renal Workforce Planning Group (2002) recommended the following nurse patient ratios:

- 1 WTE nurse per 4.5 HD patient
- Skill mix 1.5 nurses: 1 healthcare assistant (HCA).

This workforce plan is based on patient-centred care, integrated multiprofessional working, and current best practice.

Renal nurses

Renal nurses must have the educational and clinical knowledge, skill, and expertise in renal nursing to manage renal patients in different stages of their illness and on particular RRT modalities to maintain a high standard of patient care. Nurses must have excellent communication skills, and develop their individual leadership and management abilities. Nurses play an important role in the decision-making of patient care with the multiprofessional team where decisions are made about the care and changes to patient treatment. In addition, nurses require the knowledge and skills in recognizing the physical, psychological, and psychosocial needs of haemodialysis patients and families and implement appropriate actions to enhance care delivery.

Nursing assistants

HCAs work within the nursing team in skilled roles, such as performing physiological measurements, machine preparation, stock control of unit supplies, and maintaining a safe working environment for attending patients and staff. In-house teaching programmes for nursing assistants are commonly used, and in the UK a National Vocational Qualification (2004) level 3 in renal support is available.

Technical staff

Are vital for equipment maintenance and repair, water treatment monitoring and surveillance, and assist in plumbing requirements for preparation of patients' homes for home haemodialysis.

Counsellors and social workers

Should be available to offer guidance and provide personal, emotional, and practical support for patients at all stages of their pre-dialysis and dialysis care.

Dieticians

Each dialysis unit should have access to dedicated renal dieticians to assess, provide specialist advice, and review patients' nutritional requirements. Dieticians should maintain a proactive education programme for patients.

Satellite dialysis facilities

Previously all patients commenced dialysis in a central hospital-based unit and did not move to a satellite unit until they were well established on the HD programme. Currently many patients are now transferring to satellite units following a short time in the main units or are commencing dialysis immediately in the satellite unit. This change in practice and ethos of the satellite unit requires the healthcare professionals to have excellent nursing skills and a sound knowledge base to enable staff to meet the complex medical and psychosocial needs and provide comprehensive clinical support during dialysis treatment for this patient group.

Staff working in a satellite unit are expected to be autonomous practitioners and manage the common complications that patients' experience during treatment. Nursing staff must be experienced and skilled in patient assessment and decision making, as medical staff are often not available on site. Dialysis patients are now seen and care reviewed in haemodialysis nurse-led clinics based at satellite units. A nephrologist may visit the satellite unit on a weekly basis to provide medical advice or see patients for care review. Good communication and IT links between the satellite and the main unit in hospital are essential.

Satellite dialysis units are expanding as main hospital sites become less accessible and increasingly busy. Advantages of satellite dialysis facilities include:

- less distance for patients to travel for treatment, less time travelling, and less waiting for transport
- enhances patient experience and quality of patients' lives
- better provision of patient-centred care
- more stable patient group
- opportunities for autonomous nursing practice as satellite units are often nurse-led.

Nursing education and audit

Education

Education within the dialysis unit is an important factor in the personal and professional development of staff. Patient care is more complex, with many patients experiencing many co-morbid diseases that impact on their health and well-being. Ideally in-house education/interprofessional learning forums should be available for all bands of staff. Staff should undertake university-accredited specialist renal and advanced renal courses. A designated education nurse/education team is of benefit to provide support to all levels of nursing staff.

Nursing audits

Are essential for the maintenance of high standards of clinical practice, and for professional development. Audits should have clear remits, identify a standard against which to assess practice, and have a mechanism for closing the audit cycle (i.e. improving and re-assessing practice). Targets should be underpinned by national and local standard setting—in the UK the Renal National Service Framework, Clinical Practice Guidelines by the Renal Association, and Infection Control Saving Lives Standards are useful documents upon which to base clinical audits.

Areas for audit by nursing staff may include:
• vascular access use, planning, and adequacy
• achievement of adequate biochemical indices
• management of anaemia, iron, and EPO
• calcium and phosphate control
• dialysis adequacy
• BP control
• infection control.

Possible components of nurse education programme on dialysis or CRRT
This is not an exhaustive list!
• What is RRT?
• Modalities
• Patient selection
• Risks and benefits
• Initiation and dose
• Basic principles of dialysis
• Diffusion and ultrafiltration
• Convection
• Fluid pathways
• Blood pathway
• Dialysate
• Basic equipment description
• Pumps
• Fluids
• Safety features
• Monitoring screens
• Interpreting pressures
• Vascular access
• Policy and procedures for placement and care of access
• Clearly identify nurse responsibilities
• Initiating therapy
• Anticoagulation
• Trouble shooting alarms
• Flushing filter/returning blood
• Terminating therapy/emergency disconnect
• Resuscitation policies and cardiac arrest calls
• Reviews of unit protocols
• Laboratory value interpretation.

Infection on the dialysis unit

Infection control

Within dialysis units, this is of paramount importance. Nursing staff must take adequate precautions and implement appropriate practices that will substantially reduce the risk of workplace transmission of infection to patients and staff within this high-risk environment. This is achieved through the use of universal precautions when handling blood and body fluids, and isolation of patients and machines, if required. Patients admitted or re-admitted to a unit or having first HD treatment should be tested for HBsAg and HCV (and HIV in some units), unless they have been tested in the month before admission. The machine must be isolated and only used for that named patient if the virology results are not available. Whenever possible, staff should nurse only infected or uninfected patients during a shift. Each dialysis unit must have local infection control policies.

Hepatitis B virus (HBV)

Patients positive for hepatitis B require treatment in isolation and with a designated machine. Protective clothing must be used at all times. Special care must be taken when dealing with blood spillages. Nursing staff who have not been vaccinated against hepatitis B should not work in a high risk area. A vaccination programme should be in place for patients (ideally pre-dialysis) and staff. Patients who are being treated in dialysis units should be tested for HBsAg ideally monthly, but at least every 3 months.

Hepatitis C virus (HCV)

Present in ~0.4–15% of patients (but much higher in some developing countries). Most renal units do not isolate patients, but dedicated machines are often used. Patient-to-patient spread can occur, so care must be taken to avoid and clear blood spillages, and prevent blood sprays. Proper cleaning and disinfection processes must be carried out between patients according to the manufacturer's instructions. All patients should be tested for HCV every 3 months.

HIV

HIV-positive patients are usually managed as for HCV-infected patients, not routinely isolated but dialysed with dedicated machines. HIV testing is not routinely performed in all units, except for patients on a transplant waiting list, or those wishing to dialyse in other units. The issues around HIV testing are sometimes controversial.

MRSA and vancomycin-resistant *Enterococcus* (VRE)

Patients positive for MRSA or VRE are not usually isolated within an outpatient dialysis area, although segregation of these patients often occur in ward areas. The risk of spread of MRSA is minimal in clothed outpatients; however, universal precautions, and especially strict hand washing between patients will minimize the spread of resistant organisms.

Infection control policies

The following is a general guide to infection control:

- Clean hands using correct handwashing technique before and after individual patient contact and between procedures on the same patient.
- A plastic apron must be worn when attending to patients and must be changed between each patient.
- Gloves must be worn whenever there is direct skin contact with blood, body fluids, or potentially infected surfaces in the working environment.
- A protective face shield must be worn when initiating and terminating dialysis and when removing used blood lines from the dialysis machine.
- Remove gloves and wash hands between patients.
- Items used on a treatment station should be either disposable or for single use, and reserved for a single patient.
- Clean areas should be designated and used for the preparation and handling of medications and should be separated from contaminated areas.
- Multidose medication vials should be prepared for use away from the patient.
- Use new external venous and arterial pressure transducer filters for each patient's treatment, to prevent blood contamination of the dialysis machine pressure monitor.
- Clean and disinfect dialysis stations between patients (including chair, table, bed, machine), and especially the dialysis machine control panel.
- Discard fluids carefully and clean/disinfect all containers.

Chapter 4

Home and frequent haemodialysis

Home haemodialysis

In most countries the number of patients on home dialysis declined over the last 25 years (currently 1% in the USA, 4% in Canada, 1% in France, and 5% in the UK), although it remains significant in New Zealand (17%) and Australia (10%). There has been a recurrence of interest more recently with developments in technology and the recognition of the significant benefits of both home-based and more frequent dialysis (for the individual and health economically). The UK NICE issued guidance in 2002 requiring all patients (in the UK) to be offered the option of home HD. Between 2011 and 2013 there was a 20% increase in patients on home HD in the UK. The introduction of the NxStage® machine has led a sustained increase in patients on home HD in the USA. Patients on home HD have better survival, lower morbidity, and greater quality of life, even after correcting for their lower age and lower incidence of co-morbidity.

Patients in whom home dialysis will be successful need:
- the ability and motivation to learn to carry out the process
- to be stable on dialysis
- to be free of complications and significant concomitant disease
- to have good vascular access (AVF is best)
- reliable equipment
- appropriate space and facilities in the home (water supply may need modifying to increase flow rates if not using NxStage®, electricity)
- the presence of a helper (spouse, partner, or friend) prepared to assist is ideal but not an absolute necessity.

The maintenance of independence is a very important part of the benefit of home HD, and patients feel much more in control of their disease and their dialysis. However, some home HD patients and their carers find the responsibility of carrying out the procedure and dealing with any potential problems to be very stressful and can feel isolated from hospital support staff. Home HD can also place a considerable long-term burden on carers both emotionally and financially if they are prevented from working. The presence of dialysis equipment in the house can be a constant reminder of the patient's illness.

Home dialysis programmes require dedicated nephrologists, technicians and nurses, and full 24h technical support. Suitable patients should be identified early, have good access fashioned, be trained, supported, and closely followed up. Motivation and a desire for independence are more important than intelligence. Instruction should be individualized, and is often accomplished in a dedicated training centre. It may take from 6 weeks to 3 months. Most patients perform standard 3× weekly dialysis, but daily home dialysis is an option with newer equipment, either long hours overnight (often 5 times a week) or daily short hours.

Benefits of home haemodialysis

Significant benefits have been shown using both conventional hours hae-modialysis and for extended hours (but most benefits probably accrued by the move to a home-based therapy rather than the extra hours—see ➔ Intensive haemodialysis regimens, p. 242):
- Improved quality of life, patient mood, sleep, depression
- Most independence and personal freedom
- Lower mortality and morbidity and hospital admissions
- Enhanced ability to work
- Improved sexual function
- Time for family and community engagement
- Reduced travel time/cost
- Improved nutritional state with reduced dietary and fluid restrictions
- Improved BP control
- Reduced drug burden (especially phosphate binders with extended hours)
- Home haemodialysis gives best opportunities for longer hours
- Lower cost.

Cost effectiveness of home HD

Home dialysis is cost-effective even allowing for the initial set-up costs. Estimated costs of home dialysis are £19,000 pa in the UK compared with £30,000 to £35,000 for hospital HD. Most patients perform stand-ard 3× weekly dialysis, but daily home dialysis is an option with newer equipment. Kidney Health Australia estimated that increasing the use of home dialysis over the next 10 years would lead to an estimated net savings of between A$378 and A$430 million for the Australian health system. (See Table 4.1.)

Table 4.1 Financial costs and savings when increasing home HD programmes rather than hospital or satellite HD

Additional costs	Savings
Consumables	Pay costs (mostly nursing staffing costs)
Machine leasing or purchase	Travel costs
Home conversions (power, water, etc.)	Pathology (blood, virology, etc. testing)
Training programmes for patients	Pharmacy (reduced drug prescriptions)
Reduced income to hospital organization providing HD	Holiday dialysis
	Capital costs of new builds for satellite centres or expansion of hospital units including loans and depreciation
	Environmental

Problems and barriers to home haemodialysis

Although the overall benefits of HD are considerable, the problems for individual patients should not be underestimated, especially psychosocial. These may be perceived as barriers to home HD but can usually be managed if recognized and planned for. They can, however, prevent successful adoption of home HD and may influence medical staff in conversations with patients. Ultimately anyone who can drive a car can undertake home HD; almost anyone can learn if motivated.

Potential barriers include:
- fear of cannulation
- worries about coping at home
- social isolation and feeling of abandonment
- out-of-pocket costs and increased water and electricity bills (should not be an issue in properly established home HD programmes)
- access infections or access failure (especially if using extended or more frequent hours dialysis)
- carer burn-out: this is a significant and under-recognized issue
- need for dedicated training units or staffing and staff who can train in hospital or satellite HD units
- space for supplies and dialysis equipment
- modifications to home electricity and water
- system funding: governments need to ensure appropriate funding arrangements for home HD programmes in order to incentivize renal units to invest appropriately.

Overcoming potential barriers requires education of patients and staff, especially those seeing patients with CKD pre-dialysis, local expertise, and local leadership for home HD:
- Excellent pre-dialysis education, and training and support materials
- Home visits, on-call systems
- Early care in a self-care satellite facility or enhanced self-care in a hospital HD facility
- Support groups.

Home dialysis machine technology

Until recently most home HD programmes used conventional HD equipment designed for home use, e.g. Fresenius 2008K@home™ or Gambro AK96®, however the introduction of the NxStage® technology has led to its rapid uptake in many countries for its ease of use, small footprint, and probable cost and clinical effectiveness. Sorbent systems were historically used in remote areas but are no longer available. Sorbent systems did not require a water source (just 6L of bottled or tap water), had no requirement for an RO system, filtration or water drainage, and were easily transportable. Their dialysis efficacy, however, was limited. Conventional HD machines require permanent plumbing, waste connections, RO systems and filters, and space for storage of consumables, dialysers, etc. Machines often have a slightly smaller footprint than those used in centre, can allow remote monitoring, and advanced alarms such as wetness monitoring for patients undertaking overnight dialysis.

The NxStage® machine is a compact single-pass system and consists of a cycler which controls the administration and monitoring of the treatment (flow, times, UF rate, etc.) and a single-use disposable drop-in cartridge containing both fluid and blood circuits and dialyser. Blood flow rates are high but dialysate low in contrast to conventional HD. Dialysate is provided either in sterile bags or generated in a batch using a dedicated system (NxStage® PureFlow™). Ultrapure batches (usually 60L, for 2–3 dialysis sessions) are produced from concentrates and tap water, generally containing lactate 45mmol/L (not bicarbonate), potassium 1mmol/L, sodium 140mmol/L, calcium 1.5mmol/L. It has a very small footprint (38 × 38 × 46cm; 34kg) and once the dialysate is made the machine can be disconnected from the water supply. PureFlow™ houses 60L of dialysate and requires a little more space (60 × 74 × 80cm). Patients would generally only use bags when travelling or away from their main home. The machine itself is portable, requires minimal plumbing, is easy and rapid to set up given the cassette-based system containing all lines and filters, does not require RO and has a reduced carbon footprint. There is a reduced requirement for anticoagulation. The cost of the PureFlow™ system for on-line dialysate generation is significant but overall costs per treatment probably comparable to conventional home HD systems.

Other new machines are in development for home dialysis therapies.

Intensive haemodialysis regimens

Daily HD (sometimes called quotidian) and/or nocturnal dialysis have been introduced because of the potential benefits of longer dialysis in addition to the benefits of home treatment. There are a number of options for more intensive or frequent dialysis:

- daily overnight (nocturnal; 8–10h 6 or 7 times per week): long frequent dialysis
- daily 4h
- daily short hours (usually 2–3h).

All are best achieved in a home dialysis setting, but can be delivered in-centre. New technologies such as the NxStage® system may allow cost-effective increased frequency of dialysis.

Duration of dialysis may be an important predictor of survival independent of dialysis dose, although similar benefits can accrue with shorter hour dialysis when done daily, e.g. 2h 6–7 times per week. The benefits are similar to those seen with long hours hospital HD (e.g. 8h 3×/week) as practised in Tassin, France, with lower morbidity and mortality, normal BPs, less restricted diet, lower phosphate, and lower β_2m. There is a theoretical concern about the loss of essential solutes, catabolism, and immune stimulation with daily HD.

Daily dialysis is cost-effective, costing only ~US$25,000 pa in the USA (cost savings because of reduced morbidity, hospital admissions, fewer drugs, etc.). Problems include time for machine set-up daily, travel time and costs if not done at home, and risks from increased access manipulations. (See Table 4.2.)

Table 4.2 Various home HD regimens

	Frequency (sessions/ week)	Duration (hours)	Dialysate flow (mL/min)	Blood flow (mL/min)	sKt/V urea weekly
Conventional HD	3	4	500–800	250–450	2.5
Short daily HD	5+	2.5–3	500–800	400	3.75
Long hours HD	3–4	>5.5	300–500	250–400	3.75
Long frequent HD	5+	>5.5	300–500	200–300	5.8
NxStage®	5+	2.5–3.5	400	150–200	–

Daily overnight dialysis

Patients can be monitored remotely. In small studies, patients report significantly improved quality of life, symptoms, and sleep patterns, have a daily Kt/V of 1.0, better BP control, less need for antihypertensive medication, lower serum phosphate (and often need phosphate supplementation), improved nutritional state, increased serum albumin, and can have relaxed dietary restrictions. Cardiac morphology improves, EPO requirements are reduced, higher Hb, improved mental functioning and sexual activity, improved endocrine function, bone disease, access functioning and overall patient survival. Calcium depletion can occur. These results have not all be borne out in randomized trials or larger cohorts. Patients also have fewer intradialytic complications including hypotension, cramps, and fatigue. Smaller needles and often single needles, and slower blood flow rates (150mL/min) can be used. Extra monitors may be required or alterations in connectors to reduce the risk from disconnection during sleep.

Small cohort studies have shown that patients dialysing in centre for 7–8h 3× per week can accrue similar advantages but this is not commonly available.

Short daily dialysis

Session lengths vary from 1.5 to 3h 6 times per week, and may offer similar advantages to nocturnal dialysis (but not proven yet and see ➔ Frequent dialysis outcomes, p. 244). Blood and dialysate flows are the same as in conventional HD when using conventional equipment. Phosphate control is not markedly improved in short dialysis (unless total dialysis time is increased) since patients gain an increase in appetite which offsets the small increase in phosphate clearance.

New technologies such as the NxStage® dialysis system might offer major advantages. This provides a very small footprint machine, single-use cartridges containing the filter and tubing hence easy set-up, and lactate-based dialysate either generated from a second module or provided in pre-filled bags (for travel), low dialysate flow rates and volumes (generally between 10 and 25L).

Frequent dialysis outcomes

It is often claimed all regimens increasing dialysis frequency (i.e. long frequent and short daily) improve outcomes with fewer hospitalizations, less medication, fewer symptoms between and during dialysis, less restless leg syndrome, less tiredness, better toleration of dialysis, better BP, anaemia and phosphate control, better appetite, nutrition, sleep, sexual function, and energy. However it is critical to separate the effects of home therapy itself from the effect of increasing dialysis frequency, since many studies have shown that patients on home HD 3×/week conventionally also have significantly improved outcomes compared to patients dialysing in centre. Furthermore the benefits of prolonged duration and frequency may not be the same as short daily dialysis. Two major trials have reported the effects of increasing dialysis frequency (from the Frequent Hemodialysis Network (FHN))[1,2] and a large number of studies based on these two trials reported during 2011–2014. Both trials were affected by difficulties in recruitment and an atypical population of patients.

- Australian cohort data show no mortality benefit of frequent or extended home dialysis over conventional home dialysis, but significant benefits over conventional in-centre HD.
- US cohort studies have sometimes shown mortality benefits of daily home HD versus conventional 3× weekly in-centre HD, but not consistently, and a large multinational cohort of 318 patients showed increased mortality.
- Cohort studies have shown both frequent and extended dialysis reduce left ventricular mass index (LVMI).
- The FHN in-centre daily study[1] showed NO difference in patient survival but LVMI and a composite physical health score did improve in patients on daily HD, and predialysis phosphate and BP were much lower.
- The FHN nocturnal dialysis study[2] could only recruit 87 patients, and showed NO benefit on mortality, LVMI or a physical health score, and only beneficial effects on phosphate and BP.
- Nocturnal home dialysis (but not daily short hours HD) led to much more rapid loss of residual renal function than conventional HD, which might be detrimental.
- Neither FHN trial showed benefits on cognitive function, depression or on hospitalization rates.
- Both trials showed increased adverse access events (thrombosis, access interventions needed).
- Patients in all studies report high levels of perceived caregiver burdens.

Complications from more frequent dialysis

- Hypophosphataemia even with relaxed diet may need phosphate replenishment.
- Access thrombosis, stenosis, aneurysms.
- Risk of catastrophic events (blood line disconnection) rare but increased.
- Extra cost for water, power, dialysate, and disposables.
- Depression, anxiety, and burden on caregivers.

Increasing dialysis frequency conclusions

Dialysing at home offers substantial benefits on a variety of outcome measures and is cost-effective.

Increasing the frequency of dialysis either by long hours nocturnal dialysis or short daily dialysis has not been proven to offer additional widespread benefits, will not increase life expectancy, will significantly improve phosphate control and BP, but may cause accelerated loss of residual renal function and access failure. Effects on longer-term outcomes such as amyloid, neuropathy, etc. not yet demonstrated: modalities with increased convective clearance may achieve this.

References

1. Chertow GM et al. In-center hemodialysis six times per week versus three times per week. N Engl J Med 2010; 363: 2287–300.
2. Rocco M et al. The effects of frequent nocturnal home hemodialysis: the FHN nocturnal trial. Kidney Int 2011; 80: 108092.

Monitoring home haemodialysis patients

Dialysis at home must be as safe as in hospital. Attention to emergency procedures and appropriate training is paramount. Patients need support for initial set-up (including all technical aspects related to water, electricity etc.) and ongoing delivery of consumables and supplies (usually done monthly). Patients need a proper assessment to ensure they will be safe and competent to dialyse at home, and administer medications such as iron and EPO. Home visits will be needed, more in the first year, and this needs a clear system with expert home haemodialysis nurses and supporting physicians, dieticians, and social workers. Much support can be provided by telephone, email, virtual clinics, etc. as well as direct face-to-face visiting. A 24h on-call facility must be available, which might be based around an inpatient dialysis provider or renal unit/ward. Support groups can provide key support and friendship from expert patients. Patients need clear plans for disaster management (e.g. power failure, flooding, etc.). Units should monitor drop-out rates, dialysis adequacy, and infection rates as in hospital based dialysis.

Routine monitoring is much the same as for all HD patients with identical monthly blood testing, and monitoring of BP, dry weight, and access at each dialysis session. Monitoring during extended hours (especially overnight) dialysis requires extra consideration of security of access needles, monitoring for line disconnection, and possibly remote monitoring of machine alarms.

Environmental issues

HD has significant environmental impacts, some of which may be increased in home settings depending on the technology used. Environmental foot-print caused by:

- high power usage (~1000 kilowatt hours (kWh) per year per patient): in Australia a solar power solution for dialysis may be income generating
- high water usage and wastage (producing 120L of dialysate requires ~400L of main water, 'reject' water often lost to drain); high energy costs of producing RO water. 5–6 home based HD sessions may 'waste' > 2000L water per week. NxStage® equipment uses significantly less water, less power, and produces less waste water
- high carbon costs (~7 tonnes CO_2 equivalent per year) from lighting, heating, staff and patient travel, paper and printers etc. Likely to be lower in home HD mostly from reduced travel for both patients and staff
- waste disposal (packaging) requiring incineration or landfill
- patient costs: depending on reimbursement for electricity and water.

Nursing patients on home haemodialysis

Most home HD patients are either referred by the pre-dialysis team, consultant nephrologists, managers of dialysis units, or referrals of failed transplant patients who need to resume dialysis. Ideally of course this should be done pre-dialysis. Most dialysis centres should have a 'Home Therapy Clinic' for the patients to be seen by a team to consider all home therapies (home HD, peritoneal dialysis).

Key considerations:

• Patient interest to undertake treatment at home.
• Patient's ability to learn to carry out procedure independently or must have a carer committed to help with the HD treatment.
• Excellent HD access and able to maintain a stable condition whilst on treatment.
• Free from other illness or diseases that could affect their ability to carry out safe treatment at home.
• Suitable home environment with adequate space to accommodate the kidney machine and treatment equipment.

A designated home dialysis nurse has an initial consultation with the patient to provide information on the different home therapy options and what home dialysis involves. Once the patient is identified as suitable for home HD, training commences in the main or satellite unit where the patient dialyses, or less commonly in a dedicated training centre. A named nurse provides the patient training at each dialysis session covering all aspects of haemodialysis. Other key team members include the nephrologist, dietician, social worker, and usually a home care partner who should train with the patient so they can assist them.

Complications of home haemodialysis

Serious adverse events are very uncommon in home HD programmes. One study from Canada of the experience of 190 patients over more than 10 years and 500 patient-years of treatments reported 1 death and 6 serious adverse events, giving a crude rate of 0.06 events per 1000 dialysis treatments. 6 of the 7 events involved significant blood loss almost all from patient error in setting up the equipment. 1 was an air embolism from failure to clamp a CVC.

Education and training of patient must include recognition of possible complications, without frightening patients! Most patients undertaking home HD do it safely for many years without any problems, but training is key.

Machine complications

- Clotting of circuit
- Air entry into extracorporeal circuit
- Temperature and conductivity alarms
- Loss of water or electrical power during the dialysis session
- High/low venous pressure
- Low arterial pressure
- Blood leak especially from needle or line disconnections.

Patient complications

- Hypotension
- Cramps
- Nausea and vomiting
- Headache and fever
- Chest pain
- Problems with fistula/graft or vascular catheter during dialysis.

Education and training for home haemodialysis

Education and training of patient will include:

Haemodialysis machine

- Identification of all functional parts of the machine
- Water and electricity connection
- Assemble the necessary supplies and prepare equipment for use
- Function check of machine to confirm its safety
- Lining and priming of machine safely and independently
- Ensure correct use of dialysate solution
- Conduct alarm tests to ensure safety
- Disinfection of machine
- Trouble shooting of machine alarms.

Haemodialysis prescription

- Understand concept of dry weight
- Perform and record vital signs (temperature, BP, weight)
- Calculation of intradialytic weight gain for fluid removal
- Accurate programming of time, total fluid loss, dialysate flow, heparin prescription, and dialysate concentration on machine.

Care and management of vascular access

Vascular catheter

- Clean and perform dressing of vascular catheter using strict aseptic technique
- Able to recognize signs and symptoms of line infection
- Recognizes further complications such as poor flows, displacement, cracks or holes, and take appropriate action.

Arteriovenous fistula or graft

- Preparation and cannulation of AVF/AVG
- Able to obtain blood sample from AVF/AVG
- Able to recognize complications associated with AVF/AVG and take appropriate action
- Understanding of looking after AVF/AVG.

Haemodialysis treatment

- Safely initiate and discontinue treatment adhering to strict asepsis.
- Perform and record intradialytic monitoring of observations.
- Demonstrate awareness of actions to any unexpected outcomes.
- Able to maintain record of observations and dialysis parameters.

Summary of home HD training programme for patients:
- How to monitor and care for your access
- How to take your blood pressure and record it
- Set up a place in your home to do your treatments
- Set your fluid removal goal, based on your weight and BP
- Set up the dialysis machine and test all of the alarms
- Insert and tape down the needles or attach lines
- Monitor the treatment and keep good treatment records
- Clean the filter on the water treatment system
- Take water samples to test the safety of your water
- Order enough supplies of each type to last you a month
- Recognize problems to report to your home dialysis team
- What to do in case you have a problem with your machine
- Safely dispose of medical wastes.

The training programme is tailored to suit individual patient's needs. Duration of training is variable but normally takes 3–6 months. Once a patient has successfully completed training and been assessed as competent in carrying out treatment independently they can start home HD.

The first few HD sessions at home are overseen by the home dialysis nurse from start to finish to support the patient/family/carer.

Education resources should be available including leaflets, contact numbers, audio-visual guides, and patient information websites. Regular communication through visits and phone calls are made so patients continue to feel supported at home.

Other general education
- Teach patient about their disease and its treatment.
- Teach patient how to administer injections of EPO, iron, and LMWH.
- Importance of fluid and dietary prescriptions/advice.
- Importance of adhering to medication regimen.
- Importance of adhering to treatment regimen.
- Lifestyle changes.
- Employment and income loss support.
- Provide information on what actions to take when unwell and to report to home HD nurse/local renal unit or hospital.

A multidisciplinary approach is necessary for the successful management of a patient on home HD. Care and education must be patient centred to support patient independence and to help patients take an active role in their own care which will impact on their overall health and well-being to maintain a better quality of life.

Peritoneal dialysis

Principles of peritoneal dialysis

In PD, solute and fluid exchange occur between peritoneal capillary blood and dialysis solution in the peritoneal cavity. The 'membrane' lining this cavity consists of a vascular wall, interstitium, mesothelium, and adjacent fluid films. Only about one-third of visceral peritoneum is in contact with dialysis fluid, and it is therefore the parietal peritoneum that is primarily involved in peritoneal transport.

Three-pore model of solute transport

Evidence suggests that there are 3 sizes of pores in the capillary wall:
- Small pores (average radius 40–50Å) for transport of small molecular weight solutes
- Large pores (average radius >150Å) for transport of large molecules such as albumin
- Ultrasmall pores (3–5Å), or aquaporin-1, are permeable only to water and are the major water channels.

Small molecular weight solute transfer

Occurs by diffusion down a concentration gradient or by convection.

Diffusion

- Solute transport occurs down a concentration gradient, e.g. phosphate ions diffuse from a high concentration in plasma to dialysate which has no phosphate.
- Occurs through small pores described above.
- Small solutes diffuse at a faster rate than larger ones.
- Rate of transport depends on concentration gradient, peritoneal surface area, and number of small pores, i.e. membrane permeability.
- Rate of transport will be fastest at the beginning of a fluid exchange when the concentration gradient is the greatest. With increasing dwell time, equilibration will occur between dialysate and plasma, thereby reducing the concentration gradient and therefore the rate of solute transport. The speed at which this occurs will depend on the rate of transport.
- Concentration gradient can also be from dialysate to plasma, e.g. lactate in dialysate diffuses across the peritoneal membrane from dialysate into plasma.

Convection

- Also known as solute drag.
- Occurs with UF (i.e. water transport down an osmotic gradient).
- Amount of solute transported by this means depends on the sieving coefficient (ratio of solute concentration in ultrafiltrate compared with plasma).
- Large molecules, e.g. albumin, predominantly cross the peritoneal membrane by convection and utilize the large pores.

Fluid movement

- Net fluid movement, or UF, is determined by the difference between fluid transferred into the peritoneal cavity by UF and the uptake of fluid out of the peritoneum through peritoneal lymphatics.
- Water transport occurs across both small and ultrasmall pores.
- Ultrasmall pores—or aquaporin-1—account for ~40% total water transport.
- UF rate is governed by Starling's law and is therefore determined by net difference of osmotic and hydraulic pressures:
  - Osmotic pressure is determined by osmotic agent used in dialysate—usually glucose but alternative agents, e.g. amino acids, are used, and more are being developed.
  - Hydraulic pressure is determined by the intraperitoneal pressure which depends on the exchange volume and posture; it is higher when standing upright compared with lying flat.

Factors affecting efficiency of peritoneal dialysis

Efficiency of PD, as with HD, depends on the total time on dialysis and the dwell time of each exchange, blood flow, surface area and permeability of the peritoneal membrane, dialysate flow, and UF rates.

Time on dialysis

Dialysis does not happen when the abdomen is empty of fluid. Thus PD regimens which include dry periods are not so efficient, but can be used if the patient has significant residual renal function

Dwell time

The amount of solute and fluid transported across the peritoneal membrane depends on the dwell time of each exchange. See ➔ Effect of dwell time on solute and fluid transfer, p. 259.

Blood flow

Occurs through peritoneal capillaries and is therefore not as controllable as in HD. Adequacy of PD is reduced when blood flow is reduced in low cardiac output states (hypotension, heart failure). Blood flow through peritoneal capillaries can be increased by vasodilators. In experimental animals, IV or intraperitoneal (IP) vasodilators increase PD clearances. Their use in patients is limited by hypotension.

Peritoneal surface area

This is similar to the surface area of the skin: $1.7–2.0m^2$ in an adult. The thickness is highly variable. Effective surface for dialysis also depends on the blood supply. In low cardiac output states, less membrane is perfused, reducing dialysis efficiency.

Membrane permeability

Membrane permeability, or effective pore size and numbers, depends on ultrastructural differences in the various components (particularly capillaries and mesothelium) and changes over time. Introducing dialysis fluid into the peritoneal cavity has profound ultrastructural effects, including development of mesothelial intracellular oedema, destruction of organelles, interstitial oedema, diminished numbers of microvilli, and submesothelial deposition of collagen fibres. After an episode of peritonitis, further dramatic changes occur. The mesothelium becomes devoid of microvilli, and in severe episodes there may be accompanying layers of surface fibrin. There is partial recovery after a single episode, but repeated episodes of peritonitis result in irreversible damage to the membrane with changes in permeability characteristics.

Effect of dwell time on solute and fluid transfer

Differing amounts of solute and fluid are transferred with different dwell times of dialysate. This is summarized in the table. For simplicity, only two examples of membrane permeability (low and high permeability) are given, although four grades of permeability are defined by the peritoneal equilibration test (PET). It can be seen that for patients with high membrane permeability, PD is more efficient using rapid exchanges with short dwell times, and for patients with low membrane permeability, long dwell times. (See Table 5.1.)

Table 5.1 Dwell time

Dwell time	Low permeability membrane	High permeability membrane
Short (1–2h)	Solute+	Solute++
	Water+	Water+++
Medium (4–6h)	Solute++	Solute+++
	Water+++	Water+
Long (10–12h)	Solute+++	Solute++++
	Water++	Water+/–

Modes of peritoneal dialysis

Different methods of delivering PD have evolved both for the social convenience of the patient and to maximize the efficiency of PD in terms of both solute (clearance) and fluid (UF) transfer.

Intermittent peritoneal dialysis (IPD)

This was the original form of PD developed mainly for the treatment of AKI at a time when HD was not readily available. Dialysis most commonly takes place for 24h twice a week using rapid exchanges each of 1–2h duration. The exchanges are usually done via an automatic cycling machine, but can be done manually.

A regimen commonly used is 20L of dialysate over 20h with 2L exchanges of 2h duration (10min for running in, 90min dwell time, and 20min for draining). This regimen maximizes UF by using short exchanges, but solute transfer is rarely sufficient for long-term management. IPD is therefore mostly restricted as a temporary form of dialysis (AKI, waiting for training for PD, as part of the management of fluid leaks, after abdominal surgery).

Continuous ambulatory peritoneal dialysis (CAPD)

This consists of 3–5 exchanges over 24h (see Fig 5.1).

CAPD was first introduced in the 1980s when it was shown theoretically that four 2L exchanges over 24h, with 2L of UF, would enable a patient to maintain a steady blood urea level of ~30mmol/L. Although small MW solutes, such as urea, equilibrate rapidly between plasma and dialysate during the long dwell times of CAPD, larger MW substances, such as creatinine or middle molecules, are dialysed continuously, as the concentration gradient between blood and dialysate is maintained throughout the dwell time. PD removes large MW substances more efficiently than HD.

Automated peritoneal dialysis (APD)

Uses an automatic cycling device to perform rapid exchanges overnight. There are different modes of APD depending on whether fluid is left in the peritoneum or an extra manual exchange is performed during the day (see Fig 5.2).
* *Night-time IPD (NIPD)* consists of rapid exchanges overnight with a 'dry' peritoneum during the day.
* *Continuous cycling PD (CCPD)* consists of rapid exchanges overnight with one fluid exchange during the day (at various times).

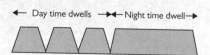

Fig. 5.1 Graphical representation of a typical CAPD regimen.

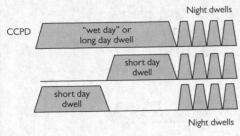

Fig. 5.2 Examples of different APD regimens using rapid overnight exchanges and a single daytime exchange (CCPD).

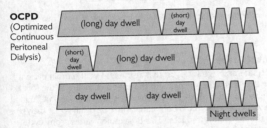

Fig. 5.3 Examples of OCPD regimens.

Optimized continuous peritoneal dialysis

This is used when maximal solute transfer is needed, e.g. once the patient has become anuric. Optimized continuous PD (OCPD) consists of rapid exchanges overnight, a long day dwell, and an extra exchange that is usually done manually at a time of day convenient for the patient. (See Fig 5.3.)

Tidal peritoneal dialysis

This is a form of APD where only a percentage (usually 50–85%) of the total volume of dialysate run into the peritoneum is exchanged at each cycle. The patient is attached to the cycling machine for the usual time overnight, but there are more frequent, incompletely exchanging, cycles than with other forms of APD. Tidal PD is particularly useful for patients who complain of pain during inflow. There is no evidence that this technique increases clearance. (See Fig 5.4.)

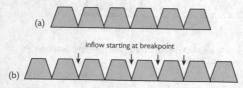

Fig. 5.4 Night-time incomplete exchanges on tidal PD.

Fig. 5.5 Breakpoint therapy. (a) Normal APD. (b) Breakpoint—achieves two more cycles.

Breakpoint therapy

Speed of dialysate drainage varies so that at the end of the drain cycle it is much slower than at the beginning, with the speed changing at the 'breakpoint'. The initial speed is ~200–300mL/min dropping to 30–60mL/min at the end. Dialysis efficiency would be greater if the next inflow of dialysate starts when the drain flow reduces. The breakpoint varies from cycle to cycle so that using a fixed tidal regimen may not be as 'efficient' as using a machine that detects the breakpoint. (See Fig 5.5.)

CAPD technique and systems

Dialysate is run into the peritoneum via an in-dwelling silastic catheter, where it dwells for a variable length of time before being drained out and fresh fluid run in. When CAPD was first developed in the USA, sterile fluid was only available in glass bottles. As patients could not walk round with glass bottles attached to them all the time, multiple connections and disconnections had to be made, resulting in an unacceptably high rate of peritonitis. CAPD as we know it today was initially developed in Canada where plastic bags were available for sterile fluid.

The historic systems

This system consisted of a bag of dialysate (1.5–3.0L for adults) connected to a line attached to the peritoneal catheter.
- Dialysate was run into the peritoneum.
- The plastic bag was rolled up and hidden under the patient's clothes.
- At the end of the dwell time the bag was unrolled and placed on the floor for the dialysate to drain out under gravity.
- The line was disconnected and a fresh bag of dialysate was attached.

The connection between the bag and line was therefore broken 3–5 times a day (depending on the number of exchanges performed). The usual connection was a spike or Luer lock device. Although patients are trained to do each bag change using a no-touch sterile technique, there was still a high peritonitis rate of about one episode per 9 patient-months. Various devices were produced to decrease bacterial contamination during the connection process, using ultraviolet light, heat sterilization, or bacterial filters, but none was particularly effective in reducing the peritonitis rate. (The use of ultraviolet sterilization can be useful as an aid for poorly sighted individuals.)

The Y-system or disconnect system

This has reduced peritonitis rates and also increased the acceptability of CAPD to patients, as they no longer have a plastic bag attached to themselves all day. The bag containing the dialysate comes already attached to a Y-shaped giving set and a sterilized empty bag attached to the other arm of the 'Y'.
- The patient connects the short arm of the Y-tubing to his/her catheter.
- A small amount of fluid from the new bag is drained directly into the empty bag—'flush before fill'.
- In principle, any bacteria at the end of the catheter are flushed away, and not into the patient.
- The patient drains out the old dialysate from the peritoneum into the empty bag.
- When completed (~20min), the line to the drainage bag is clamped and the new fluid is run into the peritoneum.
- At the end of the exchange, the patient disconnects the tubing and places a sterile cap at the end of the catheter.

Different manufacturers of PD equipment use slight variations of the disconnect system. The peritonitis rates are similar (1 in 24–30 patient-months), and are uniformly better than with the standard system (1 in 9–12 patient-months). (See Fig 5.6.)

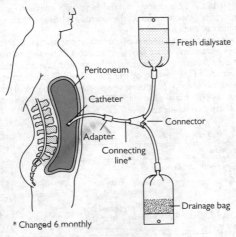

* Changed 6 monthly

Fig. 5.6 Disconnect PD system.

Peritoneal dialysis catheters

Several types of catheters are available. Most are made of silastic rubber with two Dacron® cuffs, which are placed at either end of a subcutaneous tunnel. The tunnel increases the distance that bacteria have to migrate from the skin into the peritoneum. The Dacron® cuffs physically anchor the catheter so it can't be dislodged, and block the migration of bacteria along the tunnel. Double-cuffed catheters have a lower infection rate than single-cuffed catheters.

Exit site infection remains one of the major complications of catheters. Newer designs aim to reduce this, e.g. the Scott–Moncrieff catheter, which is buried subcutaneously at time of insertion with the end released and brought out on to the surface of the skin when PD needs to start. New materials such as silver-impregnated silastic may inhibit bacterial growth, but are not yet widely available. Recent RCTs have not confirmed the benefit of either of these developments. (See Table 5.2.)

Table 5.2 Peritoneal dialysis catheters

Type of catheter	Advantages	Disadvantages
Straight Tenckhoff catheter		
100mm section containing 1mm side-holes	Simplest catheter to insert	Relatively high risk of catheter migration
Straight subcutaneous portion between peritoneal entry and skin exit	Can be inserted by variety of techniques	
Coiled Tenckhoff catheter		
Coiled 200mm section containing 1mm side-holes	Slightly reduced risk of catheter migration	Migration of coiled end can cause abdominal pain
Straight subcutaneous portion between peritoneal entry and skin exit	Can be inserted by variety of techniques	Insertion is more complicated
Swan-necked catheter		
150° bend in subcutaneous portion between peritoneal entry and skin exit	Incidence of exit site infections may be reduced	Can only be inserted surgically
		Less commonly available so can only be inserted by specialized personnel
Scott-Moncrief or buried catheter		
Same as Tenckhoff or swan-neck catheter but subcutaneous portion buried until PD needs to commence when catheter is exteriorised with simple skin incision	Inserted electively before dialysis is needed. Starting PD therefore not dependent on access to surgical lists and no wait needed for exit site healing	Requires general anaesthetic for insertion. Rarely catheter is blocked when exteriorised

Insertion of peritoneal dialysis catheters

PD catheters can be inserted percutaneously using a Seldinger technique (with or without a laparoscope or peritoneoscope) or surgically. (See Table 5.3.)

Table 5.3 Insertion of peritoneal dialysis catheters

Insertion technique	Advantages	Disadvantages
Percutaneous Seldinger technique	Performed under local anaesthetic Minimizes hospital stay Operating theatre not required Can be performed by physician. Incision sites small allowing early use of catheter	'Blind' technique so no control of catheter position Not suitable in presence of intra-abdominal adhesions. Not suitable for more complex catheters, e.g. Swan-necked
Laparoscopic	Catheter tip can be positioned. Incision sites small allowing early use of catheter Suitable for all types of catheter Catheter tip can be sutured into pelvis Omentectomy can be performed if needed	Equipment expensive Specialized personnel required
Surgical	Catheter tip can be positioned Suitable for all types of catheter Essential in presence of adhesions. Old PD catheter can be removed at same time	Requires surgical and theatre time General anaesthetic needed Larger incisions so ↑risk of incisional hernia or fluid leak if catheter used early

Pre-operative preparation for peritoneal catheter insertion

This is identical for all modes of catheter insertion:

- Ensure that patient requires the catheter, will be able to undertake PD, and that he/she understands the principles of catheter care.
- Obtain consent for the procedure.
- Patient should bath using an antiseptic soap, e.g. chlorhexidine scrub.
- Discuss with patient where he/she would like the exit site placed (usually in iliac fossa below insertion site). Avoid belt-line of trousers. Should be easily accessible for the patient to care for the exit site. The exit site should not be under an abdominal overhang in obese patients.
- Mark exit site with indelible ink with patient sitting.
- Powerful aperient, e.g. Picolax®, should be taken the night before catheter insertion to decrease risk of bowel perforation and eases placing of catheter IP.
- Give prophylactic antibiotics ~1h before catheter insertion (see Table 5.4). There is evidence for use of:
  - vancomycin
  - cephalosporins—these avoid risk of vancomycin resistance but should not be used in units with high prevalence of *Clostridium difficile*.
- The patient must empty their bladder immediately before catheter insertion (to avoid accidental bladder perforation). Palpate abdomen carefully before insertion to ensure no palpable bladder, loaded colon, or other abdominal masses
- If general anaesthetic is to be used, patient should be starved and an ECG and CXR performed.

Table 5.4 Reduction of peritonitis risk using prophylactic antibiotics

Peritonitis within 14 days of catheter insertion	Noprophylaxis	Vancomycin 1g	Cefazolin 1g
Risk of peritonitis (%)	12	1	7

Peritoneal dialysis catheter insertion technique

Percutaneous Seldinger insertion technique

This technique is simple to learn and can be done easily by physicians. This obviates the need for theatre time and general anaesthetic. Although the procedure can be carried out by the bedside in the ward, it is sensible to move the patient to a 'clean' room. The nurse assisting should have experience with PD. Full facilities for managing sedated patients should be available including suction, oxygen, BP, SaO_2, and, ideally, end-tidal CO_2 monitoring, and resuscitation equipment close to hand.

- Pre-operative patient management as above.
- Ensure the sheets on the bed are clean.
- The patient should be lying flat with one pillow.
- Tell the patient what will happen at each stage of the procedure.
- Give IV sedation *slowly*, e.g. metoclopramide 10mg, fentanyl 25–100mcg, and midazolam or diazepam (depending on patient response).
- Scrub up and lay out catheter insertion set on trolley.
- Anaesthetize area 2–3cm below umbilicus (usually with lidocaine) injecting down towards peritoneum.
- Make 2–3cm vertical incision in midline and dissect bluntly down to the linea alba).
- Insert 16–18-gauge introducing needle—it is safest to use a needle with a plastic outer sheath, which can be advanced over the sharp inner needle; if in the peritoneum, the plastic sheath should be advanced very easily. The inner needle is then removed. This technique minimizes risk of bowel perforation.
- Attach sterile giving set to the hub on the plastic sheath and run in ~500mL warm saline: this also minimizes risk of bowel perforation.
- Advance guidewire through the introducing sheath. The wire should feed in very easily. *If there is any resistance to inserting the guidewire, the procedure should be abandoned.* The most common cause for this is a loop of bowel loaded with faeces, or the existence of adhesions.
- Remove outer sheath over the wire.
- Use rigid dilator over guidewire to make a track for the catheter.
- Insert a larger dilator with a 'peel-away' sheath over the guidewire trying to angle it down into the pelvis. Remove the guidewire and dilator together leaving the large sheath.
- Insert the catheter through the sheath, which is then peeled off.
- Make sure that the first Dacron® cuff is buried deep in the skin incision site.
- Make the exit site (the spot should be marked). It should be at least 3cm from the site where the distal cuff will be in the subcutaneous tunnel to avoid subsequent extrusion of the cuff through the exit site.

- As small an incision as possible should be used to make the exit site to avoid fluid leakage and the need for sutures.
- Attach a tunnelling device to the catheter to create the subcutaneous tunnel and bring out the catheter.
- Attach a connector to the catheter, and then a short line to the connection device to enable dialysate bags to be attached. These actual devices will vary depending on the manufacture of the dialysate bags.
- Suture the original insertion site. Sutures are not needed and should be avoided at the exit site as they increase the risk of early exit site infection.

Laparoscopic peritoneal dialysis catheter insertion

- A specially designed peritoneoscope or standard laparoscope can be used.
- The peritoneoscope is a small optical instrument (2.2mm diameter) used to choose the optimal location within the peritoneum, while the catheter is being inserted percutaneously.
- Peritoneoscopic insertion can be performed under local anaesthetic, can therefore be done by a physician, and does not require operating theatre time.
- Laparoscopic techniques are also used for catheter insertion, using standard 5–10mm diameter trocars. There is excellent visualization of the peritoneum, allowing the catheter to be sutured into the pelvis, division of adhesions, and omentectomy as required.
- Incisions using both techniques are small, thereby reducing post-operative pain and minimizing the risk of fluid leaks, allowing early use of the PD catheter.

See Table 5.5 for complications.

Table 5.5 Complications of peritoneal dialysis catheter insertion

Complication	Diagnosis	How to avoid	Management
Bladder perforation	Urine drains from catheter	Ensure that bladder is empty prior to catheter insertion	Re-site PD catheter Catheterize bladder for several days
Bowel perforation	Solid particles in PD effluent	Bowel evacuation prior to catheter insertion	Laparotomy to identify and repair perforation. It is often possible to leave the PD catheter *in situ* Appropriate antibiotics
	Abdominal pain with multiple Gram −ve organisms in PD fluid	Run in 500–1000mL fluid prior to catheter insertion if using 'blind' technique	
		Avoid 'blind' percutaneous technique if high risk of adhesions. Do not persist with percutaneous technique if there is resistance to advancing guidewire	
Intraperitoneal bleed	Blood in PD effluent	Same as above	Conservative management if haemodynamically stable
	Change in patient's haemodynamic status depending on amount of blood loss	'Blind' percutaneous technique should not be used in patients known to have bleeding disorder	Heparanize catheter to avoid its clotting
			If patient unstable, laparotomy
Fluid leak	Fluid draining from exit site	Make all incisions as small as possible	Drain out PD fluid
		Limit volume of PD exchanges if using catheter early	Avoid any further PD until exit site healed
Exit site infection	Red exit site with or without pus	Prophylactic antibiotics	Appropriate antibiotics

Malfunctioning catheters

A well-functioning PD catheter will enable the dialysate exchange (usually 1.5–2L) to be run in over 5–10min and drained out over 15–20min under the force of gravity alone. Disadvantages of a slower dialysate flow rate are:

- inconvenience for patient—CAPD exchanges take too long or the APD machine will alarm (interrupting sleep)
- decreased efficiency of PD as exchange dwell time will be decreased.

Poorly functioning catheters

Usually present with poor drainage (outflow failure), though there can be problems with inflow. If the patient continues to perform their exchanges without full drainage of fluid, abdominal distension, fluid leaks, and hernias secondary to increased intra-abdominal pressure can occur.

Early non-functioning

Occurs from the time of catheter insertion until the patient has completed their training and is established on PD. About 30–50% of new catheters will have some problem with drainage and ~10% will need replacing for complete non-function. Rarely, PD catheters may fail to function at all in an individual even after several attempts.

Late non-functioning

Can also occur in patients on maintenance PD, but this is much less common. The most common causes are shown in Table 5.6.

Table 5.6 Malfunctioning catheters

Cause	Mechanisms	Early or late	Inflow or drainage problems
Constipation	Stagnant loops of bowel loaded with faeces preventing free flow of fluid Catheter adheres to bowel wall	Both	Predominantly drainage, but on occasion poor inflow
Intra-abdominal adhesions from previous surgery	Loculated areas of IP fluid Catheter tip trapped so only small volume of fluid can be infused	Early	Both
Intra-abdominal adhesions from peritonitis	Loculated areas of IP fluid Catheter tip trapped so only small volume of fluid can be infused	Late	Both
Catheter migration up to diaphragm	Catheter tip no longer in pelvis where fluid pools (by gravity); can be caused or complicated by constipation	Both	Drainage
Catheter kinking	More commonly in catheters stitched into the peritoneum	Both	Both (more commonly drainage)
Blood in peritoneum	Blood clot blocks catheter	Early	Both
Fibrin formation	Catheter blocked by fibrin	Late	Both
Peritonitis	Catheter blocked by pus	Late	Both
Hernias (if large)	Loculated fluid	Late	Drainage

Investigation and management of malfunctioning catheters

Depends on the likely cause. (See Table 5.7.)

- The first step is to exclude blockage by blood, fibrin, or as a complication of peritonitis. The diagnosis is therefore usually fairly obvious.
- Abdominal X-ray will show the position of the catheter and the presence of any significant faecal loading of the large bowel.
- X-ray screening while infusing dialysate to which IV X-ray contrast material (e.g. Omnipaque®) has been added will show whether the fluid becomes loculated or moves freely into the abdominal cavity.
- CT peritoneogram with contrast injected down the catheter can also show loculated fluid, catheters leaks, hernias, etc.
- MRI scanning can be used as above and avoids injection of contrast material down the catheter.
- Ultrasound can demonstrate subcutaneous fluid leaks and hernias.
- Peritoneal scintigraphy using radiolabelled isotopes is sometimes used.
- Management is successful in 60–90% of malfunctioning catheters.

Table 5.7 Investigation and management of malfunctioning catheters

Cause	Diagnosis	Management
Constipation	History; confirmed on X-ray	Aperients and regular laxatives
Intra-abdominal adhesions from previous surgery	History of previous surgery; only small amounts of fluid can be infused.	Re-site catheter under direct vision into area free of adhesions.
	X-ray with contrast material	Consider stitching catheter into pelvis
		Remove catheter if further attempts at PD fail or if adhesions thought to be widespread
Intra-abdominal adhesions from peritonitis	As above	Catheter removal—adhesions usually too widespread to re-site catheter
Catheter migration up to diaphragm	Occasionally history of episode of abdominal pain when catheter moved.	Use aperients if any faecal loading on X-ray
	Confirmed on X-ray	Encourage patient to walk around
		If simple methods fail, either re-site catheter or exchange for Oreopoulos catheter
Blood in peritoneum	Usually occurs after catheter insertion	Fill catheter with heparin or urokinase
		Infuse urokinase solution through pump (5000–10000U in 50mL saline at 10mL/h)
Fibrin formation	Can occur at any time on PD	Add heparin to dialysate (1000U/exchange) for few days
Peritonitis	Blockage occurs if peritonitis severe	Add heparin to dialysate (1000U/exchange)
		Consider catheter removal if peritonitis not improving
Hernias (if large)	Clinically obvious. X-ray needed to check for other causes of malfunctioning	Repair hernia if technically possible

Repositioning peritoneal dialysis catheters

Up to 15% of new catheters need to be repositioned, though this is less frequent when the catheter is sutured directly into the pelvis at insertion. There are various techniques of manipulating the catheter back into the pelvis.

- Surgical: the catheter can be freed from any adhesions and then replaced into the pelvis, where it should be sutured into position to avoid further migration.
- Laparoscopic repositioning: preferable to laparotomy because of reduced post-operative morbidity, less pain, and a smaller incision site, allowing earlier use of the catheter.
- Guidewire manipulation under X-ray control: is done at a few centres depending on local expertise and availability of fluoroscopic screening. There is a high risk of re-migration of the catheter.

UK Renal Association standards for PD catheter insertion

The Renal Association published standards for PD catheter insertion in 2010.[1] These include (with level of evidence in brackets):

- Each centre should have a dedicated team involved in the implantation and care of peritoneal catheters (1C).
- Catheter insertion should be performed at least 2 weeks before starting PD. Small dialysate volumes in the supine position can be used if dialysis is required earlier (2B).
- Renal units should have clear protocols for peri-operative catheters.
- Local expertise at individual centres should govern the choice of method of PD catheter (1B).
- Each PD unit should have the ability to manipulate or re-implant PD catheters when necessary (1B).
- Urgent removal of PD catheters should be available where necessary (1A).
- A dedicated area should be used for catheter insertion with appropriate staffing, suction, oxygen, and patient monitoring facilities (1A).
- No particular catheter type is proven to be better than another (2C).
- PD catheters should be inserted as day case procedures as long as this does not compromise the quality of care (2C).
- PD catheter insertion training should be available to all trainees with an interest (1C).
- PD catheter insertion should not be delegated to inexperienced unsupervised operators (1A).
- There should be regular audit at not less than 12-monthly intervals of the outcome of catheter insertion.

Summary of audit measures

- More than 80% catheters should be patent at 1 year (censoring for death and elective modality change).
- Complications following catheter insertion:
  - Bowel perforation < 1%
  - Significant haemorrhage <1%
  - Exit site infection within 2 weeks of catheter insertion <5%
  - Peritonitis within 2 weeks of catheter insertion <5%
  - Functional catheter problem requiring manipulation or replacement or leading to technique failure <20%.

Constipation in peritoneal dialysis patients

Management of constipation is key to preventing and managing malfunctioning catheters. Heavily loaded loops of bowel prevent the movement of fluid through the peritoneal cavity, resulting in pools of loculated fluid and hence poor drainage. Catheter migration towards the diaphragm is more likely as the loaded loops of bowel push the catheter up out of the pelvis. The risk of migration at the start of PD is reduced by the use of aperients prior to catheter insertion, between insertion and regular use, and by patients taking regular laxatives while they are on PD. Patients should be educated in the importance of avoiding constipation to improve compliance (usually poor for aperients). Constipation is more common in patients when starting PD, at the time when they are most at risk of catheter malfunction. Regular exercise also helps to avoid constipation and encourages the catheter to remain in the pelvis.

Causes of constipation at the start of PD include:
• reduced fibre in diet—patients are often anorectic or are placed on a diet with less fibre, particularly if potassium is restricted
• reduced exercise
• use of phosphate binders, most of which are constipating
• iron supplements can cause constipation
• many patients are elderly in whom there is already an increased risk of constipation.

Peritoneal dialysate: standard fluid composition

PD depends on removal of waste products and excess fluid from blood by diffusion and UF across the peritoneal membrane. Both are two-way processes, with molecules being able to pass from blood to dialysate or vice versa. The type of dialysate used in PD controls all the functions of dialysis—solute removal, equilibration of electrolytes and acid–base, and fluid removal. The composition of peritoneal dialysate can be varied but is designed to maximize diffusive solute loss from blood, and allow some degree of control over UF. It is possible to add potentially beneficial substances to dialysate that may diffuse into the blood, e.g. amino acids to improve nutrition. (See Table 5.8.)

Ultrafiltration

The passage of fluid between blood and dialysate compartments is usually controlled by the relative tonicity of the two solutions. Dialysate tonicity is varied by altering the glucose concentration, which increases the osmotic gradient between plasma and dialysate, resulting in increased fluid removal. Glucose can also diffuse from the dialysate into the blood compartment where it is metabolized into glucose. Approximately 100–200g glucose is absorbed per day. This can make blood glucose control difficult in diabetics, and can cause obesity if too many hypertonic glucose bags are used. Can also cause hyperinsulinaemia, hypertriglyceridaemia, appetite suppression, and contribute to peritoneal membrane sclerosis.

Table 5.8 Electrolyte composition of standard commercially available dialysate

Electrolyte	Concentration	Function
Sodium	130–134mmol/L	Equilibrate with plasma sodium
Potassium	1.5mmol/L	Lower plasma potassium level to normal range
Calcium (ionized)	Old standard— 1.75mmol/L	Maintain plasma calcium at upper level of normal range. Maintain plasma calcium at lower range of normal allowing for use of calcium salts to lower plasma phosphate levels
	Reduced or current standard— 1.25mmol/L	
	Low—1.0mmol/L	Lowers high plasma calcium levels to normal range
Magnesium	0.25–0.75mmol/L	Equilibrate with plasma magnesium
Lactate	35–40mmol/L	Diffuses into blood and metabolized to pyruvate (generating bicarbonate) to normalize acid–base balance. Higher concentrations result in higher plasma bicarbonate levels. Lowers dialysate pH
pH	5.2–5.5 in glucose bags	Low pH prevents glucose caramelization during heat sterilization and inhibits bacterial growth

Peritoneal dialysate: problems with lactate/glucose

Standard PD fluids contain lactate and glucose, as these are easier to manufacture and provide good dialysis and UF. There are, however, potential problems with these components:

- As glucose has to be sterilized at low pH to prevent caramelization, dialysate pH is low at ~5; this causes abdominal pain on inflow in some patients and directly contributes to neoangiogenesis and mesothelial cell damage.
- *Glucose degradation products (GDPs)* formed during the sterilization process, as well as the low pH of the fluid, contribute to bioincompatibility of standard dialysate.
- GDPs also enhance local and systemic production of AGEs; these are implicated in:
  - development of structural damage to peritoneal membrane and blood vessels
  - impairment of peritoneal defences to infection.
- Glucose is metabolized into glucose when absorbed. This has adverse metabolic consequences, particularly when high glucose concentrations are used to achieve UF:
  - new-onset diabetes
  - difficulty in controlling pre-existing diabetes
  - obesity
  - exacerbation of hyperlipidaemia.
- The rate of rise of peritoneal membrane transport is related to use of hypertonic glucose dialysate; patients who use more hypertonic fluid to achieve UF are at increased risk of developing high transport membranes. This has detrimental medium- and long-term consequences (see Peritoneal equilibration test and modelling, p. 297).

Peritoneal dialysate: alternative fluids

Peritoneal dialysate: alternative fluids

Over the last few years, several new solutions have been developed with the aim of minimizing the metabolic and biocompatibility problems of standard dextrose/lactate dialysate.

Icodextrin

A glucose polymer, to achieve UF. This is a very large polymeric glucopyranose molecule produced by hydrolysis of starch and has a similar structure to glycogen. Each molecule contains between 20 and >500 glucose molecules linked together. It is isosmotic with human serum (~282mosmol/kg) and allows UF to occur over a long period of time by 'dragging' water molecules through the peritoneal membrane. Little back diffusion from the intraperitoneal cavity into the circulation occurs, thereby making it suitable for long dwells.

Ultrafiltration with icodextrin
- UF with icodextrin is slow and occurs evenly through a long dwell, which should be >8h to get maximal effect. Icodextrin is therefore used for the overnight dwell in CAPD or the daytime dwell in APD.
- Provides the same UF after 8–12h as 3.86% dextrose, and 3.5–5.5 times more than 1.36% dextrose.

Advantages of icodextrin
- Sustained UF.
- Replacing hypertonic glucose reduces hyperglycaemia and hyperlipidaemia.
- Lower GDP content than conventional lactate-buffered dialysate.

Disadvantages of icodextrin
- Contains lactate and is therefore acidic with pH of 5; some patients on bicarbonate-buffered fluids notice the difference and can find the icodextrin exchange relatively uncomfortable.
- Metabolized to maltose; use is therefore limited to a single daily exchange because of concerns of high circulating plasma maltose levels.
- Can cause hypersensitivity reactions; transient skin rashes are not uncommon; exfoliative dermatitis can rarely occur.
- Can cause sterile peritonitis with predominantly mononuclear cells in the dialysate:
  - an outbreak of this in 2003/4 was due to a fault in the manufacturing process, resulting in contamination with a bacterial wall product.
- Licensed to a single manufacturer (Baxter)—it is therefore expensive if using alternative PD products

Amino acid dialysate

1.1% amino acid-containing solution is produced by Baxter as Nutrineal®. It is presented in a single bag, is lactate buffered, and has the equivalent UF capacity of 1.36% glucose dialysate. It is promoted predominantly to improve nutrition. It must be given at the same time as calories or the amino acids are not taken up by the peripheral tissues; in CAPD, it is used at the same time as the main meal; in APD, it is used as part of the overnight exchanges so given with a lot of glucose.

Advantages of amino acid dialysate
- No GDPs.
- Avoids peritoneal and systemic glucose exposure with metabolic advantages of less hyperglycaemia and hyperlipidaemia.
- May improve nutrition.

Disadvantages of amino acid dialysate
- Low pH.
- Licensed for single daily use only as absorption of amino acids can exacerbate uraemic symptoms and acidosis.
- Expensive—it has been difficult to prove clinically important improvement in nutrition, and it is much cheaper to use oral nutritional supplements.

Low-sodium dialysate

Reducing sodium concentration of dialysate would increase sodium diffusion from plasma; this increase in sodium removal should improve BP control. Trials are currently taking place, but it will be some time before low sodium dialysate will be commercially available.

Biocompatible dialysate: new bag designs

Double-chamber bags

New technology has allowed the development of double- or triple-chamber bags:

- Allows low pH dextrose solution to be in a separate compartment when sterilized, preventing formation of GDPs.
- Enables storage of glucose at a low pH, thereby minimizing formation of GDPs during protracted storage.
- Allows use of bicarbonate as alternative buffer to lactate.
- Multibag systems prevent the precipitation that would occur when mixing bicarbonate buffer with calcium and magnesium in solution; the two solutions are separated in storage, with a connecting seal being broken just before running the dialysate into the peritoneum.
- Each of the main PD manufacturers produce low GDP fluids using different versions of the multibag:
  - *Physioneal®* (Baxter) uses a lactate/bicarbonate mixed buffer (25mmol/L bicarbonate with 15mmol/L lactate, pH 7–7.4). This was developed rather than using pure bicarbonate because of lower scoring for abdominal pain on inflow of fluid
  - *Stay Safe Balance®* (Fresenius) separates glucose and electrolytes from a lactate buffer and achieves a neutral pH when mixed
  - *BicaVera®* (Fresenius) uses pure bicarbonate buffer (34mmol/L); does not result in neutral pH but avoids using lactate.

Potential advantages of biocompatible dialysate

Despite the fact that biocompatible dialysate fluids have been available for some years, there is still very limited evidence of benefit to justify the increased cost. There are several theoretical advantages and a few observational studies to support their benefit, and limited RCT evidence.

- Reduces abdominal pain on inflow (RCT evidence for Physioneal®).
- Patients who have never complained of pain often feel more comfortable when using these fluids.
- Improved peritoneal defence mechanisms in animal studies.
- Conflicting evidence about peritonitis rates and outcomes from RCTs and observational studies.
- Improved peritoneal membrane biocompatibility with less inflammation and eventual sclerosis—this has been demonstrated in animal studies but remains to be proven in patients.
- Lower UF rates possibly due to less peritoneal inflammation demonstrated in several studies comparing biocompatible fluids with standard fluids.
- Reduction in peritoneal inflammation may reduce systemic inflammation and thereby preserve residual renal function longer; conflicting evidence from RCTs.
  - It is possible that any observed increase in urine output could be related to increased fluid load related to lower ultrafiltration rate

Potential disadvantages of biocompatible dialysate

- More expensive with little hard evidence of benefit.
- Technically, multibags are more difficult to manufacture, and in particular the larger 5L bags for APD are just becoming available; this means that double the number of connections are sometimes needed when using 2.5L bags.
- Still contain dextrose with all its metabolic complications.
- Some evidence that UF may be slightly lower than using standard fluids.
- Not all are at physiological pH and most still contain lactate.
- RCT data mostly from small under-powered and short-term studies. Large trials determining difference in technique and patient survival, or effect on long-term complications such as EPS, are unlikely to be done.

See Table 5.9 for advantages and disadvantages of different dialysates.

Table 5.9 The various dialysates available have different advantages and complications.

Agent	Mechanism of action	Advantage	Disadvantage
Dextrose	Increases osmotic gradient between blood and dialysate. Greatest effect during beginning of exchange when osmotic gradient at its peak	Cheap; readily commercially available UF controlled by changing glucose concentration	Adverse metabolic effects; adverse effects on membrane permeability; need for low pH to prevent formation of GDPs during sterilization; net absorption of fluid from dialysate during long dwells
Icodextrin	Presence of large molecule in dialysate drags water across peritoneal membrane; UF dependent on time and not on diffusion gradient	Reduces dependence on high-concentration glucose solutions; effective in patients with poor UF even when using high-concentration glucose; long duration of UF particularly useful for daytime dwell of APD or overnight exchange of CAPD	Very expensive; not commercially available from all manufacturers; metabolized to maltose, resulting in high maltose levels—long-term consequences (over years) still not known
Lactate	Metabolized to form bicarbonate and therefore normalize acid–base status	Cheap; easy to produce commercially available fluid; long experience of use	Acidic, so low dialysate pH; bioincompatible fluid; can cause pain on dialysate inflow

(continued)

Table 1.6 (*Contd.*)

Agent	Mechanism of action	Advantage	Disadvantage
Bicarbonate or bicarbonate/lactate	Normalizes acid–base status	Biocompatible; no pain on inflow; patients with no history of pain also feel more comfortable and less bloated; less GDPs as glucose sterilized in separate compartment; theoretically long-term benefits for membrane function and maybe peritonitis outcomes	Needs double-chamber bag; expensive; no long-term data of effects on membrane function or peritonitis outcomes
Amino acids	Alternative osmotic agent; marketed as nutritional agent	Less hyperlipidaemia; absorption of amino acids may improve nutrition	Expensive; can only be used for 1 exchange as otherwise causes acidosis and rise in plasma urea; effect on nutrition not impressive in trials or in clinical practice

Prescribing CAPD

Adequate dialysis can only be assured if dialysis adequacy is measured. Underprovision of PD is common, particularly as residual function declines. Adequacy should be measured within the first 2 weeks of starting CAPD, and regularly thereafter.

An initial regimen is, however, required, and should be individualized for each patient. The variables to be considered are:

- volume of exchange
- number of exchanges
- timing of exchanges
- possibility of days off dialysis
- UF requirements and therefore glucose concentration for each exchange
- residual renal function
- size of patient.

The initial CAPD prescription

This should provide adequate dialysis and sufficient UF. Membrane permeability characteristics vary enormously between patients, and cannot be predicted prior to starting CAPD. Residual renal function also plays a crucial part at the onset of dialysis. Many patients will need less PD (number or volume of exchanges) at the start of dialysis than later, once residual renal function declines.

A standard daily CAPD regimen is four 2L exchanges, three during the day and one overnight.

Individual patient requirements vary widely. Patients starting dialysis will often need only three exchanges. However, as they lose renal function they will inevitably need four or more exchanges, and it is usually easier (psychologically) to adapt a regimen if they commence on a standard four-exchange regimen that can then be altered as necessary.

Volumes and ultrafiltration requirements

Exchange volume

This is determined principally by the size of the patient. Small patients tolerate smaller volumes. Too large a volume can cause high intra-abdominal pressure, which increases the risk of developing hernias or fluid leaks. If a catheter has to be used within the first 2 weeks, a smaller volume of fluid (1–1.5L) should initially be used to minimize the risk of fluid leaks. It is often psychologically easier to start a patient on a larger volume of fluid than they might need (e.g. 2.5L).

Ultrafiltration requirements

Also vary from patient to patient and depend mainly on urine output and fluid intake. Most patients commencing PD will still be passing reasonable urine volumes, and so UF will not be as important during the first few months. Not all patients can restrict their fluid intake, and some with even a large urine output may require significant UF from dialysate.

Table 5.10 Recommendations for initial CAPD prescription

Exchange volume	Small size patient—1.5L
	Standard size patient—2L
	Large size patient—2.5L
	All should be reduced by 0.5L if catheter used within first 2 weeks
Number of exchanges	Four (3×4–5h, 1×8–10h)
Type of dialysate	Glucose containing
Glucose concentration during day	No UF requirements: all 'week' (1.36% glucose)
	UF needed: 1–2 'medium' (2.27% glucose)
Dextrose concentration overnight	'Weak' (1.36% glucose)

Initial choice of dialysate dextrose concentration to achieve adequate UF is by trial and error, as the permeability of a patient's membrane will not be known. Care is needed particularly after the long overnight exchange as some patients absorb fluid. This can result in fluid overload in patients who were euvolaemic prior to starting dialysis. (See Table 5.10.)

Dialysis adequacy should be measured soon after a patient is established on CAPD, ideally within the first 2–3 weeks. It may then be possible to reduce the number of exchanges to three per day.

Adequacy of peritoneal dialysis

The aims of dialysis of any sort include maintenance of normal body fluid status, normal electrolyte and acid–base balance, and removal of nitrogenous and other waste products. Clinical observations and biochemical measurements can monitor the first two. The degree of adequacy of removing nitrogenous waste products is more difficult to determine. Subjectively the patient should feel well. However, as many factors other than dialysis adequacy determine patient well-being (e.g. depression causes tiredness, loss of appetite, and poor sleep), objective measurements are needed. Urea and creatinine kinetics (weekly Kt/V and C_{crea}) are an attempt to measure dialysis adequacy objectively. These measurements only reflect clearance of small MW substances, so it is important to include a measure of protein intake, such as PCR, to assess appetite and nutritional status, important end-products of dialysis.

Body fluid status

- Subjectively: presence or absence of shortness of breath and oedema.
- Objectively: presence or absence of oedema, difference between actual and 'dry' weight, raised JVP and raised BP.
- Aim for normality, as chronic fluid overload causes hypertension and LVH (independent risk factors for cardiovascular morbidity).

Electrolyte and acid–base balance

- Aim for sodium, potassium, and bicarbonate levels in normal range.
- Calcium and phosphate levels should also be in normal range, but their levels are determined by factors other than dialysis.

Nitrogenous waste products

Measurements of dialysate Kt/V (urea clearance) and Ccrea are based on the volume of dialysate effluent, and urea and creatinine concentration, over 24h. There are two methods:

- collect all dialysate effluent during 24h in a large container, mix, and take a sample
- measure volume of effluent and take a sample from each exchange (or overnight drainage bag if on APD).

The first method is cumbersome for the patient, but calculation is straightforward. The second method is easier for the patient, but the calculation is more complex, particularly for APD.

Residual renal function is particularly important in PD, which is less efficient at removing small molecules than HD. It is not practical to use repeated isotopic measurements of residual GFR. Methods based on 24h urine collections are used. At low GFR, C_{crea} overestimates GFR, and urea clearance underestimates GFR. A reasonably accurate estimate of GFR can be obtained by measuring both urea and C_{crea} and using the average of the two results.

Weekly Kt/V (dialysate+renal) is estimated from:

- Kt—sum of daily peritoneal and renal urea clearance
- V—volume of distribution of urea (approximately equal to body water).

Weekly C_{crea} (dialysate+renal) is estimated from:

- dialysate/plasma (D/P) creatinine ratio

- 24h dialysate volume
- add in residual renal function
- correct for BSA—divide result by patient's BSA and multiply by 1.73m²

Weekly dialysis $C_{crea} = (D_{crea} \times \text{Dialysate vol.} \times 1.73 \times 7)/(P_{crea} \times BSA)$

PCR is an estimate of the daily protein intake, calculated from urea losses in dialysate and urine, assuming the patient is in nitrogen balance:
- Urea appearance, g/day = $(Vu \times Cu)+(Vd \times Cd)$, where V and C represent volume and urea concentration in urine (u) and dialysate (d);
- PCR = $6.25 \times$ (Urea appearance+1.81+[0.031 $\times$ lean body weight, kg]);
- Increasing dialysis dose results in a rise in PCR; although this could be due to the mathematical similarities in calculating Kt/V and PCR, independent measures of nutrition also improve.

Kt/V, C_{crea}, and PCR can be calculated using commercially available computer programs such as PD Adequest™ (Baxter) using a 24h urine collection, 24h dialysate collection, or samples from individual exchanges, and blood sampling. All calculations need mean dialysate concentration over 24h—this is calculated differently for CAPD and APD:

$$\text{Mean dialysate solute concentration in CASPD} = \frac{\text{Sum of solute concentration for each exchange}}{\text{Number of exchanges}}$$

Mean dialysate solute concentration in APD

= (Overnight V $\times$ C)+ (daytime dwell V $\times$ C)+(manual exchange V $\times$ C)/Overnight V+ daytime dwell V+manual exchange V

where V = volume, C = concentration.

Kt/V and C_{crea} may not correlate in patients on PD mostly because peritoneal clearance is predominantly by diffusion. Smaller molecules (urea) are cleared better, especially in low transporters. High transpor-ters have better C_{crea} because of increased convective clearance with increased UF.

Goals

Guidelines for minimum dialysis adequacy for PD have changed over recent years with results from recent trials such as ADEMEX[3] and EAPOS[4] (see later in this topic). Earlier guidelines were based on the CANUSA[2] study, a prospective multicentre study of 600 patients in Canada and the USA evaluating the relationship of dialysis adequacy and nutritional status to mortality, morbidity, and technique failure.

Although the CANUSA study suggested a positive relationship between outcome on PD and dialysis adequacy, all patients studied were new to PD, many of whom had residual renal function. All patients were on a fixed regimen (mostly 4 $\times$ 2L exchanges) so dialysis dose was not increased if a patient was clinically underdialysed, and the relationship between outcome and adequacy was determined by the initial measurement of adequacy.

The conclusion from CANUSA, that the higher the dialysis dose, the better the outcome, therefore reflected the fact that a higher residual renal function at the onset of dialysis improves prognosis. This has been confirmed by re-analysis of the data. Other studies have also shown that residual renal function predicts better survival.

Both ADEMEX and EAPOS suggest that survival on PD is not determined by small solute clearance. Indeed, EAPOS suggested that UF may be a better predictor of outcome.

Key trials

CANUSA

- Observational study of survival over 2 years.[2]
- All patients on CAPD in Canada and the USA.
- All patients on $4 \times 2L$ exchanges with no change as residual renal function declined.
- Showed that baseline C_{crea} and Kt/V determined survival, but as there was no change in PD prescription, re-analysis has shown that outcome depended on residual renal function at baseline and not on PD adequacy.

ADEMEX

- Randomized, active controlled, prospective trial.[3]
- Hypothesis tested: increases in peritoneal clearance of small solutes improves patient survival.
- Primary outcome was mortality.
- 965 Mexican CAPD patients randomized:
  - control group—standard therapy of $4 \times 2L$/day
  - intervention group—two prescription adjustments aiming for peritoneal C_{crea} >60L/week/1.73m^2.
- Successful study design—mean difference between two groups in peritoneal C_{crea} of 11L/week/1.73m^2.
- No difference in patient survival between the two groups, even after adjusting for factors known to be associated with mortality in patients on PD (age, diabetes, albumin, protein intake, anuria).

EAPOS

- European, multicentre, 2-year prospective observational study of survival of anuric patients on APD: 177 patients enrolled.[4]
- APD prescription adjusted to achieve targets for C_{crea} of 60L/week/1.73m^2 and UF of 750mL/24h.
- At 1 year, 78% and 74% achieved C_{crea} and UF targets, respectively; median drained dialysate volume was 16.2L/24h with 50% patients using icodextrin.
- At 2 years, patient survival on APD was 78% and technique survival 62%.
- Age (>65 years), poor nutrition, diabetic status and UF <750mL at baseline were predictors of worse patient survival.
- Baseline C_{crea}, time-averaged C_{crea} and baseline D/P had no effect on patient or technique survival.
- Study showed that anuric patients can be successfully maintained on APD; survival is affected by baseline UF and not by C_{crea} or membrane permeability.

Targets

Previous PD adequacy guidelines were based on the CANUSA[2] study and used to recommend relatively high clearance targets (weekly Kt/V >2.0 and

C_{crea} >60L/week/1.73m^2. The UK Renal Association guidelines (2007) and American K/DOQI guidelines (2006) have incorporated the trial evidence that survival is not determined by low solute clearance and therefore recommend lower (and therefore more achievable) adequacy targets.

Small solute clearance target

The Renal Association and K/DOQI guidelines for total peritoneal and renal small solute clearance targets are very similar:

$$Kt/V >1.7$$

$$C_{crea} >50L/week/1.73m^2$$

Measuring small solute clearance is only one method of assessing dialysis adequacy. It is also important to check whether the patient has any uraemic symptoms—if they do, the dialysis dose should be increased, whatever the measured small solute clearance; the amount of symptoms for given levels of clearance varies with individuals.

Adjusting for residual renal function

Residual function of 2mL/min equates to 70.4 units Kt/V per week. Residual renal function continues to decline after a patient starts on dialysis. Thus C_{crea} and Kt/V will fall with the risk that the patient may become clinically underdialysed developing uraemic symptoms. It is therefore essential to increase the dialysis dose as residual function declines. Once a patient becomes anuric, it is difficult to achieve adequate dialysis with CAPD alone, and it is often necessary to change to APD, or even HD.

Ultrafiltration

UF through PD is only one way of achieving euvolaemia. It is also important to encourage patients to limit sodium intake to enable control of fluid intake, consider use of loop diuretics to increase urine output, and to use treatment strategies, e.g. use of ACEIs to preserve residual renal function. When patients are anuric, amount of UF is the only way of removing fluid. It then becomes particularly important to avoid regimens that result in fluid reabsorption. The UK Renal Association guidelines suggest a target of 750mL/24h in anuric patients (based on EAPOS study).

Comparison with HD

Urea clearance achieved on PD is much less than on HD (target Kt/V of 1.7 for PD compared with weekly Kt/V of 3.6 for thrice-weekly HD), but both achieve similar clinical outcomes. One explanation is that middle and large molecule clearance is higher on PD compared with HD. Another factor is probably the continuous nature of PD which thereby avoids the peaks in uraemic solute levels related to the intermittent nature of HD.

A practical approach to peritoneal dialysis adequacy

- Adequacy should be measured within a month of starting PD, with repeated measurements at 6-month intervals, so that PD regimen can be adjusted for decline in residual renal function and changes in membrane function.
- More frequent measurements of adequacy are needed if:
  - changes are made to PD regimen
  - significant rise in plasma creatinine occurs, suggesting declining residual renal function
  - patient becomes symptomatically uraemic.
- Membrane transport status should be measured within 6 months of starting PD:
  - ideally measurements should be repeated annually
  - patients transferring to APD should have a membrane transport status measurement if one has not been done within the previous 6 months
  - measurement should be repeated in anuric patients if declining C_{crea} or UF.
- All patients should have a minimum fluid removal target of 750mL/day (combination of urine output and UF).
- Careful attention should be given to patients with C_{crea} 50–60L/week/1.73m^2:
  - if patient clinically well and fluid removal >750mL/day, no change to dialysis regimen is needed;
  - if evidence of symptomatic uraemia and/or fluid overload, dialysis regimen needs to be changed;
  - if dialysis adequacy and/or UF is deteriorating on repeat measurements, and there is little room for manoeuvre with PD regimen, then an AVF should be created so that patient can be electively transferred to HD
- If C_{crea} <50L/week/1.73m^2, dialysis prescription should be increased. If this is not feasible, patient should be transferred to HD.

Peritoneal equilibration test and modelling

The *PET* is a semiquantitative test of peritoneal membrane permeability. Membrane permeability of an individual patient can be classified as high (H), high average (HA), low average (LA), or low (L). This is important to:

- determine the optimal mode of PD:
  - long dwells (i.e. CAPD) are needed for optimal diffusion in low or low average transporters, particularly those with a large BSA
  - clearance can be increased in high average or high transporters by increasing the number of exchanges overnight with APD, as adequate diffusion will occur in shorter periods of time
- determine the cause of poor UF and its possible correction:
  - high transporters will have poor UF on CAPD, particularly with long overnight exchange, because of reabsorption of glucose and water; on APD with short dwells overnight, UF will be better
  - poor UF in low or low average transporters suggests drainage problems
- *allow calculation of predicted clearance with a given PD regimen* (the only other factor needed is the patient's BSA):
  - can be useful to check on patient compliance
  - calculating the potential clearance with different PD regimens, also known as modelling, can be used to predict the optimal regimen for a patient, particularly when measured clearance appears to be inadequate—this can be done with the aid of a computer program, such as PD Adequest™.

Technique for performing the peritoneal equilibration test

- To standardize the results, the PET test is always performed in the morning after a 2L overnight exchange using 2.27% dextrose dialysate. The patient must not drain out the overnight exchange prior to the test.
- After draining out the overnight exchange, 2L of 2.27% glucose dialysate are infused into the patient while supine; the patient should be rolled from side to side after every 400mL infusion.
- At time 0 after all the dialysate has been run in, and at 120min, 200mL of dialysate is drained out; 190mL is run back into the peritoneal cavity, and a 10mL sample is collected for measurement of glucose, urea, and creatinine concentrations.
- A blood sample is taken at 120min for measurement of glucose, urea, and creatinine concentrations.
- The patient is allowed to walk around during the 4h test.
- The fluid is drained out at 240min over 20min; the volume is measured and a 10mL sample is collected for analysis.
- The lab needs to be warned about the high glucose concentration in the dialysate samples, as this may interfere with creatinine measurements.

Calculation of permeability from PET

- Dialysate/plasma (D/P) ratios for urea and creatinine concentrations are determined for the three time points.
- Dialysate in/dialysate out (D/DO) ratios for glucose concentrations are determined for the time points.
- The calculation can be done manually or by various computer programs.
- The D/P creatinine at 4h is used for membrane classification.

Peritoneal equilibration test results

Peritoneal equilibration test results

Results from PET tests can be shown graphically or simply as the 4h D/P. Examples of PET test results are shown in Figs 5.7 and 5.8 and Tables 5.11 and 5.12.

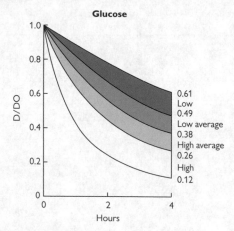

Fig. 5.7 Glucose test results.

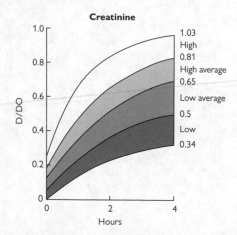

Fig. 5.8 Creatinine test results.

Table 5.11 Transport classifications

Transport classification	D/P urea	D/P creatinine	D/DO glucose	Drain volume
High (H)	0.98–1.09	0.82–1.03	0.12–0.25	1580–2084
High average (HA)	0.91–0.97	0.65–0.81	0.26–0.38	2085–2368
Low average (LA)	0.84–0.90	0.50–0.64	0.39–0.49	2369–2650
Low (L)	0.75–0.83	0.34–0.49	0.50–0.61	2651–3326

Originally published in Twardowski ZJ et al. Peritoneal equilibration test. *Peritoneal Dialysis International* 1987; 7(3): 138–47.

Table 5.12 Example of PET test result

Time (min)	D/P urea	D/P creatinine	D/DO glucose	Drain volume (mL)
0	0.09	LA0.15 H	1.00	
120	0.82	HA0.72 H	0.44 H	
240	0.99 H	0.95 H	0.22 H	2200.0 HA

Other measures of peritoneal membrane function

Several new tests are being developed and undergoing evaluation. Any test has to be simple to perform and give membrane transport status results similar to the standard PET both for clinical purposes and to provide uniformity for studies. Mostly these tests are not yet used in clinical practice. Most studies provide cross-sectional comparisons and there are limited data from the newer tests used longitudinally in individual patients. The following tests are now being used clinically by some units as they give more information about UF compared with the standard PET.

Peritoneal equilibration test using 3.86% glucose

This is also called the *standard peritoneal permeability assessment or SPA*. It is performed in an identical manner to the standard 4h PET using 2.27% glucose. It provides better information on UF as the larger drained volume results in fewer measurement errors and is more sensitive to detect significant UF failure (defined as <400mL). Comparisons with the standard 4h PET using 2.27% glucose show no effect of dialysate glucose concentration on D/P creatinine and therefore no impact on transport group categorization.

One-hour 'mini' peritoneal equilibration test

A 1h PET using 3.86% glucose may enable the evaluation of free water transport across the peritoneal membrane as well as estimating UF and transporter status as in the standard PET. This is based on the following surmise:

- UF has two principal components:
  - water passing across small pores accompanied by proportionate amounts of small solutes
  - water travelling, free of solute, via the peritoneal aquaporins
- Sodium removal in the short 1h dwell is almost all accounted for by convection through the small pores with little contribution from diffusion. By measuring the sodium removal, the proportionate amount of water accompanying it across the small pores can be calculated
- Subtracting this value from total ultrafiltrate gives an estimate of free water transport via the aquaporins.

Results show that, on average, just under half of the ultrafiltrate generated in 1h is due to free water transport. Comparison with the results from a 4h PET using 3.86% glucose shows similar transport group categorization using the D/P creatinine ratio. Interestingly, free water transport correlates with the total ultrafiltrate from a hypertonic 4h PET on the same patient; this suggests that variation in free water transport is an important factor determining the total UF.

Personal dialysis capacity (PDC™) test

- Developed by Gambro (Lund, Sweden) to give more information than the standard PET.
- Describes peritoneal membrane characteristics using 3 parameters:
  - surface area over diffusion distance—represents the effective surface area available for diffusion; thought to be roughly comparable with D/P obtained from the PET test
  - reabsorption parameter—measures reabsorption of fluid from the peritoneal cavity after the osmotic gradient has disappeared—represents mainly lymphatic flow
  - large pore flow—related to 'leakiness' of membrane and thus potentially to inflammation
- Parameters calculated using mathematical model based on 3-pore theory of membrane characteristics ($\bigodot$ Principles of peritoneal dialysis, p. 256).
- Enthusiasts for this test claim it is superior to PET-derived D/P_{crea} to describe transport of small solutes through the peritoneal membrane.
- Patients may find test cumbersome—samples have to be collected from 5 exchanges of variable duration (3, 4, 5, 2, then 10h). These are done at home with patient noting the exact time of start of drainage, total drained volume, and time of start of inflow.
- Glucose concentration of exchanges also variable—2.27% for 4h dwell, and 1.36% for exchange before; glucose concentration for other exchanges depends on volume status of patient.
- Patient visits hospital twice for blood samples before and after test.
- Patients on APD are converted to CAPD for duration of PDC™ test.
- Residual renal function determined by collection of 24h urine sample and calculated using urea and creatinine clearance.
- Advantages of PDC™ are:
  - test mostly done at home and patient does not have to spend 4h in hospital
  - calculated large pore flux is related to inflammation and has been shown to be a prognostic marker.
- However, PDC™ conceptually more difficult test to understand, and 4h of PET provide time for nurses to reinforce education and for patient to see other members of the multidisciplinary team.
- Some claim that the same information can be obtained by combining standard PET with a measure of inflammation such as CRP.
- D/P_{crea} derived from PET remains standard for following patients' membrane characteristics and for research studies.

Increasing dialysis delivered by CAPD

To increase amount of dialysis delivered or ultrafiltration rate

In PD, unlike HD, blood flow, membrane permeability, and surface area are fixed. In CAPD, hours are also fixed as the process is continuous throughout 24h. The only factors that can be increased are dialysate flow rates and the amount of UF.

Exchange volume and number determine dialysis flow rates

Increasing the exchange volume by >0.5L at a time is not usually acceptable to the patient because of abdominal discomfort and/or distension. The increase in intra-abdominal pressure, particularly when ambulant, increases the risk of fluid leak and hernias. It is also difficult to increase the number of exchanges. By starting a patient on four exchanges a day and reducing to three after a couple of weeks (if possible), it is usually acceptable to patients to increase again from three to four exchanges per day. Most patients will not or cannot increase to five exchanges a day because of the time commitment. There is therefore a practical limit to the amount of dialysis that can be delivered by CAPD.

Increased ultrafiltration

This is indicated if the patient becomes fluid overloaded while complying with their fluid restriction. Initially the number of medium (2.27%) or strong (3.86%) glucose exchanges should be increased. In some patients, reabsorption of fluid occurs from the overnight bag, thereby decreasing the net amount of fluid removed during the day. In this case, a medium glucose bag should be used overnight. Icodextrin should be used for the long overnight exchange if UF remains poor, or an excessive number of hypertonic exchanges are needed (e.g. regimens using two strong or three medium exchanges), or if patients are becoming fat from the glucose caloric load because of the increased use of hypertonic dextrose to control fluid status.

Examples of alterations in CAPD prescription follow:

Reduction to three exchanges at the start of dialysis

A 64-year-old diabetic man starting on CAPD with symptomatic uraemia.
- Initial prescription: $4 \times 1.36\%$ dextrose exchanges.
- Assessment at 2 weeks:
  - plasma creatinine   316µmol/L
  - urine volume   610mL/24h
  - UF   800mL/24h
  - residual renal function   8.3mL/min
  - Kt/V   2.9
  - C_{crea} 122L/week/1.73m².
- Interpretation: good residual function.
- Action: regimen changed to $3 \times 1.36\%$ glucose exchanges.
- Some units would leave the regimen unchanged on the basis of more dialysis being better. However, patients often feel happier if they can have the number of exchanges reduced, even if it will be increased later.

Underdialysis—need to increase exchange volume and number

A 31-year-old man with failing renal transplant.
- After initial assessment: established on 3 × 2L 1.36% glucose exchanges.
- Assessment at 6 months:
  - plasma creatinine $\qquad$ 1272µmol/L
  - urine volume $\qquad$ 0mL
  - UF $\qquad$ 400mL/24h
  - Kt/V $\qquad$ 1.3
  - C_{crea} $\qquad$ 44L/week/1.73m^2.
- Interpretation: inadequate dialysis and UF.
- Action: regimen changed to 5 × 2L exchanges.
- Assessment 2 months later:
  - plasma creatinine $\qquad$ 1000µmol/L
  - urine volume $\qquad$ 0mL
  - UF $\qquad$ 600mL/24h
  - Kt/V $\qquad$ 1.7
  - C_{crea} $\qquad$ 50L/week/1.73m^2.
- Interpretation: improved but dialysis and fluid loss still inadequate.
- Action: increase volume to 2.5L. Use Quantum exchange device at night to increase compliance.
- Assessment 2 months later:
  - plasma creatinine $\qquad$ 961µmol/L
  - urine volume $\qquad$ 0mL
  - UF $\qquad$ 400mL/24h
  - Kt/V $\qquad$ 2.2
  - C_{crea} $\qquad$ 62L/week/1.73m^2.
- Interpretation: dialysis now adequate but fluid removal remains inadequate. Check PET, consider APD, unlikely to last long on PD, consider early AVF formation for HD.
- If dialysis had remained inadequate would need to change to APD or HD.

Prescribing automated peritoneal dialysis

The principal differences between APD and CAPD are:
- most of the exchanges are done by machine at night
- there is more flexibility in prescribing APD than CAPD
- the dialysate volume at night, while the patient is supine, can be larger than during the day, as the rise in intra-abdominal pressure is less
- the number of exchanges can be increased more easily as they are done by machine and not by the patient

The limiting factors to overnight dialysis are:
- the number of hours the patient is prepared to remain attached to a machine
- short dwell times which require rapid solute diffusion
- cost of dialysate—the greater the quantity used, the more expensive is the dialysis. A regimen using 20L of dialysate overnight will provide the same amount of dialysis, and may be more comfortable for the patient, as a regimen using 10L overnight and 2L during the day (long day dwell), but is considerably more expensive. APD regimens may have to restrict the amount of dialysate used to keep costs in a realistic range
- patients need to be able to carry the large volume APD bags of dialysate (5L)
- most patients do not get sufficient dialysis from overnight APD alone, and require additional daytime exchanges (see → Increasing delivered dialysis and ultrafiltration in automated peritoneal dialysis, p. 307).

Ultrafiltration

This is generally greater on APD than on CAPD because there is less absorption of fluid from the peritoneum during the short duration cycles. Icodextrin can be used for the long day dwell in patients who would otherwise reabsorb fluid. Some patients become volume depleted when changing to APD from CAPD, and many can reduce antihypertensive drugs because of improved fluid control.

The cycles used overnight can either be $4 \times 2.5L$, $5 \times 2L$, or $6 \times 1.5L$ depending on the size of the patient and the permeability of the membrane. The larger the patient, the larger should be the volume of each exchange. The more permeable the membrane, the shorter should be the duration of each exchange. Larger volume bags are safer to use (less connections) and more economical—5L bags are therefore generally used for the overnight exchanges. (See Table 5.13.)

Table 5.13 Recommendations for initial APD prescription

Residual renal function	Night-time exchanges	Daytime exchanges
>7mL/min	10L over 8h	None
4–7mL/min	10L over 8h	1.5–2.5L long day dwell
2–4mL/min	10L over 9h	1.5–2.5L long day dwell
<2mL/min	10L over 9h	1.5–2.5L long day dwell and 1.5–2.5L manual exchange

Increasing delivered dialysis and ultrafiltration in automated peritoneal dialysis

Variables that can be changed to increase adequacy of APD

- Volume and number of exchanges overnight
- Hours attached to machine overnight
- Volume and duration of long day dwell
- Introduction of manual exchange during day (usually at tea-time when patient comes home)
- Volume and duration of manual exchange.

Variables that can be changed to increase UF in APD

- Dextrose concentration of fluid used at night and during day
- Use of short, frequent exchanges overnight, particularly for patients with high permeability peritoneal membranes
- Use of icodextrin in long day dwell.

Tidal PD

Theoretically this should result in greater adequacy as the cycles are shorter and the residual fluid volume between cycles should allow slower diffusion. However, there is no difference in small solute clearance when tidal regimes have been compared with standard cycles with the same total volume of dialysate being used overnight. The indications for tidal PD are therefore when the patient experiences pain at the end of drainage or when poor drainage at the end of cycles results in alarms disturbing the patient's sleep.

APD is only really suited to patients with more permeable peritoneal membranes, as most of the dialysis is done overnight with short frequent exchanges. Patients with a low permeability membrane are not suitable for APD, as insufficient diffusion will occur during a short exchange (cycle), unless they have significant residual renal function. Thus a PET should be performed ideally before starting APD (if being changed from CAPD), or as soon as possible after commencing APD. Dialysis adequacy should be measured within 2 weeks of beginning APD (preferably) and alterations made to the dialysis prescription as needed. Larger patients will also have difficulty achieving adequate dialysis with APD, and require increased fill volumes.

Examples of alterations in automated peritoneal dialysis prescription

Increase hours on machine

A 48-year-old man on APD. Because of shift work he was unwilling to be on machine for more than 8h. PET testing—HA transporter.

- Initial prescription:
  - 5 × 2L exchanges over 8h at night
  - 2L × 2.27% glucose daytime dwell
  - 2L × 2.27% glucose manual exchange.
- Assessment:
  - plasma creatinine 1463µmol/L
  - residual renal function 0.8mL/min
  - Kt/V 2.2
  - C_{crea} 47L/week/1.73m².
- Interpretation: underdialysed.
- Action: increase hours on machine to 9h.
- Repeat assessment:
  - plasma creatinine 1337µmol/L
  - residual renal function 1.0mL/min
  - Kt/V 1.8
  - C_{crea} 59L/week/1.73m².

Adding daytime exchanges

A 63-year-old woman on APD because of incisional hernia. PET—HA transporter.

- Initial prescription:
  - 9L (6 × 1.5L exchanges) over 9h at night
  - no daytime fills (because of hernia).
- Assessment:
  - plasma creatinine 558µmol/L
  - residual renal function 2.5mL/min
  - Kt/V 2.1
  - C_{crea} 55L/week/1.73m².
- Assessment 6 months later:
  - plasma creatinine 764µmol/L
  - residual renal function 0.9mL/min
  - Kt/V 1.5
  - C_{crea} 37L/week/1.73m².
- Interpretation: loss of residual function.
- Action: agreed to hernia repair to allow daytime exchanges and larger fill volumes overnight.

- New prescription:
  - 5 × 2L exchanges over 9h at night
  - 1.5L × 2.27% glucose daytime dwell
  - 1.5L × 1.36% glucose tea-time exchange.
- Repeat assessment:
  - plasma creatinine   593μmol/L
  - residual renal function   0.5mL/min
  - Kt/V   2.2
  - C_{crea} 62L/week/1.73m^2.
- Interpretation: improved solute clearance despite loss of residual function.

Peritoneal dialysis in anuric patients

One of the major hurdles for PD is to provide adequate dialysis in the patient with little or no residual renal function. Using CAPD, it is difficult to increase the number and/or volume of exchanges. APD can overcome this difficulty as it is easier to increase the number and frequency of exchanges. The prescription should be individualized to the patient's BSA and membrane permeability (D/P). Patients often need a daytime exchange as well as a long day dwell (with fluid left in the peritoneum after disconnection from the machine). (See Table 5.14.)

- Patients with higher D/P ratio require increased number of exchanges at night.
- Patients with higher BSA require higher fill volume per exchange.
- Icodextrin should be considered for the long daytime dwell as it can improve UF and clearance.

Individualizing APD treatment:

- Assess membrane permeability by performing a PET test before starting APD.
- Assess patient's lifestyle to determine how long they can stay on the machine at night.
- Most anuric patients will require an extra daytime exchange—this can be performed manually or automatically through the machine (depending on the type of machine). All anuric patients should begin with an extra exchange that can be dropped if overachieving on clearance and UF targets.
- UF—a minimum of 1000mL daily is recommended. This can be achieved by using icodextrin for the long daytime exchange and/or by altering dwell times overnight. Higher glucose concentrations can also be used to increase UF.

Survival

EAPOS has shown that anuric patients can be successfully maintained on APD with the same survival as with other modes of dialysis. This is important, not just for patients already on PD, but also for HD patients who have no further vascular access.

Monitoring treatment

- Measure clearance at least every 6 months; more frequently if the patient is symptomatic of underdialysis or changes have been made to the dialysis regimen.
- If clearance is not reaching target, alterations can be made to number of hours on the machine overnight, total volume of dialysate, volume and number of exchanges overnight, volume of daytime exchanges.
- UF can be increased by using more overnight exchanges (i.e. decreasing cycle length) in high transporters (who tend to absorb peritoneal fluid), by increasing the glucose concentration of night and day exchanges, or by using icodextrin as the long day dwell.
- Sometimes it is helpful to repeat the PET and 'remodel' the patient.

Table 5.14 Peritoneal dialysis in anuric patients

Patient surface area	Permeability (D/P)			
	Low	Low average	High average	High
<1.71 BSA	CAPD	3×2.5L (9–10h o/n) *Plus* 2×2L daytime	4×2L (8h o/n) *Plus* 2×2L daytime	4×2.5L (8h o/n) *Plus* 2×2L daytime
1.71–2.0 BSA	CAPD or HD APD 3×2L (9–10h) *Plus* 2×2L daytime	3×3L (9–10h o/n) *Plus* 2×2.5L daytime	4×2.5L (8h o/n) *Plus* 2×2.5L Daytime	4×2.5L or 5×2L (8h o/n) *Plus* 2×2.5L daytime
>2.0 BSA	CAPD or HD APD 3×2L (9–10h o/n) *Plus* 2×3L daytime	CAPD or HD	4×3L (8h o/n) *Plus* 2×2.5L daytime	4–5×2.5L (8h o/n) *Plus* 2×2.5L daytime

o/n, overnight. BSA= 0.007184 × (patient's height, cm)$^{0.725}$ × (patient's weight, kg)$^{0.425}$.

Residual renal function

There is increasing evidence that preserving renal function impacts on dialysis outcomes beyond the higher clearances achieved. When looking at these studies, it is important to remember that the dialysis prescription has not always been increased to allow for the decline in renal function, sometimes because the study has been done in countries where there are economic limitations and HD is not an option.

- Important for fluid and solute removal.
- Salt and water removal important predictors of survival for patients on PD.
- Evidence of increased inflammation with declining residual renal function—higher inflammatory cytokine and CRP levels.
- Higher left ventricular mass has been found in patients with lower residual renal function due to hypervolaemia and worse BP control.
- Cohort studies in PD patients have shown that predictors of survival include residual renal function independently of other factors.
- Important for nutrition—worse nutrition has been observed in patients with lower residual renal function, presumably because of increased inflammation and need for fluid restriction.
- EPO dose required to maintain a stable Hb increases with declining residual renal function, partly because of increased inflammatory state and partly because of increasing uraemia.

Preserving residual renal function

Residual renal function persists for longer in patients on PD compared with HD due to the different effect of the two modalities on haemodynamic function. Furthermore, there are many ways of preserving residual renal function for longer in patients on PD.

- Use of ACEIs or ARBs—this is supported by some small RCTs.
- Avoid use of nephrotoxic agents:
  - X-ray contrast agents—make sure patient is well hydrated and consider using acetylcysteine beforehand (no good evidence for benefit)
  - aminoglycosides—only use when essential and monitor levels.
- Loop diuretics will increase urine output (but not GFR). There is one randomized study showing greater urine output in patients taking furosemide 250mg once daily compared with those taking no diuretic.
- Avoid fluid depletion—there is a risk of decline in residual renal function if fluid removal is increased too much in the quest for BP control.
- Some evidence that loss of residual renal function is greater in patients starting on APD compared with CAPD. This is not confirmed in all studies and may relate to the use of very rapid cycles, thereby increasing fluid loss on the overnight regime.
- There is very limited evidence that use of more biocompatible fluids may result in slower decline—theoretically this may be possible because of the reduction in inflammatory state. Randomized control evidence is awaited!

Causes of underdialysis

Feature of underdialysis include uraemic symptoms, hyperphosphataemia, and fluid overload. The principal reasons for this occurring are:

- Loss of residual renal function without increasing PD prescription:
  - Usually occurs at a steady rate so underdialysis can be avoided by pre-emptively increasing the PD prescription
  - Exposure to nephrotoxic agent, e.g. X-ray contrast material, nephrotoxic drugs
  - Fluid depletion
  - Hypotension
  - Cardiac event.
- Patient compliance—patients who choose PD value their independence and ability to take control. There are many reasons why patients do not carry out their prescribed regimen:
  - Denial of their need for dialysis
  - Social factors that make it difficult for them to do any sort of dialysis
  - Work demands, particularly shift patterns, making it difficult to keep to a regular regimen
  - Willing to do a limited regimen, e.g. 3 exchanges a day on CAPD or night exchanges on APD, but not to expand prescription as residual function declines.
- Poor compliance should be suspected under the following circumstances:
  - Plasma creatinine higher than expected for measured clearance
  - Fluid overload despite adequate UF
  - Evidence of poor compliance with medications—high BP, high phosphate, poorly controlled diabetes, etc.
- Peritoneal membrane factors:
  - *Low membrane transport* results in slow diffusion rates and a requirement for long exchanges. This makes it difficult to increase peritoneal clearance
  - *High membrane transport* causes poor UF when using long exchanges
  - *Loss of UF* can occur with prolonged time on PD.
- Patient factors:
  - Unable to increase volume of exchanges because of history of hernias or fluid leaks
  - Large body size—once anuric, it can be difficult to expand the PD regimen sufficiently for really large patients (BSA >2m^2)
  - Difficulty in fitting PD regimen round work, social, family demands
  - Patient does not want to transfer to HD—or cannot, if no vascular access.

Some patient examples

Patient 1

Sonia is 45 years old and started on CAPD 12 months ago. She is a single mother and lives with her 14-year-old daughter, and does not want HD. She still has some residual renal function and is meant to be doing 3 exchanges a day. She often misses clinic appointments and her blood test results are always high. On a rare visit, she looked clinically uraemic, BP was high at 173/112mmHg and Hb was 8.5g/dL despite being on EPO. She was not on the transplant list as she had no telephone. A few weeks later she told the PD team that her daughter was having drug problems, was known to the police, and had stolen her mobile phone. With help from social workers, these problems gradually resolved and Sonia found it easier to undertake her PD regimen.

Patient 2

Mr S was 82 years old. He had been on PD for 7 years. He had started on CAPD and for the first few years coped well despite chronic obstructive airways disease. When he became anuric he changed to APD with C_{crea} of 65L/week/1.73m^2, but he lost UF and became increasingly short of breath. He was also finding it difficult to cope with the PD himself. An AVF was therefore created but, prior to starting HD, he was admitted with an acute coronary event and pulmonary oedema. He had to have HD for fluid removal, but he had a cardiac arrest on his second dialysis. After this event the family decided it was best for him to stay on PD and his son helped with the APD. This went well for some months but unfortunately the son suddenly died from an MI. Following this Mr S returned to CAPD as this was easier for him and his wife. C_{crea} was low at 45L/week/1.73m^2, but Mr S did not want to transfer to HD. He stopped dialysis a few months later when he developed an ischaemic foot ulcer and would have required an amputation.

Patient 3

Sarah was a 42-year-old woman who had recently commenced on CAPD after being transplanted for 10 years and had been on PD prior to the transplant. She lost her residual renal function very quickly and was anuric within 6 months of starting PD. Initially she had been well, but then started losing her appetite and lost several kg in weight. A PET showed that she had low average membrane transport. Despite this she was transferred to APD, but despite increasing time on the machine to 10h, doing 6 × 2L exchanges overnight, using a daytime dwell and a daytime exchange, her clearance remained low at ~50L/week/1.73m^2 and she was clinically uraemic. Although she was not keen, she agreed to have an AVF and was transferred to HD.

Peritoneal dialysis-related infections

Infection in peritoneal dialysis can be divided into:
- exit site infection
- peritonitis.

Peritonitis continues to be a major cause of morbidity and technique failure for patients on PD and can directly lead to or contribute to mortality, particularly in patients with multiple comorbidity. Protocols for the prevention and management of infection are therefore essential for any PD unit. PD units should also regularly audit their infection rates, nature of infections, cure rates, and complications.

Reporting infection rates

Methods for reporting PD-related infections

- As rates (calculated for all infections and each organism):
  - Months of PD at risk, divided by number of episodes and expressed as interval in months between episodes.
  - Number of infections by organism for a time period, divided by dialysis-years' time at risk, and expressed as episodes per year.
- As percentage of patients who are peritonitis free per period of time.
- As median peritonitis rate for the programme (calculate peritonitis rate for each patient and then obtain the median of these rates).
- Relapsing episodes should not be counted as another peritonitis when calculating peritonitis rates; recurrent and repeat episodes should be counted.

Audit standards for peritonitis

- The International Society of Peritoneal Dialysis (ISPD) recommendation is for 1 episode/18 patient months (0.67 episodes/year at risk).[5]
- The UK Renal Association audit standards[6] are:
  - peritonitis rates of <1 episode per 18 months in adults and 12 months in children
  - a primary cure rate of ≥80%
  - a primary cure rate of ≥80%.
- Overall rates as low as 1 episode every 41–52 months (0.29–0.23/year) have been reported from some centres, e.g. from Hong Kong and Korea.

Terminology regarding peritonitis

The ISPD guidelines include the following definitions of peritonitis-related terminology:

- *Recurrent peritonitis:* an episode that occurs within 4 weeks of completion of therapy of a prior episode but with a different organism.
- *Relapsing peritonitis:* an episode that occurs within 4 weeks of completion of therapy of a prior episode with the same organism or 1 sterile episode.
- *Repeat peritonitis:* an episode that occurs more than 4 weeks after completion of therapy of a prior episode with the same organism.
- *Refractory peritonitis:* failure of the effluent to clear after 5 days of appropriate antibiotics.
- *Catheter-related peritonitis:* peritonitis in conjunction with an exit-site or tunnel infection with the same organism.

Exit site infections

Presentation

Infection round the PD catheter exit site can occur at any time from insertion of the catheter. Can be graded as:
- grade 1: area of redness round exit site
- grade 2: redness plus small amount of exudate on dressing, or crusting round exit site
- grade 3: frank pus exuding from exit site
- grade 4: abscess at exit site
- grade 5: tunnel infection—redness and tenderness on palpation over subcutaneous tunnel; the diagnosis of tunnel infection can be confirmed by US if necessary, which will show areas of loculated fluid along tunnel.

Cause

Most common organisms are *Staphylococcus aureus* and *Pseudomonas* spp. Incidence ~1 episode per 27 patient months. Increased risk in nasal *Staphylococcus* carriers (2- to 3-fold).

Treatment protocol

Redness alone

No treatment required. If redness persists, or is associated with itching, consider allergy to the cleaning fluid or dressing and change to saline alone.

Exudate or pus

It is essential to take a swab for culture before cleaning the exit site. The protocol on ➔ Performing an exit site dressing, p. 322 should then be followed.

Note
- Other organisms can also be found—follow culture results.
- If no improvement in infection consider catheter removal.
- If tunnel infection present, catheter is more likely to need removal, particularly if peritonitis also present.
- If infection recurs, consider removal of catheter, particularly if poor response to another course of antibiotics. (See Table 5.15.)
- If severe subcutaneous infection, patient should be placed on HD and another PD catheter should not be inserted until infection eradicated.
- If catheter being removed for recurrent infection, removal should be done after course of antibiotics—another PD catheter can then be inserted at same time (using a different exit site), thereby avoiding the need for HD. Some units have tried re-siting the extraperitoneal tunnel only, with some success.
- Exit site infection can progress to infection of the subcutaneous cuff. This can sometimes be successfully treated by deroofing over the cuff site, shaving of the cuff from the catheter (avoiding puncture of the tube itself), or complete catheter change. Cuff shaving usually ineffective for Gram-negative infections. (See Fig. 5.9.)

Table 5.15 Oral antibiotics used in exit-site and tunnel infection[7]

Amoxicillin	250–500mg bd
Cefalexin	500mg bd to tds
Ciprofloxacin	250mg bd
Clarithromycin	500mg loading dose, then 250mg bd
Erythromycin	500mg qds
Flucloxacillin	250–500mg qds
Fluconazole	200mg od for 2 days, then 100mg od
Flucytosine	0.5–1g/day
Linezolid	400–600mg bd
Metronidazole	400mg tds

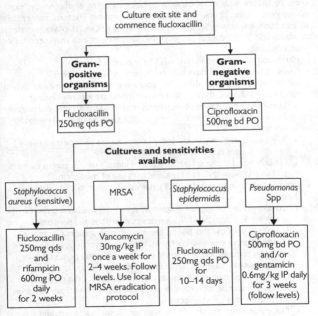

Fig. 5.9 Treatment of exit site infection.

Prevention of exit site infections

- Prophylactic antibiotics given at the time of catheter insertion reduce the risk of early infections. Vancomycin has been shown to be effective, but some units prefer not to use it because of the threat of emergence of vancomycin resistance. Good prophylaxis can also be achieved with cephalosporins, e.g. cefuroxime 1.5g.
- Good catheter exit site care will minimize exit site infections.
- It is important to reduce the number of *S. aureus* and *Pseudomonas* exit site infections as these can result in peritonitis, recurrent exit site infections, tunnel infections, and catheter loss.
- If MRSA is grown, patient should be placed on full local MRSA eradication protocol and should be isolated from other PD patients.

Topical mupirocin

Mupirocin is a naturally occurring antibiotic used topically as either a cream or ointment. It inhibits bacterial protein synthesis and shows no cross-resistance with most other antibiotics, including erythromycin, penicillins, gentamicin. There is no systemic absorption. Bacteria susceptible to its action are *Staphylococcus aureus* including MRSA, *Staphylococcus epidermidis*, and *Streptococcus pyogenes*. Mupirocin resistance may occur after prolonged use.

Mupirocin can be used in two ways to prevent infection:
- *Nasal application* for 5 days in patients known to be *S. aureus* carriers—this has been shown to reduce the risk of exit site infections in randomized studies, though data on peritonitis are less convincing:
  - Less risk of resistance as mupirocin is used intermittently, particularly if use is confined to patients known to have positive nasal swabs for *S. aureus*.
  - Regimen is cumbersome—5-day course has to be repeated every month; patient compliance is poor.
  - Patients need repeated nasal swabs to identify new *S. aureus* carriers and to motivate them to continue with use of mupirocin.
- *Topical application to exit site* in all patients whenever exit site dressing is changed:
  - Continued use of topical mupirocin at exit site has been shown to eradicate *S. aureus* and MRSA exit site infections and peritonitis.
  - In units that follow this policy, there is often an apparent increase in Gram-negative exit site infections. However, overall Gram-negative infection rates appear to remain constant while the percentage of infections rises (due to overall lower infection rates).
  - Emergence of mupirocin resistance has not been a clinical problem although it can be identified, probably because patients are at home so there is little cross-infection.
  - Mupirocin ointment should be used for Silastic® catheters and mupirocin cream for polyurethane catheters.

Topical gentamicin cream

Gentamicin is active against Gram-positive and Gram-negative organisms. One RCT has shown that exit site infection rates are lower in patients using topical gentamicin cream at the exit site compared with those using mupirocin, probably because there was a reduction in Gram-negative as well as Gram-positive infections. Patient numbers, however, were low and follow-up was only for 6 months. There are therefore no data on the emergence of gentamicin resistance. Gentamicin cream is not licensed in the UK though it can be obtained by hospital pharmacies. General use of topical gentamicin cream is therefore not recommended, but some units are using it in patients after a *Pseudomonas* exit site infection or when patients are known to be carriers of *Pseudomonas*.

Performing an exit site dressing

Supplies
- Absorbent perforated dressings
- Surgical adhesive tape
- 1 sterile gallipot
- Normal saline
- 1 packet sterile gauze swabs
- 1 alcohol wipe
- Alcohol gel
- Mupirocin nasal ointment or gentamicin cream.

Start of procedure
1. Wash hands with surgical scrub for 1min
2. Clean work surface with alcowipe
3. Open new dressing (leave inside wrapper)
4. Open gauze (leave inside wrapper)
5. Open gallipot (leave inside wrapper)
6. Fill gallipot with saline solution
7. Remove old dressing.

Looking for infection
1. Observe dressing—see if there is any staining.
2. Observe catheter exit site for sign of infection: redness, swelling, pus or bleeding, tenderness/pain.
3. Contact PD unit if present.

Completing dressing change
1. Apply hand gel and allow to dry.
2. Without touching the centre of the gauze square, join all 4 corners together and dip it in to the saline solution.
3. Using one circular movement, clean around the catheter, discard gauze.
4. Repeat steps 2 and 3 twice, every time using a new piece of gauze.
5. Without touching the centre of the gauze square, join all 4 corners together and using one circular movement dry around the catheter.
6. Using 5th piece of gauze squeeze some of the mupirocin ointment (or gentamicin cream) on to the gauze and apply around the exit site.
7. Apply new dressing over the catheter exit site.
8. Carefully anchor catheter with tape so that catheter is well immobilized.

Peritonitis

Peritonitis is one of the major risks of PD causing significant morbidity and in some instances mortality. It is one of the principal causes of dropout to HD. Peritonitis rates have fallen over the last 15 years from ~1 episode per 9 patient-months (single-bag system) to 1 episode per 24 patient-months (disconnect systems). A suggestion that lower rates of peritonitis can be achieved using APD probably reflects patient selection rather than a true benefit.

Aetiology

Two major routes of infection in the peritoneum:
- skin contaminants
- from within the peritoneum via the bowel.

Skin contaminants

These are introduced at the time of connections or via an infected exit site. *Staphylococcus aureus*, MRSA, and *S. epidermidis* (coagulase-negative staphylococcus) are the most common. Staphylococci adhere to the catheter, which can make eradication difficult. This is often the underlying cause of recurrent infections. *S. aureus* usually causes a more severe peritonitis than *S. epidermidis*. Frequency of *S. epidermidis* has decreased with increased use of disconnect systems, and *S. aureus* increased.

Pseudomonas infections can also occur via skin contamination, and are often associated with exit site infections.

Gram-negative infections

These are due to bowel organisms introduced into the peritoneum either by poor hygiene or directly from the bowel. Any pathological process increasing bowel permeability can cause peritonitis, most commonly episodes of diarrhoea or diverticulitis. Often mixed organisms are found. Bowel perforation (e.g. appendicitis) should also be considered with mixed Gram-negative peritonitis, especially if bacterial counts are high.

Other types of infection

- Fungal infections can occur following recent prolonged courses of antibiotics.
- TB in immunosuppressed individuals.
- Water-borne atypical mycobacteria very rarely.

Risk factors and prevention of peritonitis

Risk factors for development of peritonitis
- Number of connections and disconnections made each day between catheter or its attached line.
- Poor hand washing.
- Patient ability to carry out connections using sterile non-touch technique.
- Exit site infections, particularly tunnel infections.
- In hospital, exchanges being carried out by poorly trained personnel.
- Lack of clean area in home or at work to carry out exchanges.
- Poor eyesight unless special connection devices are used.
- Patients disconnecting themselves from APD machine at night (toilet, care for children, etc.).
- Diarrhoea, particularly if associated with poor hand washing.
- Diverticular disease, particularly if complicated by diverticulitis.
- Frequent use of IP antibiotics predisposes to fungal peritonitis.
- Peritonitis rates are not increased in diabetics or the elderly.

Prevention of peritonitis
Units should consider all the above factors. Prevention is also achieved by:
- careful selection of patients
- patient education and training
- training of carers (family members, paid individuals) who may help with exchanges
- avoiding constipation—many patients are elderly and will therefore have diverticular disease, and diverticulitis is more common when constipated
- use of antibiotic creams, e.g. mupirocin, gentamicin, at exit site
- repeated training of ward nurses about PD—this is essential given the frequent turnover of nurses
- isolating patients who are carriers of antibiotic-resistant bacteria, such as MRSA or VRE
- ensuring that exchanges are only done by trained personnel when patients are admitted for intercurrent illness or surgery.

Clinical features of peritonitis

- Abdominal pain (80% of patients)
- Cloudy fluid on drainage
- Fever (50%)
- Nausea (30%) and diarrhoea (7–10%)
- Poor drainage
- Loss of UF.

The severity of an episode of peritonitis depends on the causative organism. The need for hospitalization depends on the severity, and on the ability of the patient to carry out the treatment regimen. No organisms are grown from ~20% episodes (usually mild). *Staphylococcus epidermidis* peritonitis often clinically mild. Episodes due to *S. aureus* or Gram-negative infections are much more severe and have a worse prognosis.

Abdominal pain is a key symptom but very variable, and in some patients is not a feature until the bags have been cloudy for some days. Patients should be trained to report a cloudy bag as soon as they see one regardless of whether they have any other symptoms. Abdominal pain can be severe and require opiate analgesia. Fever occurs in more severe cases. If there is delay in diagnosis, or failure to respond to treatment, the fluid becomes increasingly turbid and eventually looks like 'pea soup'. Drainage can then become poor as the catheter becomes blocked. Even in milder cases, fibrin can form and block the catheter. Loss of UF is also a feature of peritonitis, and may persist even after the episode has cleared.

Complications

Most cases are mild and respond quickly to antibiotics. Complications occur when the diagnosis is delayed, or there is a poor response to treatment. They include:

- failure to respond, necessitating catheter removal and transfer to HD
- loss of UF
- loss of appetite and increased catabolism resulting in malnutrition
- fungal peritonitis after repeated courses of IP antibiotics
- persistent intra-abdominal sepsis requiring laparotomy and drainage
- formation of adhesions and later catheter malfunction
- ileus (in severe infections)
- death (rare).

Diagnosis of peritonitis

- Key investigation is microscopy and culture of drained peritoneal dialysate.
- Dialogue with microbiology laboratory is important to maximize culture positivity rates.
- Whole PD bags should be sent to the bacteriology laboratory. Fluid is either centrifuged or filtered to increase positive culture rates.
- Fluid sample can be obtained by aspirating with a syringe from a freshly drained bag, but may have a lower chance of positive culture.
- Fluid should not be obtained directly from the catheter as any break in the system carries the risk of introducing infection.
- The diagnosis of peritonitis is based on the number of white blood cells (WBC) found on microscopy alone: either >50 or >100WBC/mm^3.
- A Gram stain should be done if any organisms are seen on microscopy.
- Bacteria are present in low concentrations in PD fluid, so culture can be negative (~20% cases).
- Yield of positive cultures increased by inoculating fluid into blood culture bottles, or concentrating bacteria from whole PD bags.
- Positive cultures, in the absence of WBC on microscopy, usually represent contaminants and should therefore not be treated. Causes of sterile culture: antibiotics, poor culture technique, early sampling (bacterial count too low for isolation).

Differential diagnosis of cloudy fluid

- Bacterial peritonitis with positive cultures
- Bacterial peritonitis with negative cultures
- Chemical peritonitis, e.g. endotoxin
- Eosinophilic fluid
- Chylous fluid (rare)
- First sample drained after fluid flush of 'dry' abdomen
- Haemoperitoneum.

Treatment of peritonitis

Treatment of peritonitis

Principles

The recommendations made here are based on current guidelines from the International Society of Peritoneal Dialysis.

Treatment with antibiotics should be commenced at once in all patients with a cloudy bag and in those with positive microscopy—culture results should not be awaited. Most units treat peritonitis with IP antibiotics. The advantages are:

- high antibiotic concentration in peritoneum
- no IV access needed
- patients can administer antibiotics themselves, minimizing need for hospitalization.

IP antibiotics are systemically absorbed and blood levels of potentially toxic antibiotics such as vancomycin and aminoglycosides need to be monitored.

Numerous different antibiotic regimens have been developed in different hospitals. There is no evidence that one is any better than another as long as the following rules are followed:

- initial antibiotics with broad Gram-positive and Gram-negative cover
- peritoneal concentration of antibiotic high enough to eradicate infection (particularly important with oral antibiotics)
- follow-up of culture results and appropriate adjustments made to antibiotics
- allowance for renal excretion of antibiotics if there is residual renal function
- measurement of vancomycin and aminoglycoside blood levels (as appropriate) to avoid underdosing if patients have residual renal function, and overdosing with the potential side effects of nephrotoxicity and ototoxicity
- sufficient duration of treatment to avoid recurrence of infection
- ease of administration, especially by patients, to avoid need for admission to hospital.

Patient-friendly regimens are based on once-daily addition of antibiotics to dialysate. Antibiotic stability depends on the type of dialysate; it can be >48h with standard dialysate, but is much shorter in bicarbonate-based fluids. Patients therefore need to be trained to add antibiotics to dialysate bags or need to come up to the PD Unit to collect a pre-injected bag for immediate use. For patients on APD, the antibiotics are added to a bag that is given when the patient comes off the machine and then allowed to dwell for 6h.

Vancomycin and aminoglycosides

Traditionally, many regimens have been based on vancomycin and an aminoglycoside, e.g. gentamicin. Both are renally excreted and therefore need only intermittent administration—weekly with vancomycin (depending on residual renal function) and daily with gentamicin. Because of the emergence of VRE and the risk of development of vancomycin-resistant staphlycocci, the ISPD recommended in both their 1996 and 2000 guidelines that the use of vancomycin should be restricted in the treatment of peritonitis to those cases failing to respond to other standard treatment. These guidelines depended on the use of cefalotin or cefazolin (first-generation cephalosporins).

ISPD guidelines

Guidelines for management of peritoneal infection are published by the ISPD every 4–5 years. The most recent were published in 2010. The mainstay of treatment is for the initial antibiotic regimen to provide cover against Gram-positive and Gram-negative organisms. Traditionally this has been achieved by the use of vancomycin and aminoglycosides, usually gentamicin. There have been changes over the years owing to concerns about the development of vancomycin resistance and nephrotoxicity-related aminoglycosides.

- 1996—avoidance of vancomycin with initial treatment based on first-generation cephalosporins, such as cefazolin, added to each exchange, with gentamicin added to one exchange each day.
- 2000—recommendation changed to avoid aminoglycoside use in patients with residual renal function; cefazolin and ceftazidime were the initial antibiotics in patients with residual renal function, and cefazolin and gentamicin if no residual renal function. However, there was little evidence to support this view, and evidence in larger groups of patients suggested that the use of gentamicin for treatment of peritonitis did not affect residual renal function if blood levels were monitored and dose adjusted as needed.
- 2005—recognizes that no hard evidence for any particular regimen, that vancomycin resistance has not proved (so far) to be as major a problem as originally feared, and that, as discussed above, gentamicin can be used if carefully monitored. No hard guidance therefore given for particular antibiotics, but rather advice that antibiotics used should cover local antibiotic sensitivities of common organisms.
- 2010—empiric antibiotics must cover both Gram-positive and Gram-negative organisms. Selection of empiric therapy should be centre-specific dependent on the local history of sensitivities of organisms causing peritonitis. Gram-positive organisms may be covered by vancomycin or a cephalosporin, and Gram-negative organisms by a third-generation cephalosporin or aminoglycoside.

ISPD guidelines 2010

Initial treatment with vancomycin/gentamicin.

Cefazolin is no longer licensed in the UK—this plus the fact that bioavailability is <24h in bicarbonate-based fluids has resulted in more units using a vancomycin-based regimen. Fortunately, vancomycin-resistant enterococci have not become as common as feared when first detected in the 1990s.

Day 1	Send PD fluid for micro and culture; clean up exit site if inflamed
	Treatment:
	Vancomycin 30mg/kg IP up to total dose of 2g
	Gentamicin 1.5mg/kg IP (if urine output >500mL/24h)
	0.6mg/kg IP (if urine output <500mL/24h)
	Allow exchange with antibiotics to dwell for 6h
	Then gentamicin 0.6mg/kg to be given daily until cultures available
	Patient must return on a daily basis for administration of gentamicin or be trained to inject antibiotics into dialysate fluid immediately prior to use
	If patient on APD, antibiotics should be added to 1.5 or 2L bag which should be allowed to dwell for a minimum of 6h
Day 4	Patient returns to PD unit—change treatment according to PD fluid culture result and response to treatment

Treatment based on microbiology

Treatment changes based on microbiological diagnosis. (See Table 5.16.)

Table 5.16 Treatment based on organisms

Organism	Treatment	Duration
Staphylococcus epidermidis	Stop gentamicin Continue *vancomycin* according to levels	14 days
Staphylococcus aureus	Stop gentamicin Continue *vancomycin* according to levels Consider adding rifampicin 300mg bd orally (discuss with microbiologists)	21 days
Enterococcus spp.	Continue *gentamicin* 0.6mg/kg IP daily (according to levels) Add *amoxicillin* 125mg/L to each exchange Patient needs to inject these themselves just before use. If patient unable to inject own bags, further treatment should be *vancomycin* alone	14 days
Culture negative	Continue *vancomycin* according to levels Stop *gentamicin* Start *ciprofloxacin 500mg bd orally*	14 days
Gram-negative rod	Continue *gentamicin* 0.6mg/kg IP daily (according to levels)	14 days
Pseudomonas spp.	ADMIT TO HOSPITAL Continue *gentamicin* (according to levels) AND discuss with microbiologists to choose appropriate 2nd agent Consider catheter removal	21 days
Fungal	ADMIT TO HOSPITAL Flucytosine loading dose 50mg/kg orally in 4 divided doses and then 500mg bd (monitor blood levels) AND fluconazole, 200mg orally or IP daily If no improvement by day 3, remove catheter If improving continue antifungal treatment (with low threshold for catheter removal)	4–6 weeks or 7 days after catheter removal

Monitoring and response to treatment

If patient ill, admit to hospital—monitor temperature, WBC, CRP, appearance of dialysate

Day 2—if poor clinical response, reculture

Day 3—if poor clinical response, check cultures and change antibiotics if appropriate

Day 4—*if still poor response (persistent cloudy fluid, high CRP and WBC), REMOVE CATHETER*

Clinical monitoring

Patients and their treatment need close monitoring during an episode of peritonitis.

- If patient ill: admit to hospital immediately, monitor temperature, WBC, CRP, appearance of dialysate.
- Day 2: if poor clinical response, re-culture PD fluid and blood.
- Day 3: if poor clinical response, check cultures and change antibiotics if appropriate.
- Day 4: if still poor response (persistent cloudy PD fluid, high CRP and WBC), *remove catheter*. Do not delay further.

Prescribing vancomycin

- Dose: 30mg/kg IP (round to nearest 250mg; max dose 2g).
- Frequency: every 5–7 days depending on blood levels.
- Patients with residual renal function or on APD will need more frequent dosing.
- Repeat doses: aim to maintain blood level ≥10mg/L. Higher blood levels may be indicated in units with significant prevalence of intermediate vancomycin resistance.
- Check blood levels when patient returns at 4 days:
  - if ≤12mg/L, bring patient back next day (day 5) for repeat dose
  - if 13–15mg/L, repeat dose 2 days later (day 6)
  - if 15mg/L, take blood level and give repeat dose 3 days later (day 7)
  - if repeat dose given at day 5, bring back for repeat blood level on day 9 and give further dose according to above schedule
  - if repeat dose given at day 6, bring back for repeat blood level on day 11 and give further dose according to above schedule.

Prescribing gentamicin

- Dose: 0.6mg/kg IP.
- Frequency: daily, but dose may need to be changed according to blood levels.
- Repeat doses: aim to maintain blood level 2–4mg/L.
- Check blood levels every 3–4 days when patient returns to collect pre-injected dialysate bags:
  - if ≤2mg/L, give new supply of bags with dose increased by 0.2mg/kg (patient must start on fresh supply of bags with new dose within 24h)
  - if 2–4 mg/L, no change
  - if 4–5mg/L, reduce dose by 0.2mg/kg with supply of bags given at next visit
  - if 5–6mg/L, give new supply of bags with dose decreased by 0.2mg/kg (patient must start on fresh supply of bags with new dose within 24h)
  - if ≥7 mg/L, miss a day and reduce dose.
- Blood levels *must* be checked at every visit.

TB peritonitis

- Should be suspected if patient comes from endemic area with culture-negative peritonitis and mostly lymphocytes in PD effluent. Also occurs in immigrants from developing countries.
- Can also be associated with refractory bacterial peritonitis.
- Can be caused by atypical *Mycobacterium* spp.
- Most patients respond to triple antituberculous therapy, though catheter removal may be needed, particularly if atypical *Mycobacterium* spp.
- TB peritonitis is not necessarily associated with long-term morbidity, and many patients will be able to continue with PD or return to PD after treatment.

Treatment of automated peritoneal dialysis peritonitis

- Patients can continue on usual APD regimen with antibiotics added to daytime exchange.
- Some units have a policy that patients are changed to CAPD for treatment of peritonitis—this is unnecessary and can be inconvenient for the patient requiring long hospital stays if they do not have CAPD stocks at home and/or are not familiar with performing CAPD.
- There have been concerns that patients may present late, as cloudy fluid could be missed, as the PD fluid drained from the machine is much more dilute than in CAPD (larger volumes). This might be a problem particularly if overnight fluid is drained directly into waste (e.g. a drain) and not into a bag.
- Cure rates of APD peritonitis treated by adding antibiotics to the day time dwell are the same as for CAPD (i.e. ~80%).
- Use of rapid exchanges may affect antibiotic pharmacokinetics, with need to increase dose (with once-daily antibiotic) or frequency of dosing (with vancomycin).

Treatment of refractory peritonitis

Peritonitis failing to respond to treatment

Patient should symptomatically feel better and fluid should be clear within 2–3 days of starting treatment.

If not:
- Check antibiotic sensitivities and re-culture fluid.
- Consider removal of PD catheter if:
  - patient remains symptomatically unwell, i.e. remains febrile or no improvement in abdominal pain
  - evidence of increasing sepsis, i.e. hypotension, fever, etc.
  - fluid fails to clear despite appropriate treatment for 4 days
  - fluid becomes increasingly turbid
  - catheter becomes blocked by thick fluid
  - exit site infection or tunnel infection due to same organism as peritonitis
  - peritonitis has become recurrent, i.e. repeat infection due to same organism within 4 weeks of original infection.

Removal of PD catheter

- This should not be delayed beyond 4 days from onset of non-responsive peritonitis as delay results in increased morbidity after catheter removal.
- Usually a simple procedure, but will need a general anaesthetic as Dacron® cuffs of catheter will be surrounded by fibrous tissue.
- Consider laparotomy if increasing sepsis, or in presence of ≥2 Gram-negative organisms, suggesting a possible bowel lesion.

Reinsertion of PD catheter

Many patients want to restart PD even after a severe episode of peritonitis requiring catheter removal. Patients may have poor vascular access necessitating a further attempt at PD.
- Allow at least 4 weeks before reinserting catheter.
- The catheter should be inserted surgically or laparoscopically because of the risk of adhesions, except after relatively mild peritonitis (catheter removed only because of persistently turbid fluid, or because of recurrent peritonitis with the last episode being treatable).
- The catheter should be sutured into the pelvis at the first attempt at reinsertion, so that it is placed appropriately if there are any adhesions.
- Consider forming an AVF for HD at same time the patient is having a general anaesthetic, as there is an increased risk of catheter malfunction.
- Retrain patient when recommencing PD to ensure there are no technique problems.

Complications of peritonitis

Peritonitis remains a major cause of dropout from PD to HD. 20% of patients with peritonitis do not respond to antibiotic treatment. Even if the episode has been fully treated without catheter removal, long-term morbidity can result:

- poor nutrition due to the catabolic state associated with peritonitis
- loss of UF during and after an episode
- repeated episodes of peritonitis can cause long-term UF failure necessitating transfer to HD
- use of broad-spectrum antibiotics can cause diarrhoea from *Clostridium difficile* infection
- fungal peritonitis may develop after repeated courses of IP antibiotics
- intra-abdominal adhesions making further PD difficult
- ileus, fluid collections, and/or abscess formation, especially if catheter removal is delayed
- ascites—this can be massive and can persist for months after catheter removal; frequent drainage may be required, with associated loss of protein resulting in worsening nutritional state
- encapsulating peritoneal sclerosis
- death—there is a mortality rate of 2–5% with peritonitis, particularly in patients with multiple co-morbidities and the elderly.

Encapsulating peritoneal sclerosis

Clinical features

Encapsulating peritoneal sclerosis (EPS) is a devastating complication of long-term PD. Prevalence is ~2% in patients on PD for 4 years and ~10% in patients on PD for 8 years. Peritoneal biopsy studies suggest that peritoneal fibrosis and sclerosis occurs with increased time on dialysis; a small proportion will then progress on to EPS, when a thick-walled membranous cocoon wraps itself round loops of bowel causing intestinal obstruction and subsequent malnutrition.

Clinical course

- Clinical symptoms at presentation include symptoms suggestive of bowel obstruction (abdominal pain, intermittent constipation, vomiting), weight loss, ascites (which can be haemorrhagic).
- Most commonly symptoms occur after PD is discontinued and patient transferred to HD or transplanted.
- Onset can be very rapid particularly after severe peritonitis.
- An inflammatory process occurs in some patients prior to onset of EPS with abdominal pain, sterile peritonitis, or ascites and raised CRP.
- Determinants of developing EPS appear to be:
  - UF failure
  - length of time on PD
  - loss of residual renal function
  - change in membrane transport status to 'high'
  - severe peritonitis.
- Clinical course is variable:
  - *Severe cases* progress rapidly over weeks/months to complete bowel obstruction with severe malnutrition and eventual death, though some patients can be maintained on parenteral nutrition.
  - *Moderate cases* have a less progressive and more intermittent course with nutrition maintained by patients learning to eat small amounts frequently and the use of oral nutritional supplements.
  - *Mild cases* can lose all their symptoms over time and not require any dietary manipulations.
- With increasing awareness of EPS as a complication of PD and increasing numbers of long-term PD patients, the diagnosis is being made more frequently, resulting in an apparent increase in EPS.

Diagnosis

Ideally the diagnosis should be made early during the inflammatory stage or before the patient becomes severely malnourished from recurrent bowel obstruction.

- *Clinical features:* a high index of suspicion is needed to make diagnosis at early stages, particularly in patients who have recently changed to HD or been transplanted after many years on PD:
  - unexplained haemorrhagic ascites
  - unexplained high CRP with abdominal pain
  - unexplained weight loss.

- *Abdominal X-ray* is not particularly helpful but may show peritoneal calcification in more advanced cases.
- *Abdominal CT scan* (with contrast to show peritoneal thickening more easily) is becoming the standard method of diagnosing EPS. Abnormalities on CT scan consist of:
  - peritoneal thickening
  - peritoneal calcification
  - thickened bowel loops
  - dilated bowel
  - abnormal bowel distribution with bowel pulled into centre of abdominal cavity ('fist sign')
  - presence of ascites which is often loculated (if patient now on HD or transplanted).
- *MRI scan* has been suggested as a useful tool, but there is little experience of its use:
  - Fast scans have to be used because of bowel movement.
  - Does not demonstrate peritoneal calcification.
- *Surgery* demonstrating classical fibrous cocoon encasing bowel remains the gold standard method of making diagnosis, but is not indicated in majority of patients and carries high risk of bowel perforation. Should generally be avoided unless carried out in specialized centres

Treatment

As EPS is rare, reports of treatment outcomes are anecdotal; there are no randomized clinical trials.

- *Drug treatment:*
  - Immunosuppression—prednisolone, ciclosporin, tamoxifen have all been used; may be useful if evidence of inflammation, e.g. raised CRP. Onset of EPS after transplantation when patients already on large doses of immunosuppression does suggest that this approach is not an effective treatment.
  - Tamoxifen (antifibrotic and reduces transforming growth factor-β) has been reported as effective in some case reports, though not confirmed in all series. Tamoxifen is prothrombotic, and calciphylaxis has been reported as a life-threatening complication of its use in EPS.
  - Sirolimus has been tried because of its antifibrotic actions—however, also immunosuppressive with high risk of infection, and no convincing evidence of any benefit.
- *Surgery* to release loops of bowel from the fibrous cocoon has high morbidity and mortality because of risk of perforating bowel unless done by experienced teams:
  - Adhesionolysis with careful dissection and removal of the fibrous cocoon and freeing up of the bowel loops can be effective for obstructive disease but has to be done by an enthusiast—operation takes hours and may need to be redone as there is a significant relapse rate.
  - Success higher if patient not malnourished—some time on parenteral nutrition may therefore be beneficial before undertaking surgery.

Nutritional support

This is probably the most effective method of reducing mortality and morbidity associated with EPS.
• All patients should have regular dietetic review.
• Patient should be educated to eat small amounts frequently.
• *Oral supplements* should be started if food intake thought to be inadequate or if weight loss occurs.
• *Parenteral nutrition* should be considered if severe symptoms of bowel obstruction and/or weight loss continues despite oral food supplements:
  • High risk of infection from central lines used for parenteral nutrition. Decision of starting parenteral nutrition should therefore not be taken lightly.
  • This is particularly true for patients who are immunosuppressed post transplantation.
  • Dedicated feeding line must therefore be used—avoid temptation to use it for drugs, other fluids, blood-taking just because patient has bad veins (not uncommon in patients who have been on dialysis for years!).
  • If patient on HD, volume control is often difficult.
  • Despite all this, some patients do well on home parenteral nutrition and can survive for years.
  • Some patients can manage to return to oral nutrition after a period of bowel rest on parenteral nutrition.

Causes and prevention of EPS

The abdomen is not designed for PD—it is therefore hardly surprising that carrying out PD for years can result in this potentially devastating complication. The factors in peritoneal dialysate thought to cause EPS include:
• high glucose concentration—particularly use of 3.86% glucose
• bioincompatibility:
  • low pH
  • presence of GDPs.

Use of more biocompatible, pH neutral, bicarbonate-based fluids appears to cause a smaller rise in inflammatory cytokines and may therefore delay the onset of changes leading to EPS. Animal studies appear to confirm this possibility, but the new fluids have not yet been used for long enough in patients to determine whether they prevent or delay the onset of EPS and thereby enable patients to remain on PD for longer.

Screening for EPS

Ideally, patients should be screened for EPS and stop PD if any suggestion of its development. However, there is no good screening method, though some units now do routine CT scans at 4–5 years.
• Changes on CT scan seem to appear at a late stage in the development of EPS; patients can have a 'normal' scan and develop EPS weeks to months later.

- MRI scan has been suggested as a screening tool, but it is expensive, fast scans are needed and peritoneal calcification would be missed.
- Clinical markers such as declining UF, rising D/P on PET, no residual renal function, are often found but may just be markers of time on PD. EPS can certainly occur in patients with none of these features.
- If EPS is suspected, transfer to HD may not be optimal management as stopping PD is well known to provoke the onset of EPS.

Length of time on peritoneal dialysis: ISPD position paper

In 2009, the ISPD convened an international working party to determine whether the length of time on PD should be limited because of the risk of EPS.[8] The working party concluded that there was a need to avoid blanket rules:

- EPS occurs in minority of long-term patients
- With good nutritional management and/or surgery, morbidity and mortality reduced
- Taking patients off PD may precipitate EPS and symptoms usually milder on PD
- Need to take into account patient quality of life, preferences, and life expectancy.

Recommendations of ISPD working party

- Risk for developing EPS is considered to be extremely low during first 3 years of PD, and low for patients <5 years on PD.
- The development of EPS should be considered as a potential risk after 3–5 years on PD.
- There is no benefit of screening for a 'pre-EPS' state by using the clinical indicators mentioned above, or by radiology using CT scanning
- *For patients who want to remain on PD for as long as possible, recommendations are:*
  - discussion about potential risks of continuing PD (UF failure, EPS) and of starting HD (vascular access, endocarditis, osteomyelitis, haemodynamic intolerance)
  - vascular access should be discussed and planned with the patient prior to transfer to HD
  - ensure that eligible patients are on a transplant list as soon as possible after starting dialysis. Possible living donors should be discussed annually with all patients.
- *Older patients and those with comorbidities have a limited life expectancy when starting dialysis.*
  - Few will therefore survive long enough on PD to be at risk of developing EPS.
  - Such patients are unlikely to be candidates for transplantation so their quality of life on dialysis is very important.
  - Important to consider realistically life expectancy, feasibility of HD for that patient and how this would affect their quality of life.

Discussions with the patient should be part of a shared decision making process about overall prognosis and future goals of care.

Hernias, leaks, and other complications

Although peritonitis is always considered to be the main complication of PD, there are many others. (See Table 5.17.)

Table 5.17 Complications of PD

Cause of complication	Complication
Presence of intra-abdominal fluid	Hernias
	Fluid leaks
	Rectal prolapse
	Vaginal prolapse
	Lumbar back pain
	Pain on inflow of fluid into peritoneum
	Decrease in appetite
Infection	Exit site infection
	Tunnel infection
	Peritonitis
Catheter migration	Poor drainage
Protein losses into dialysate	Hypoalbuminaemia
	Poor nutrition
Membrane changes	Loss of UF
Social factors	Social isolation
	PD 'burn-out'

Hernias

Occur in up to 15–20% of patients. The most common are incisional (related to catheter insertion or to previous abdominal operations), inguinal, and umbilical. Hernias can occur at many other orifices, and all have been reported in patients on PD. They are usually reducible, but can strangulate if the orifice is small. They are caused by increased intra-abdominal pressure and are more common with higher volume exchanges, and when dialysate volume is increased to improve adequacy. In men, a patent processus vaginalis can allow fluid to track into the scrotum, mimicking a hernia.

Any hernia detected before the onset of PD should be repaired prior to (or at same time as) PD catheter insertion.

Management

- Surgical repair of hernia.
- Reduction in exchange volume, conversion to APD overnight, or IPD if there is any delay in surgery (lower intra-abdominal pressure when patient is supine).
- HD (or IPD if HD not possible) for 2–3 weeks after surgery—hernia is more likely to recur if CAPD or daytime exchanges of APD started too early.
- Delay in using full exchange volume for first 2 weeks of CAPD or APD, to reduce risk of recurrence. If hernia recurs after surgical repair:
  - consider repeat surgery with longer period on HD after repair—depends on size and location of hernia
  - if there is residual renal function, change from CAPD to APD at night only (i.e. no daytime exchange)—dialysis adequacy will need to be carefully monitored
  - consider use of elasticated support girdle with abdominal hernia or truss with inguinal hernia
  - patient may have to be converted to HD.

Fluid leaks

Can be early or late.

Early

Immediately after catheter insertion, fluid leaks through the exit site if it is not yet fully healed. This carries a risk of exit site infection.

Management

Discontinue dialysis until exit site is fully healed. Lower volume exchanges should then be used to ensure that no fluid leakage occurs before the patient is established on a standard regimen.

Late

Once the exit site has healed, fluid can still leak from the peritoneum, but as there is no passage through the skin, the fluid will pool in subcutaneous tissues. Patients present with, often massive, abdominal wall and leg oedema. In men, fluid can track into the scrotum causing hydrocoeles. Patients often notice poor fluid drainage. Although the defect in the peritoneum is often at the site of catheter insertion, fluid can also leak into the scrotum if there is a defect in the inguinal canal. These leaks are most frequent within the first month of a new catheter, but can occur at any time, particularly if exchange volume is increased.

Management

- If leak is into lower abdominal wall only, discontinue PD for 2–3 weeks. No other dialysis may be needed if there is adequate residual renal function, otherwise HD or IPD (lower intra-abdominal pressure when supine).
- Use lower volume daytime exchanges for first 2 weeks of recommencing PD.
- If there is scrotal swelling, or the abdominal wall leak recurs, the patient should be investigated to look for hernias.
    - *Ultrasound* with fluid in peritoneum; site of leak and any hernia are easily delineated—best test to use as non-invasive and can be done very quickly, but operator dependent.
    - *CT scan* with contrast material injected into peritoneum—invasive so risk of peritonitis—but good visualization of leak and/or hernia.
    - *MRI scan* gives good visualization and is non-invasive—more expensive and not always readily available.
- While waiting for surgical repair, patient should be changed to night-time exchanges only if on APD, or if on CAPD, low volume exchanges or no dialysis if adequate residual renal function. Dialysis adequacy needs to be carefully monitored.

Pleuroperitoneal leak

Occurs in 1–10% of patients, presents with pleural effusion (with high glucose content), and can be confirmed by contrast peritoneography or radiolabelled albumin or sulphur colloid instilled into the peritoneum. Treatment (drainage, pleuradhesis) usually unsuccessful. Resolve spontaneously in 40% of cases.

Prolapses and pain

Prolapses

Rectal and vaginal prolapse are not common but are related to increased intra-abdominal pressure. Management is similar to that of herniae, i.e. surgical repair if possible, followed by a period of HD and then reduced exchange volumes to minimize risk of recurrence.

Back pain

Lumbar back pain is usually caused by development of a lumbar lordosis from the weight and volume of fluid in the abdomen. The pain is usually mild, but can be severe enough to discontinue PD and change to HD.

Inflow pain

Pain on inflow of fluid is not uncommon in the first 2 weeks of PD and usually resolves spontaneously. Check line position, constipation, and dialysate temperature. Pain is often reduced if a clamp is put on the line to reduce the rate of dialysate inflow. Persistent pain is usually caused by irritation of the peritoneum by the acidic dialysate fluid. Inflow pain is much less frequent when using biocompatible dialysate.

Other complications of peritoneal dialysis

Malnutrition

Poor nutrition is a feature of both HD and PD. The contributing factors on PD include:

- decreased appetite in some patients because of a feeling of abdominal fullness—sometimes patients can eat more if they drain out before a meal
- protein losses in dialysate, particularly during peritonitis
- loss in dialysis adequacy as residual renal function declines.

Membrane changes

Occur with time on PD. Often the permeability increases with resultant loss of UF. This can be managed by changing to APD and/or using icodextrin. UF failure is an important cause of dropout to HD.

Haemoperitoneum

Occurs in 6–50% of patients and is usually transient. Can occur in menstruating women. May require additional catheter flushes to prevent blockage, and occasionally heparin instillation into catheter. Also caused by pancreatitis, ruptured ovarian or hepatic cysts, sclerosing peritonitis, and other intra-abdominal pathology.

Eosinophilic peritonitis

Rare, usually sterile, and often caused by reaction to the PD catheter itself. Rare causes are fungal peritonitis, or allergic reactions to vancomycin or icodextrin.

Social complications of PD

Should not be underestimated. If a patient feels isolated or develops burnout, their technique will be less good, with the risk of developing peritonitis. Anorexia and poor nutrition will also occur if the patient becomes isolated or depressed. Social factors contribute significantly to dropout from PD to HD.

Pre-operative assessment for peritoneal dialysis patients

PD is a continuous treatment not requiring anticoagulation or vascular access, and so the timing of surgery and pre-operative care is much simpler than for patients on HD.

Pre-operative assessment and management:

- Full blood count, plasma potassium, ECG, and CXR.
- Insulin infusion should be commenced in diabetics.
- PD should be adjusted to ensure that patient is euvolaemic at time of surgery.
- If blood transfusion is required, ensure that volume overload does not occur by using higher strength glucose dialysate, or by transferring patient to IPD for the transfusion (to increase UF).
- Dialysate should be drained so that abdomen is empty prior to surgery:
  - essential for any abdominal surgery
  - prevents limitation to movement of diaphragm and respiratory compromise by high intra-abdominal pressure.
- IV cannulae should not be placed in either forearm—the patient may need a fistula in the future so all potential veins should be preserved.
- If it is anticipated that HD will be needed post-operatively, an internal jugular CVC should be inserted while the patient is anaesthetized.

Post-operative management for peritoneal dialysis patients

- Plasma potassium should be checked as soon as possible after surgery (potassium increased by tissue trauma, blood transfusions, haematomas, potassium-containing infusions).
- PD can be restarted immediately after non-abdominal surgery (use smaller volumes if respiratory problems).
- Avoid PD completely for a few days after abdominal surgery because of the risk of fluid leakage.
- Recommence PD a week after abdominal surgery (assuming any drains have been removed), preferably using IPD or daytime dwells of APD, to avoid prolonged periods of raised intra-abdominal pressure that may occur with CAPD.
- Patients with little or no residual renal function will need HD in the early post-operative period after abdominal surgery.
- Patients with significant residual renal function (GFR >5mL/min) may not need any dialysis until it is safe to recommence PD. The patient must be closely monitored during this time, especially volume status and potassium.
- CAPD or the daytime exchanges of APD can be restarted once abdominal wounds are completely healed (usually ~2 weeks). Restart with small volume exchanges, e.g. 1.5L for the first week.
- After extensive bowel surgery it may not be possible to return the patient to PD due to the formation of adhesions causing poor drainage. PD must be discontinued if a colostomy or ileostomy is formed.
- Avoid nephrotoxins (NSAIDs, gentamicin, X-ray contrast) as residual renal function of crucial importance in overall adequacy of PD.

Peritoneal dialysis and transplantation

PD has no influence on graft survival. Some units continue patients on PD if dialysis is required post-transplantation, while others transfer patients to HD. Transplant surgery is usually extraperitoneal so there is little risk of fluid leakage post-transplantation. If the peritoneum has been breached PD should be withheld for 1–2 weeks. Even when HD is used post-transplantation, the PD catheter can be left *in situ*. Provided the exit site is regularly dressed, the risk of developing exit site infection is minimal. The catheter can then be removed once transplant function is established. If the transplant fails and the patient has to return to dialysis, PD can be re-established with minimal trauma (physical and psychological). (See Table 5.18.)

Table 5.18 Advantages and disadvantages of PD and HD post-transplantation in PD patients

	PD	HD
Advantages	Avoids insertion of neck vein catheter	Most transplant nurses trained in HD
	Continuous dialysis with minimal fluid shifts and reduced risk of hypotension	Dialysis adequacy and fluid removal more easily controlled
	Avoids use of heparin, so reduced risk of bleeding post-operatively or after transplant biopsy	
Disadvantages	Transplant nursing staff need to be trained in PD	Risks of central venous catheterization
	Risk of peritonitis in immunosuppressed patient	Risk of septicaemia from temporary neck line
	Dialysis adequacy in PD depends on residual renal function, which may fall post-transplant if patient becomes hypotensive or septicaemic	Risk to transplant of episodic hypotension

Transfer of PD patient to HD

Successful transfer to HD after a period of time on PD is a feature of integrated care. Outcomes, including survival, are obviously better if this transfer is achieved in a planned manner and not precipitated by an acute event. The need for transfer should therefore be anticipated and discussed with the patient and his/her family so there is time to create functional vascular access.

Indications for elective transfer to HD

Medical
- Difficulty in achieving small solute clearance despite increasing dialysis prescription and changing PD modality (if appropriate)
- Difficulty in achieving adequate UF to maintain euvolaemia
- Recurrent catheter problems
- Anticipated decline in residual renal function that would result in underdialysis and patient already using maximal PD prescription
- Increasing risk of EPS—see ⊃ Encapsulating peritoneal sclerosis, p. 335.

Psychosocial
- Increasing difficulty in performing PD because of changing social factors or physical disability of patient (e.g. deteriorating vision, decreased hand dexterity, decreased mobility)
- Depression
- Burnout of patient and/or family after long period of time on PD
- Poor compliance, though many such patients will comply equally poorly with HD.

Acute transfer to HD

Acute unplanned transfer to HD means that the patient is usually sicker and acute vascular access with CVCs is required. It is therefore not surprising that such transfers are associated with extended hospital stays and/or mortality. Transfer to HD is usually multifactorial, and the acute event comes as no surprise and could have been avoided if elective vascular access had been created.

Causes of acute transfer
- Peritonitis not responding to treatment and needing catheter removal. This can be unexpected but can be anticipated to occur more frequently in patients who are unwell because of poor dialysis or other illness, or who have the psychosocial problems listed above.
- Symptomatic underdialysis and/or fluid overload; both of these can usually be anticipated unless there has been an unexpected rapid decline in residual renal function.
- Sudden change in social circumstances, e.g. death of family carer.
- Intercurrent illness preventing patient from being able to do own PD e.g. stroke, amputation.

Is there a time limit to PD?

Despite the conclusions of the ISPD position paper (see ➋ Length of time on peritoneal dialysis: ISPD position paper, p. 340) some feel that patients should electively stop PD after 5 years because of the increasing risk of EPS (see ➋ Screening for EPS, p. 337). Factors to consider for each patient include:

- overall prognosis—if patient has poor predictors for long-term survival, e.g. age, co-morbidity, other illness, then there is no indication for elective transfer to HD just because they have been on PD for a certain period of time
- risk factors for EPS—no residual renal function, rising transport status on peritoneal membrane function tests, declining UF
- changes on screening CT scan such as peritoneal calcification and/or bowel tethering or dilatation; peritoneal thickening on its own is not a good indicator for future EPS
- likelihood of transplantation—patients and families are often prepared to reconsider issue of living donation rather than transfer to HD
- patient wishes—many patients prefer to stay on PD because of the quality of life it offers rather than change to HD.

Effecting transfer to HD

Many patients are reluctant to transfer to HD as they prefer quality of life offered by PD and are used to support from PD team. Communication and joint decision making are therefore vital.

- Education and sharing information with patients about dialysis adequacy and importance of residual renal function throughout time on PD enables patient to understand why prescription needs changing and why transfer to HD may be necessary.
- AVF does not have to be used immediately—patients may accept it as an insurance policy if things change.
- Patient should be able to visit local HD unit so that links can be made with new nursing team and they can see new environment.
- Discuss possibility of home HD—enables those who can to remain on a home treatment with all its advantages.
- Some patients just refuse to transfer to HD despite all the information given to them—they cannot be forced to change, but the situation can be rediscussed.
- Initiating HD as once a week treatment while continuing on PD can be an option for the hesitant patient—enables them to become familiar with HD unit and the new healthcare team responsible for their care.
- Transfer to HD at end of life may not be appropriate; it will not improve patient survival and could have a major negative effect on quality of life. This should be discussed with the patient and family. Often, with the aid of carers (paid or family help), the patient can be maintained at home. Referral to community palliative care will improve symptom control and the patient can be enabled to die at home or in a hospice as he/she wishes.

References

1. The Renal Association (2009). *Peritoneal Access*. Available at: 🖰 www.renal.org/Clinical/GuidelinesSection/PeritonealAccess.aspx#downloads
2. Churchill DN, *et al* for CANUSA Study Group. Adequacy of dialysis and nutrition in continuous peritoneal dialysis: Association with clinical outcomes. *J Am Soc Nephrol* 1996; 7: 198–207.
3. Paniagua R, et al. Effects of increased peritoneal clearances on mortality rates in peritoneal dialysis: ADEMEX, a prospective, randomized, controlled trial. *J Am Soc Nephrol* 2002; 13: 1307–20.
4. Brown EA, *et al.* on behalf of EAPOS Group. Survival of functionally anuric patients on Automated Peritoneal Dialysis: the European APD Outcome Study (EAPOS). *J Am Soc Nephrol* 2003; 14: 2948–57.
5. Li PK *et al.* Peritoneal dialysis-related infections recommendations: 2010 Update. *Perit Dial Int* 2010; 30: 393–423.
6. The Renal Association. *Peritoneal Dialysis in CKD*, July 2010. Available at: 🖰 www.renal.org/clinical/guidelinessection/PeritonealDialysis.aspx#downloads
7. Li PK et al. Peritoneal dialysis-related infections recommendations: 2010 Update. *Perit Dial Int* 2010; 30: 393–423.
8. Brown EA et al. Length of time on peritoneal dialysis and encapsulating peritoneal sclerosis. *Perit Dial Int* 2009; 29: 595–600.

Chapter 6

Nursing issues in peritoneal dialysis

Role of the nurse in peritoneal dialysis

The best PD units are managed by multidisciplinary teams whose members have different roles but are all regarded as equals. The essential roles needed are:

- pre-dialysis education and assessment
- community assessment of home and family
- assistance, if needed, for rehousing
- assessment of other social and family needs
- psychological, nursing, and medical support of patients as they reach ESKD and require catheter insertion
- psychological support of patient and family to be independent and manage their own dialysis
- education of patient and/or family members to carry out dialysis techniques
- dietetic input regarding fluid and food intake
- home assessment—enables patient to carry out dialysis in their own environment (home and work), and help solve intercurrent problems
- assessment for long-term complications of dialysis
- assessment of dialysis adequacy
- psychosocial support of patient often over many years
- guidance over problems with dialysis, and assessment of alternative modalities, e.g. APD or HD if failing on CAPD.

In practice, most of this will be carried out by PD nurses with back-up from medical staff. Regular input is also needed from social workers, dieticians, counsellors (or rarely psychiatrists), and, on occasion, physiotherapists or occupational therapists. Many problems can be solved at regular meetings of the multidisciplinary team, but there will also be times when the patient will benefit from a case meeting involving appropriate care team members, themselves, and other family members.

Nursing care of peritoneal catheters

Nursing care of peritoneal catheters

The peritoneal catheter is the lifeline of the patient on PD—its lifespan depends on the care given to it both at insertion and after. Care is aimed at immobilization of the catheter, the exit site, prevention of contamination, and patient education.

Exit site care

This is crucial—exit site infection is one of the major causes of catheter loss. The nurse has a key role in preventing infection.

At catheter insertion

- Planning location of exit site—it is essential to avoid the belt area where the catheter exit site would be rubbed. The exit site should be marked (in indelible ink), while the patient is sitting, above or below the belt area.
- Unless using mupirocin regularly at the exit site, nose swabs should be taken at time of catheter insertion to determine whether the patient is a carrier of *Staphylococcus aureus* or MRSA; carriers should then be started on regular nasal mupirocin.
- Sutures should be avoided at the exit site, but when needed to achieve haemostasis should be removed by 3–4 days so as not to become a nidus for infection.
- Patient should not get the exit site wet until well healed (~2 weeks after insertion).
- Twice-weekly exit site dressings should be started from 5 days after catheter insertion.

Maintenance phase

- Patients should have a daily shower without soaking the exit site for prolonged periods (as in a bath).
- The exit site should be dried well, and protected with a dry gauze swab.
- The patient should be trained to detect exit site infection and inform the PD unit if there is any redness or pus.
- Routine nasal swabs should be done at clinic visits if the patient is known to be a previous *S. aureus* carrier and is not regularly using mupirocin at the exit site.
- If exit site infection is suspected, a swab should be taken for culture before antibiotics are commenced.
- The nurse should always review the patient's technique of exit site care if infection develops.

Catheter care

Catheter care is a vital part of patient training:

- Never use scissors near the catheter, especially during exit site dressings.
- Never kink the catheter.

- Never insert any object down the catheter—it has been known for patients to try to clear blocked catheters by pushing down a wire, or even sucking the catheter.
- Ensure that the catheter is well taped to the skin so that it is not inadvertently pulled—especially important with a new catheter, which can easily be pulled out.

Nursing care of the catheter is also important:
- The catheter should be flushed after insertion; dialysate (500–1000mL) should be run in and then allowed to drain once or twice (or more if the fluid is bloodstained).
- The catheter should be flushed again 1 or 2 days prior to training to ensure good function—it is a waste of training time to discover that the catheter does not function.
- The need for laxatives should be reinforced, particularly in the period immediately after catheter insertion.

Other aspects of catheter care

Swimming
A water-resistant, plastic protective dressing should be placed over the catheter and exit site; the watertight seal should keep the exit site dry. The exit site should be cleaned and a fresh dressing replaced as soon as possible afterwards.

Surgery and invasive radiology, e.g. arteriography
Fluid should be drained out prior to most procedures.

During periods when PD is discontinued
For example after transplantation, management of fluid leak, conversion to HD, it is important that exit site care continues. The catheter should be flushed a few days prior to restarting PD, to ensure that it is still patent.

Line changes

A short line (10–15cm) is fitted on to the adapter at the end of the catheter. This makes the external part of the catheter longer and so easier for the patient to handle. The line needs to be changed regularly to avoid physical damage from heavy use. Line changes are usually done every 6 months, and must be done carefully to avoid introduction of infection:

• Hands should be washed and sterile gloves worn.
• A clamp is placed across the external part of the catheter.
• The old line is closed and soaked in betadine, before being disconnected from the adapter.
• The new line is then connected to the adapter.

Training patients for CAPD

Good patient training is the cornerstone of successful PD. For training to be successful:

- there should be a pre-dialysis assessment and education programme so that patients unsuitable for PD are not selected
- there should be a dedicated training area away from the busy ward area
- training should be one-to-one with the same nurse
- the exit site should be healed
- the catheter should have been flushed within a few days of the training period to ensure patency and functioning
- a family member should also be trained if the patient is unable to carry out exchanges him/herself
- the training period is also used to 'get to know' the patient so that their queries and worries can be addressed.

The training period should also be used for:

- dietetic review and advice about appropriate changes needed when starting on PD
- dry weight assessment and review of medications by medical staff
- review of any input that may be needed by social services.

Training programme

The training programme should be structured so that there are set learning objectives, which can be assessed by the trainer as shown in Table 6.1, and to identify barriers to learning, such as language, literary skills, patient attitudes, and ability to learn.

Table 6.1 CAPD teaching programme

	Comments
Assess patient knowledge	
Kidney failure	Teaching aides used videos
Basic principles of dialysis	
Catheter insertion and position	
The peritoneal membrane	
Managing CAPD	
Practice sessions	Supervised practice
1 Preparation of equipment	
2 Connection	
3 Flush	
4 Disconnection	
Principles of home management	Transferring skills to home
Problem solving	
Recognizing problems and knowing what to do	
Drainage	
Blood	
Discomfort	
Contamination	
Fluid management	
Recognizing problems and knowing what to do	
Overload	
Dehydration	
Target and dry weight	
Managing peritonitis	
Recognizing problems and knowing what to do	
How infections occur	
Safety measures: dos and don'ts	
Exit site and wound care	
Recognizing problems and knowing what to do	
Dressing technique	
Safety measures: dos and don'ts	
Managing your medication	
Types of regular medication prescribed	
Actions and side effects	
Who prescribes	

Table 6.1 (Contd.)	
	Comments
Dietary management	
To reinforce advice from dietician	
Types of food	
Restricted foods	
Nutritional advice	
Additional information—as required	
Transplant issues covered	YES/NO
Given information about home deliveries of fluids	YES/NO
Holiday information provided	YES/NO

Training patients for APD

There are several advantages to training patients for CAPD before commencing APD:

- CAPD easier to learn.
- PET test can be done before transferring to APD—patients with low permeability characteristics are better dialysed by CAPD.
- Manual bag exchange usually needed to maintain dialysis adequacy as residual renal function declines.
- Patients have option of reverting to CAPD when travelling. There are occasions when patients need to be trained on APD directly:
  - when family member is going to perform the dialysis
  - if patient is already anuric (e.g. transferring from HD), when CAPD will probably not provide adequate dialysis
  - if CAPD is totally unsuitable for patient's lifestyle.

As with CAPD, training for APD needs to follow a structured programme. The programme shown in Table 6.2 assumes that the patient already is familiar with the basics of PD.

Table 6.2 APD teaching programme

	Comments
Understanding how the machine works	
Machine parts	
Sequence of events for each cycle	
Fluid dynamics	
Warming fluids	
Understanding the importance of safety checks	
Power failure	
Errors	
Drains	
Bypass	
Alarms	
Stopping early	
Machine settings for you and your machine	
Equipment	
APD solutions	
Cleaning the machine	
Lining the machine	
Priming the machine	
Warming the fluids	

Table 6.2 (Contd.)

	Comments
Connecting and disconnecting at the end of dialysis	
Settings check	
Programme set	
Adjustments	
Initial drain	
End programme	
Safety checks	
Personal regimen and programme explained	
Treatment	
Cycles and volumes	
Strengths of fluid	
Day exchanges	
Fluid collection for clearance tests	
Revision of general topics related to PD	
Fluid intake and diet	
Recording information	
Weight management	
Peritonitis management	
Exit site management	
Outpatient clinics	
Stock supplies and holiday information	

Organizing outpatient care of peritoneal dialysis patients

The team looking after the PD patient is multidisciplinary. (See Fig. 6.1.)

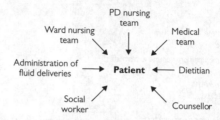

Fig. 6.1 Multidisciplinary care team.

The maintenance management of the PD patient falls into several categories:
- Telephone contact with nurses regarding drainage problems, line care, queries about fluid adjustments for weight control.
- Contact with an administrator to organize fluid supplies and holidays.
- 'Drop-in' access for exit site infections and peritonitis—both can be managed initially by PD nurses using appropriate protocols.
- Community visits by nurses to supervise first exchange or setting up of APD machine.
- Subsequent community visits can be used to assess social problems, do line changes, arrange fluid collections for clearance tests.
- Dietetic advice at onset of dialysis and then follow-up as indicated by clinical needs—each patient should be reviewed at least yearly.
- Counsellor/social worker input to aid compliance, assess for transplantation, and sort out family problems often encountered with home therapies.
- Medical/nursing review—usually every 2 months when stable.
- Medical clinic visits are a useful time for nursing, dietetic and social review.

How all of this is organized will depend on local factors such as staffing levels, geographical distribution of patients, and the need for patients to attend clinics for other medical problems. The key to successful management of PD patients depends on a well-integrated multidisciplinary team with good communication. A regular, preferably weekly, meeting of the team is a time when all aspects of each patient's care can be reviewed. Any fundamental alterations to the dialysis regimen, e.g. changing from CAPD to APD or HD, can be reviewed by all those involved.

Chapter 7

Renal replacement therapy in acute kidney injury

Indications for renal replacement therapy in AKI

Patients fall into two main groups: those with an acute presentation of single-organ kidney failure requiring RRT, who may or may not be on an ICU, and those with AKI as part of multiorgan failure who will almost inevitably be in an ICU. Serum creatinine is a very poor indicator of need for RRT, and eGFR is not meaningful or accurate in AKI. Patients with AKI have reduced creatinine generation rate, and depending on the underlying cause may have poor nutrition, low muscle mass, liver impairment, and are often elderly.

For patients with *single-organ AKI*, conventional indications for starting RRT include *hyperkalaemia* (especially if ECG changes; usually K >6.5mmol/L), *acidosis*, and *fluid overload (usually pulmonary oedema)*.

- It is difficult to define an absolute threshold of biochemical abnormality at which dialysis is always needed, and medical therapy can often stabilize a patient. The risk is that a patient with moderate hyperkalaemia, acidosis, and mild pulmonary oedema may become acutely worse or develop an arrhythmia (for example), and then be unresuscitatable.
- Distinguishing patients with ESKD from a chronic process from those with true AKI is important since patients with CKD may be much more tolerant of aberrant biochemistry than those with AKI.
- Symptomatically uraemic patients require dialysis (but not necessarily as an emergency procedure), as do those with neuropathy, pericarditis, and encephalopathy.
- Patients with rapidly declining renal function and AKI are often started on RRT before any severe metabolic complications arise in the hope that avoiding serious metabolic disturbance may improve outcome.

For patients with *multiorgan failure, sepsis syndrome*, and *post-operative renal failure* RRT is most commonly undertaken using a continuous modality of RRT (rather than dialysis) and should be begun early to minimize the deleterious effects of uraemia on myocardial function, bleeding, and wound healing (but little trial data), and to avoid severe metabolic and electrolyte disturbance.

Other indications for acute RRT include poisoning (lithium, methanol, ethylene glycol), hypothermia, hyperuricaemia, and severe metabolic alkalosis.

Contraindications

No absolute contraindications. Almost all patients can be offered RRT in AKI of some sort if it is appropriate. Relative contraindications include:
- advanced malignancy (not including myeloma)
- dementia (if definitely not an acute confusional state from uraemia or other acute illness)
- advanced cirrhosis with encephalopathy in the absence of possible liver transplantation.

Age itself should not be a contraindication to RRT in AKI.

The extent of co-morbid illness is crucially important in determining survival, morbidity, and quality of life on chronic dialysis, hence longer-term considerations may be taken into account when planning initiation of RRT in AKI. It can of course be impossible to predict the reversibility of the kidney damage in AKI. RRT can be offered to patients as a trial of therapy, and patients should aware that they can always stop at a later stage. This can, however, be difficult (especially psychologically).

Definition of AKI

The KDIGO classification for AKI is most widely used. (See Table 7.1.)

Table 7.1 KDIGO classification

Stage	Serum creatinine criteria	Urine criteria
1	Increase ≥26mcmol/L within 48h or increase ≥1.5–1.9× reference SCr	<0.5mL/kg/h for >6 consecutive hours
2	Increase ≥2–2.9× reference SCr	<0.5mL/kg/h for >12h
3	Increase ≥354mcmol/L or commenced RRT	<0.3mL/kg/h for >24h or anuria for 12h

Choice of renal replacement therapy modality in AKI

This will often depend on whether patients have single-organ kidney failure or AKI as part of multiorgan systemic illness or a post-operative complication.

Peritoneal dialysis is now very rarely used for AKI, and this is almost always only in the setting of single-organ failure within a renal unit rather than an ICU setting. Contraindications to acute PD include recent abdominal surgery, aortic vascular grafts, abdominal drains, etc., and acute PD is associated with an increased risk of morbidity (especially peritonitis). Most units caring for patients with AKI will have almost no experience of using PD for AKI.

The vast majority of RRT in AKI will be intermittent HD or a CRRT modality. CRRT is often available outside of dialysis units (on ICUs), and in hospitals without immediate nephrological support, and much expertise in using CRRT now resides with intensivists rather than nephrologists. There has been much debate as to whether intermittent HD or CRRT is the better treatment for severe AKI (where the choice is appropriate), and the evidence is conflicting: but for patients with multiorgan failure there is often really no choice other than to use CRRT. Such patients will often require completely different management overall from those with single-organ AKI. There have been randomized trials of CRRT vs intermittent HD in selected centres, but in general these have been poorly controlled and have shown equivalent results for renal recovery (for those patients who could be randomized).

Other than issues around the patient's illness, pragmatic issues also determine the precise mode of RRT available, including nursing staff, facilities, location of patient, and experience of medical staff. For patients with AKI and multiorgan failure, other factors are more important than choice of dialysis modality in determining outcome.

Continuous renal replacement therapy

Overview

CRRT strategies are particularly useful in haemodynamically compromised patients with AKI. They allow slow and gentle removal of solutes and fluid, avoiding major intravascular fluid shifts, and minimizing electrolyte disturbances, hypotension, and arrhythmias. Hypotension occurring during conventional HD may contribute further ischaemic insults to the recovering kidney in AKI. Uraemia is better controlled by CRRT than HD in catabolic patients with AKI. UF can be achieved continuously to match fluid requirements (especially enteral or parenteral nutrition, and IV drugs). Therapeutic drug levels should be more reliably maintained than with intermittent HD. Inflammatory mediators may also be continuously removed by CRRT, which has (controversially) been suggested might contribute to better haemodynamic stability. Trials do not demonstrate significant improvements in mortality compared with intermittent HD, but studies are not generally randomized, and patients with hypotension, cardiac dysfunction, sepsis syndrome, or haemodynamic instability are usually preferentially treated with CRRT. Clinical experience suggests that critically ill patients with renal failure are more easily managed by CRRT than intermittent HD. (See Fig. 7.1.)

The two most commonly used techniques are:

- CVVH (F)—continuous venovenous haemofiltration
- CVVHDF—continuous venovenous haemodiafiltration.

CVVHDF combines simple UF and solute replacement with dialysate flow through the haemofilter (dialysis). Dialysate flow is slow. Overall efficiency is increased compared to CVVH and may provide better haemodynamic stability. Most current machines offer this as the first choice of modality.

Other techniques in routine use (but less commonly) include:

- CVVHD—continuous venovenous HD
- SCUF—slow continuous UF
- SLED/EDD—sustained low efficiency dialysis or extended daily dialysis (not a 'continuous' RRT but available as a modality using most current CRRT equipment).

Arteriovenous techniques are generally no longer used but historically included:

- CAVH (F)—continuous arteriovenous haemofiltration
- CAVHD—continuous arteriovenous HD
- CAVHDF—continuous arteriovenous HDF.

The requirement for arterial access is a major drawback for arteriovenous techniques, and a major cause of complications and morbidity, although blood pumps are not required making it less dependent on specific equipment.

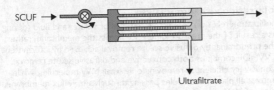

SCUF →

Ultrafiltrate

Replacement fluid

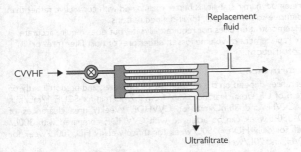

CVVHF →

Ultrafiltrate

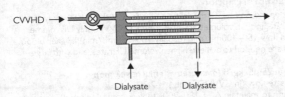

CVVHD →

Dialysate   Dialysate

Replacement fluid

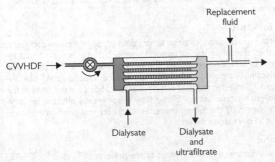

CVVHDF →

Dialysate   Dialysate and ultrafiltrate

Fig. 7.1 Principles of different CRRT modalities. Replacement fluids can be given before or after the haemofilter (pre- or post-dilution), but only shown after in these figures.

Haemofiltration vs haemodialysis

- Haemofiltration relies on convective removal of solutes and fluid (during UF), as a result of the pressure difference across the membrane, rather than the predominantly diffusive solute removal achieved by intermittent HD. CVVHDF combines both convective and diffusive solute removal.
- Diffusion is very efficient at removing only small MW molecules, while UF removes all plasma molecules passing through a high-flux membrane, regardless of MW.
- Haemodynamic stability is better maintained with convective rather than diffusive solute removal, for ill-defined reasons.
- Haemofiltration does not require dialysate, but does require accurate IV replacement of volume losses, either pre- or post-filter (pre- or post-dilution).

Performance

Clearances depend on the membrane, blood flows, and predominantly on extent of UF. Urea clearances vary from 1.7mL/min for SCUF, 17mL/min for CVVH, and 30mL/min for CVVHDF. Weekly urea clearances of 300–350L/week can be achieved with CVVHDF, compared with 300L/week for daily HD or 150L/week for thrice-weekly HD, 100L/week for CVVH, and 70L/week for PD.

Standard prescription

- Will depend on precise modality in use: for CVVHDF both dialysate flow rate and UF volumes are prescribed; in CVVH only UF volume.
- Blood flow 150–400mL/min (usually 200–250mL/min). Higher blood flows are needed to achieve higher volume UF rates, and with large filters.
- UF rate 25mL/kg/h (measured as effluent volume).
- Dialysate flow (in CVVHDF only) 1–2L/h.
- Heparin to maintain ACT 180–200s (unless contraindicated), or citrate or other anticoagulation.

Access for CRRT

Dual-lumen intravascular catheters, or double single-lumen catheters, placed in the internal jugular or femoral vein. Subclavian access should be avoided (risk of subclavian stenosis). Catheter position should be confirmed radiographically. Tunnelled catheters may reduce infection risk, but are more difficult to insert in the ICU setting. Complications are the same as for chronic dialysis vascular access. Blood flow is not greatly affected by catheter length, but is by the lumen diameter. Catheter mal-position however affects blood flow rates achieved.

Membrane

High-flux membranes (usually synthetic) are preferentially used for CRRT, given the permeability requirements of haemofiltration, however are not being used in the same manner as in high-flux HD, and have smaller surface areas. Comparisons of biocompatible and incompatible membranes have produced conflicting results on patient survival and renal recovery from AKI. Protein accumulation on membranes reduces efficacy with time.

Ultrafiltration

Controlled either volumetrically or by pressure. Pressure control can be maintained by adjusting the height of the UF collection bag in relation to the haemofilter, or by applying suction to the UF line. Simply adjusting the height of the solute collection bag below the filter will change the rate of UF. Volumetric control relies on a pump to achieve a fixed UF rate. Accurate monitoring of actual UF rate, and the pressures across the haemofilter are important. Total fluid removal of at least 10–15L/day is required to allow convective solute removal, most of which is replaced (depending on the patient's volume status). UF rate is determined by the difference between UF volume removed per hour and replacement fluid volume returned to the patient. Current recommendations are to aim for an effluent volume (UF rate) of ~25mL/kg/h.

Filtrate replacement solutions

The filtrate replacement solutions (for both CVVH and CVVHDF) and dialysate in CVVHDF are usually the same, and usually supplied as 5L sterile solutions. There are multiple formulations now available. Contain glucose, sodium, calcium, magnesium, chloride, and (usually) potassium. Buffer is conventionally provided now as bicarbonate (which has mostly superseded lactate).

- Sodium: ~140mmol/L
- Calcium: 1.6–1.8mmol/L (but some solutions calcium free)
- Potassium: 0–4mmol/L
- Magnesium: 0.5–1.5mmol/L
- Chloride: 100–115mmol/L
- Bicarbonate: ~30mmol/L.

Replacement fluids can be given either pre- or post-filter (pre- and post-dilution). Post-dilution can lead to increased Hct within the filter, reduced efficiency of UF, and filter clotting. Pre-dilution increases filter life, but slightly lowers the concentration of waste solutes within the haemofilter. Some haemofilters allow mid-dilution, which has potential benefits, but are not widely used.

Significant losses of amino acids (1–5g/day) and phosphate can occur during CRRT, but usually only with high UF rates.

Other continuous renal replacement techniques

SCUF

A form of CVVH in which no replacement fluid is given (unlike CVVH). Provides isolated UF for patients with refractory oedema (often due to heart failure), without severe renal failure. UF volume can be regulated by gravity or by pump. Electrolyte and fluid imbalances may occur, and UF volume is frequently less than anticipated due to clotting or reduced blood flow. Not widely used.

SLED/EDD

Uses HD machine generally but blood flows of 100–200mL/min and dialysate flow rates of only 100mL/min for 8–24h/day. Excellent tolerability, cardiovascular stability, and solute removal. Does not require separate CRRT equipment. Not widely used.

Dialysis adequacy in AKI

The meaning and measurement of RRT adequacy in AKI critically depends on whether the modality is intermittent HD or CRRT. For CRRT techniques, measuring Kt/V is probably not meaningful, and difficult to do.

For illustration: a 50kg catabolic patient with AKI would need at least 4.4 dialysis sessions per week to maintain a steady-state blood urea of 20mmol/L. For an 80kg patient such a steady state can only just be achieved with daily dialysis for 4h. CRRT can achieve these targets. However, the target levels of blood urea that may determine outcome have not been established.

Intermittent HD

Current guidelines (lacking real evidence) suggest that patients receiving intermittent HD in AKI should have a steady urea <25mmol/L, and a daily Kt/V of 0.9–1. Achieving prescribed dialysis in AKI can be compromised by poor access flows, low BP and cardiac output, clotting of the circuit due to lack of anticoagulation, hypercatabolism, increased oedema causing increased V. Urea generation rates also vary widely in AKI. Delivered dialysis should be checked with pre- and post-dialysis blood urea measurements, and ideally with formal UKM. The difference between prescribed and delivered Kt/V is much greater in AKI than in CKD. As a result using Kt/V is not recommended as a measure of dose of dialysis in AKI.

CRRT

Removes urea (and other small solutes) mostly by convection during UF, and by diffusion when using CVVHDF. In the short term this provides much less clearance per unit time, but over 24h and 48h more solute is removed by CRRT than conventional HD. Slow or sustained extended dialysis (SLED) achieves the same outcome using a conventional dialysis machine with low dialysate flows (100mL/min) rather than a dedicated CRRT machine. This may be more efficient but is not widely available. In general adequacy of CRRT is measured by effluent volume produced, i.e. by rate of ultrafiltration. The precise mode of CRRT will however impact on adequacy, and its measurement, which in practice mostly means the difference between pure haemofiltration (in CVVH) and haemodiafiltration (in CVVHDF).

A number of RCT have attempted to examine outcomes for patients receiving differing UF volumes ranging from 20 to 45mL/kg/h during CRRT (equivalent to ~1.4, ~2.4 and ~2.9L/h UF). Overall these studies have not shown increased benefits for increased UF volumes above 25mL/kg/h, and current recommendations are to aim for an effluent volume of 25mL/kg/h. When pre-dilution solute replacement is used in general a slightly higher UF rate is used. High volume UF (usually > 45mL/kg/h) can lead to phosphate depletion and a shortened lifespan for haemofilters.

Prescribing haemodialysis for AKI

Once dialysis has been started for a patient with AKI it is easy to forget about the dialysis itself, and simply concentrate on the many other factors involved in patient care during an acute illness (see also ➜ The first dialysis session in chronic and acute kidney disease, p. 138). However, there is increasing evidence that dialysis-related factors are important in the outcome of patients with AKI.

The following applies when using IHD in AKI:

Time

Time spent on dialysis may need changing frequently after initiation of dialysis. The first dialysis session will usually only be 2h. Over the next couple of sessions the length should be increased up to 4h for most patients. Large patients and those with hypercatabolism may need longer. Time on dialysis is often shortened because of hypotension, poor vascular access, anticoagulation problems, and difficulties in starting or completing sessions due to competing pressures on the patient (other investigations, imaging, physiotherapy, etc.). Delivered dialysis is almost always significantly less than that prescribed.

Frequency

Patients often need daily dialysis for the first few days in order to bring urea levels down into a reasonable range. Patients with marked catabolism, sepsis, fluid overload, difficult pulmonary oedema, or requiring parenteral nutrition may need daily dialysis to be continued for longer. These patients are often managed with CRRT rather than IHD.

The dialyser

Some evidence suggests that biocompatible membranes are associated with better outcomes from AKI, but this is controversial (see ➜ Biocompatibility of membranes, p. 92).

UF rate

Patients often are (or become) fluid overloaded with peripheral oedema. This is difficult to control with short dialysis sessions, due to episodic hypotension because of slow fluid redistribution. Longer sessions or continuous techniques will control fluid overload better. Patients often lose muscle mass rapidly when acutely ill, and their dry weight should be reduced appropriately. Failure to recognize this will lead to fluid overload as the difference between the target dry weight for UF and the patient's true dry weight increases.

Dialysis dose

Should be monitored and regularly reassessed, by either formal UKM, measurement of Kt/V, or at the very least by the URR, although Kt/V is not reliable in AKI, and what constitutes adequate dialysis in AKI is not clear. Most units aim for a daily Kt/V of ~1.0.

Prescribing CRRT for AKI

Most patients with multiorgan failure and AKI, or AKI requiring ITU care, will be managed with CRRT (either CVVH or CVVHDF in most cases) rather than IHD. The precise prescription will vary depending on the specific modality (CVVH or CVVHDF).

Time

Patients remain on CRRT continuously unless disconnected for imaging, surgery, other interventions, filter clot, or when patients have begun passing urine in order to determine whether sufficient recovery of renal function has occurred.

The dialyser

In CRRT the dialysers are almost all synthetic, biocompatible membranes. There is variation in dialyser size which will have an impact on solute clearance, and larger dialysers require higher blood flows.

UF rate

The UF rate is the key determinant of dose delivered in CRRT and is usually ~25mL/kg/h.

Dialysate

In CVVHDF dialysate flow rate is usually 1–2L/h (not applicable to CVVH)

Dialysis dose

This is generally monitored from frequent blood urea and creatinine measures (often twice daily), UF rate and measures of UF effluent volume. Real time urea removal can be measured but is not often undertaken. Daily true urea or creatinine clearances can be measured but again this is not common practice.

Anticoagulation for CRRT: heparin

Clotting in the extracorporeal circuit is a major problem. Haemofilters should last at least 24–36h. Pre-dilution fluid replacement will prolong filter life. Factors predisposing to increased thrombosis include:

- prothrombotic extra-corporeal circuit
- kinking of CVCs (during turning, etc.)
- hollow fibre haemofilters (rather than parallel plate)
- increased UF rates
- low blood flows
- post-dilution filtrate replacement
- reduced antithrombin III levels (and other immuno-metabolic disturbances) in critically ill patients with AKI.

Most units will use a limited number of anticoagulation techniques for which they have experience. Continuous anticoagulation increases bleeding risk but this is not usually a significant problem. Anticoagulation needs to be individualized for each patient and their comorbidities.

Monitoring

- Visual check of circuit, including bubble trap for signs of clotting.
- Regular ACT or APTT for heparin.
- Anti-Xa for LMWH and danaparoid.
- ACT and calcium for citrate.

Reduced UF rate with stable haemodynamics suggests filter or line clotting. Filtrate urea:blood urea ratio <0.6 implies poor filtration and imminent clotting. Most centres routinely change filters after 24–48h.

Heparin

Most commonly used anticoagulant. Should be included in priming solutions (1000–3000 units/L saline). Standard technique uses a loading dose of 2000–5000 units, and continuous infusion of 300–800 units/h into arterial line. A dilute solution allows better mixing with blood. Aim to maintain whole blood ACT 180–250s (or 1.5–2 × control), or APTT 40–45s, venous PTT >65s. HIT is not uncommon. Bleeding risk minimized by ACT or PTT monitoring. Clotting usually due to mechanical problems rather than too little anticoagulation.

Regional heparin

Heparin is infused pre-filter and neutralized with protamine post-filter. 1mg protamine reverses ~100 units of heparin. Avoids systemic anticoagulation, but requires close monitoring. Not widely used. Protamine can cause anaphylactoid reactions, hypotension, leucopenia, and thrombocytopenia.

Low-molecular-weight heparins

LMWHs may cause less bleeding and more predictable anticoagulation, and reduced incidence thrombocytopenia. Few controlled trials. Various regimens used:
- 2000–3000 anti-Xa units of LMWH every 20min
- 35IU/kg bolus followed by 13IU/kg infusion.

Can be monitored by antifactor X activity (aiming for 0.5–1IU/mL for patients without bleeding risk; 0.2–0.4IU/mL for patients with bleeding risk). Should not be used in patients with HIT.

Can be combined with epoprostenol.

Anticoagulation for CRRT: heparin alternatives

Heparin-free

Rarely used in CRRT on ICU since filter clotting is common, but can be implemented for patients with clotting abnormalities, thrombocytopenia, recent bleeding, or liver failure. Filters may last >24h if carefully managed, especially if small surface area filters, pre-dilution filtrate replacement, and higher blood flows. If heparin not totally contraindicated flushing circuit initially with higher heparin doses (up to 20,000 units) can help.

Epoprostenol (prostacyclin)

Inhibits platelet aggregation and adhesion. Vasodilator. Antiplatelet activity lasts 2h. Use at 4–8ng/kg/min. Trials suggest low efficacy when used alone, but prolonged filter survival when combined with (low-dose) heparin or LMWH. Can cause fall in BP.

Danaparoid

A low-MW glycosaminoglycan. Has been used in patients with HIT. Significant bleeding risk, and may still cause thrombocytopenia. Use bolus 2500U, and then 400–600U/h infusion for 1st 4h, reducing dose thereafter to 200–600U/h to maintain anti-Xa levels 500–1000U/mL.

Others

Argatroban (initially 0.5–1.0mcg/kg/min) and recombinant hirudin (initially 0.005–0.01mg/kg/h) can both be used for anticoagulation in CRRT and monitored by measuring APTT (aiming for 2× normal).

Fondaparinux (synthetic pentasaccharide) binds antithrombin and inhibits factor Xa and has been used in patients with HIT.

Anticoagulation for CRRT: regional citrate

Trisodium citrate anticoagulation

Provides no systemic anticoagulation, excellent filter life, minimal bleeding risk, but requires careful monitoring, separate calcium infusions, and non-standard replacement fluids. Citrate binds calcium, inhibiting several steps in the clotting cascade. Once returned to the patient the effect of citrate is neutralized by excess calcium in blood and hepatic metabolism to bicarbonate. Further calcium needs to be administered continuously to prevent hypocalcaemia. Replacement fluids and dialysate must be calcium free. When available, a very successful method.

One typical regimen is:
- 4% trisodium citrate infused into arterial access of haemofilter circuit (90mL of stock 46.7% trisodium citrate into 1000mL of 5% glucose)
- 0.75% calcium chloride infused into central venous access of patient (80mL of 10% calcium chloride into 1000mL of normal saline)
- trisodium citrate infused at ~190mL/h, and calcium replacement at ~60mL/h
- circuit and systemic ionized calcium monitored hourly until stable, and then 4–6h, using a blood gas analyser, and maintained at 0.25–0.35mmol/L and 0.9–1.2mmol/L, respectively
- citrate infusion is titrated to the circuit ionized calcium
- calcium infusion is titrated to systemic ionized calcium.

Patients should be monitored for alkalosis, hypocalcaemia, and hypernatraemia. Calcium and citrate infusions need to be stopped if blood or dialysate flows stop for >10min. Avoid in liver disease (risk of severe alkalosis).

Complications of CRRT

CRRT is generally well tolerated, with a similar range of complications to standard HD, most of which are uncommon. Nurses are critical in monitoring patients during CRRT for complications.

Access related

Thrombosis (in catheter or local vein), bleeding from puncture site, infection (exit site, bacteraemia, sepsis—especially Gram-positive organisms), recirculation, and poor blood flow (kinking, thrombosis). Strict aseptic techniques must be used when initiating and terminating treatments.

Circuit related

Clotting, blood loss (from disconnections, circuit clotting), disconnection (rare), sepsis, fluid balance related (excess UF or fluid replacement), and allergic reactions (to plastics, haemofilter, or sterilants). Hypovolaemia can occur easily, clotted circuits are common, and nurses need to know how to perform manual return of blood to patient.

Anticoagulation related

Local and systemic bleeding, thrombocytopenia (especially heparin induced), alkalosis, and hypocalcaemia (with regional citrate).

Others

Hypothermia (infusion fluid may need to be warmed), hypotension, fluid overload, arrhythmias, electrolyte imbalances (hypophosphataemia, hypocalcaemia, hypokalaemia, hypo- or hypernatraemia), alkalosis, bioincompatibility, air embolism (should be very rare with pump cessation on air detection), interactions with ACEIs, and nutrient losses (amino acids and trace elements).

Drugs

Dosing can be very different from intermittent HD since the continuous therapy and increased convection increases some drug losses. This may vary between CVVH and CVVHDF. May be especially important for antibiotics.

CRRT trauma

This has been described as a complication of CRRT and includes the combination of acid–base disorders, loss of heat, electrolytes (especially phosphate, also magnesium), carbohydrates, nitrogen (and amino acids), water-soluble vitamins (folic acid, vitamin B_6, thiamine, vitamin C and E), trace elements (including selenium, chromium, manganese, and copper), and antimicrobial (and other) drugs. It is increased with higher volume UF rates. Hypophosphataemia may be particularly important and can occur in 10–66% of patients on CRRT (usually those receiving higher UF rates), and has been associated with a failure to wean from mechanical ventilation.

CRRT troubleshooting guide

Machines used for CRRT vary in their specifications, but have some common alarm features. (See Table 7.2.)

Table 7.2 CRRT machine alarm features

Alarm	Cause	Action
High venous (return) pressure	Clotted circuit or filter	Change complete circuit and review heparin prescription
	Occluded blood lines	Remove occlusion
	Clot within the catheter	Unblock or remove catheter
Low arterial (access) pressure	Clot within the catheter	Unblock or remove catheter
	Occluded blood lines	Remove occlusion
	Hypovolaemia	Often due to cardiac causes, sepsis or volume depletion in patients on ICU. Treat appropriately
Air detector	Detection of air or bubbles within the venous chamber	Increase the level within the chamber if air bubbles within the circuit, disconnect the patient and recirculate until the circuit is clear
		If patient may have received air embolus place in Trendelenburg position, disconnect lines, attempt to withdraw the air from fistula needle or line, and alert the emergency team
High filter pressure	Clotted circuit or filter	Change complete circuit and review heparin prescription
	Faulty filter pressure sensor	Check sensor
Blood leakage	Defective or split filter causing leakage of blood through the filter membrane or air in effluent line causing a false alarm	If blood is present discard circuit and resume treatment

Peritoneal dialysis in AKI

PD has fallen out of favour as a means of dialysing patients with AKI with the increased availability of CRRT techniques in ICUs. Patients requiring ICU care with multiorgan failure would now rarely be thought suitable for acute PD, but it could be considered for those with single-organ failure. Acute PD is used for paediatric and neonatal AKI in some circumstances. There are potential advantages to the use of PD, especially in haemodynamically compromised patients, and acute start PD is becoming more common in many centres particularly for patients who are considered to be presenting acutely with ESKD (rather than true AKI). (See Table 7.3.)

Acute PD can be temperamental and difficult to establish. Experienced nursing is required to avoid infection, and to ensure good catheter function and use of cycling machines. Where expertise is present, PD is a useful modality in the treatment of AKI, particularly for patients with poor cardiac function in whom HD could potentially be dangerous. In general, however, CRRT techniques have superseded acute PD.

Table 7.3 Advantages vs disadvantages of PD in AKI

Advantages	Disadvantages
Widely available and easy to perform. Gentle, slow dialysis minimizing risk of disequilibrium syndrome.	PD catheters cannot be inserted in patients who are at risk of having multiple intra-abdominal adhesions
Can be done manually (although risk of infection increased compared with use of cycling machine)	Contraindicated after aortic aneurysm surgery because of risk of infecting graft
Fluid removal very gradual so minimal cardiovascular stress	Cannot be done for first few days after laparotomy because of likelihood of fluid leak
PD can be carried out more safely than HD in patients with poor cardiac function	Impairs movement of diaphragm so relative contraindication in patients on ventilators or with respiratory problems
Can be done in patients with poor vascular access PD catheters easy to place	Provides relatively small 'quantity' of dialysis in catabolic patients with AKI
No anticoagulation required	Cannot correct severe hyperkalaemia rapidly
Glucose in dialysate provides extra calories	Peritonitis in a sick patient with AKI can be fatal (as can sepsis related to line-infection in CRRT or HD)
Particularly useful in children	

Prescribing acute start PD

Exchange volume and dwell time need to be limited with new PD catheters to avoid fluid leakage. For these reasons, APD overnight with dry days or IPD for longer periods using low dwell volumes are used. (See Table 7.4.)

Monitoring of efficacy of acute PD

An accurate record needs to be kept of the UF volume during manual or automated acute PD.

- There are no guidelines for assessing adequacy of acute PD.
- Clinical observations are used to monitor the patient.
- Current PD cycling machines record ultrafiltration achieved
- Dialysis adequacy can be assessed by improvements in biochemical parameters such as plasma urea, creatinine, bicarbonate, sodium, and potassium.

Table 7.4 Variables to consider when prescribing IPD

Duration of dialysis	Usually for 10–20h each session. Session can be extended if needed to optimize biochemical or fluid control. Session can be interrupted, e.g. for X-ray, and missed time 'made up' when patient reconnected
Volume of dialysate	Usually 10 L/10h
Exchange volume	1litre for first week of new catheter. 1.5litres for second week. Can be increased to 2 or 2.5litres thereafter, depending on size of patient
Exchange frequency (or dwell time)	Dwell time determines time available for diffusion and UF
	Depends on exchange volume, so shorter dwell time used with smaller volume exchanges
	Small volumes and shorter cycles are needed to minimize intra-abdominal pressure and reduce risk of fluid leakage (for new catheters). 30–60min dwell time usually satisfactory
UF requirements	UF is determined by osmotic gradient between plasma and dialysate induced by dialysate glucose. If no fluid removal required use only 1.36% glucose
	Ratio of hypertonic (2.27 or 3.86%) glucose to isotonic (1.36%) glucose depends on UF requirement
	Amount of UF achieved varies hugely, so start gradually (e.g. 5litres 1.36% and 5litres 2.27%) and increase glucose concentration as needed
	Weigh patient (when peritoneum empty) to assess net fluid loss

Psychosocial effects of RRT in AKI

Patients with AKI face similar psychological problems to those with chronic progressive renal impairment ending in ESKD; however, they often occur in the setting of a severe acute illness, rather than during regular outpatient visits. Clearly for patients recovering renal function after an episode of AKI the impact of a brief period of RRT will be very different.

Patients will often be too ill initially to understand the potential implications of renal failure; however, the need for a visible technological intervention will not go unnoticed. Patients may not be aware from the outset that they may not recover renal function. Patients will not have had any education, counselling, or advice about dialysis, ESKD, or treatment modalities.

Patients may also be relieved to survive a severe acute illness, and thus the issue of mortality over-rides the morbidity associated with established renal failure.

Thus many of the psychological problems only manifest after the establishment of chronic dialysis, rather than in the preceding months. Patients may therefore require more counselling and education several weeks after initiation of RRT. Patients will almost always not have had the opportunity to choose PD in an acute setting, and those with ESKD should subsequently be offered the choice if appropriate to change from hospital-based haemodialysis to a home therapy (including PD).

Nurses play a crucial role, both in managing RRT safely, explaining procedures, preparing the patient (and their families) for investigations, and fluid and nutritional management.

Haemodialysis and haemoperfusion for poisoning

Dialysis can be an effective way to treat some patients exposed to poisons or drug overdoses. HD can enhance poison elimination and correct electrolyte abnormalities and metabolic acidosis rapidly. PD is much less effective and rarely used for this indication (except sometimes in small children). Haemoperfusion refers to the passage of blood through a circuit containing an adsorbent such as activated charcoal, carbon, or polystyrene resin. Drugs that bind to the adsorbent are more effectively cleared by haemoperfusion than by dialysis, but the technique is less widely available. Haemoperfusion can also eliminate protein-bound and lipophilic toxins and drugs. HD is used in 90% of patients receiving extracorporeal therapy for poisoning (<0.05% of all poisonings). Controlled studies are very rare. (See Table 7.5.)

Table 7.5 Drugs and poisons

Drugs or poisons which can be eliminated by dialysis have:	Drugs not well cleared are:
Low MW (<500Da)	Large MW
Low degree of protein binding	Protein bound
Water soluble	Lipid soluble
Small volume of distribution (<1L/kg)	
Enhanced clearance by dialysis over native clearance	

Patients who should be considered for extracorporeal therapy for poisoning have:

- severe clinical intoxication
- clinical deterioration
- prolonged coma
- poisoning with substances with delayed actions or toxic metabolites (e.g. paraquat, ethylene glycol)
- impaired native clearance (liver or renal failure)
- known toxic levels of a dialysable drug.

Performing haemodialysis for poisoning

- Usually requires percutaneous vascular access.
- A high-efficiency dialyser should be used (high KoA/urea clearance).
- Long dialysis session(s) needed (4–8h).
- Often complicated by hypophosphataemia (phosphate is not present in routine dialysate), and may require phosphate supplementation.
- Hypokalaemia may occur.
- May provoke metabolic alkalosis due to the bicarbonate in dialysate (as patients not usually acidotic).
- If patient is uraemic the dialysis necessary to eliminate a toxin may induce disequilibrium syndrome.

Haemofiltration

Less effective than HD in eliminating appropriate drugs or toxins, but may be the only technique available.

Haemoperfusion

Circuit similar to HD without dialysate, and routine dialysis pumps can often be used. Various perfusion cartridges available (no controlled comparisons). Some require priming with a dextrose solution to prevent subsequent hypoglycaemia. Circuit requires anticoagulation (usually heparin, ~6000 units per session). Some heparin is adsorbed by charcoal. Monitor anticoagulation as for HD. One session usually lasts 3h, after which charcoal is saturated. Complications include charcoal embolization, hypocalcaemia, hypoglycaemia, leucopenia, and thrombocytopenia (30% reduction in platelets common).

Drugs and toxins removed by haemodialysis

The drugs and toxins in Table 7.6 can be removed by HD.

Table 7.6 Drugs and toxins

Drug/toxin	Comments
Methanol and ethylene glycol	Dialysis will remove intact alcohols and toxic metabolites (formate, glycolate, oxalate), and correct acidosis. Should be combined with IV ethanol or fomepizole. Ethanol can be added to dialysate to maintain blood levels (at 100mg/dL). Dialysis should be continued until acidosis has resolved. May require 18–24h dialysis. Not removed by perfusion
Lithium	Poisoning common. Often precipitated by dehydration. Toxic levels >2mg/dL. Consider dialysis in all patients with levels >2.5mg/dL, or if neurological signs. Rapid rebound in lithium levels occurs after cessation of dialysis. Requires prolonged (up to 12h) or repeated dialysis
Aspirin (acetylsalicylic acid)	Poisoning usually managed with gastric lavage, oral charcoal, and alkaline diuresis. For severe poisoning (levels >80mg/dL, 4.4mmol/L), CNS symptoms, coma, or poor urine output, dialysis or haemoperfusion will remove aspirin effectively. Dialysis is preferred as it corrects the associated acidosis
Theophylline	Toxic levels >20mcg/mL. Well removed by dialysis, but better by haemoperfusion. Complication rate lower with dialysis
Barbiturates	Now rare cause of poisoning. Phenobarbital toxic levels >130µmol/L. Most patients managed with lavage, charcoal, and urinary alkalinization. Consider dialysis for prolonged coma or complications. Perfusion also effective
Phenytoin	Removed poorly by HD since protein bound, but better by haemoperfusion
Star fruit poisoning (*Averrhoa carambola*)	Causes intractable hiccups, vomiting, confusion, agitation, weakness, and death. Recovery only noted in dialysed patient

Drugs and toxins removed by haemoperfusion

The drugs and toxins in Table 7.7 can be removed by haemoperfusion.

Table 7.7 Drugs and toxins

Drug/toxin	Comments
Theophylline	Better removed by perfusion than by dialysis. Consider if levels >30mcg/mL, or earlier if liver disease or cardiac toxicity
Phenytoin	Highly protein bound, but reasonably well removed by perfusion. Only needed if severe cerebral toxicity (levels usually >30mcg/mL)
Digoxin	Severe poisoning may be accompanied by hypokalaemia, hyperkalaemia, or alkalosis. Initial treatment with oral charcoal and correction of electrolyte disturbances. Poorly removed by dialysis, but reasonably well by perfusion. Digoxin Fab antibody fragments also effective therapy for severe intoxication
Paraquat	Survival dependent on initial plasma levels. Perfusion (or dialysis) second-line therapy after repeated oral adsorbents. Prolonged therapy required
Amanita mushrooms	Benefit of perfusion (or dialysis) controversial
Carbamazepine, chloramphenicol, dapsone, disopyramide, methotrexate, paracetamol, quinine, and valproate	Have all been treated by haemoperfusion or HD
Tricyclic antidepressants and phenothiazines	Very poorly removed by extracorporeal techniques (highly protein bound)

Chapter 8

Nutrition on dialysis

Contributor

Lina Johansson
Clinical Lead Renal Dietician, Imperial College
Healthcare NHS Trust, London, UK

Protein energy wasting in ESKD

Protein energy wasting in ESKD is characterized by a progressive decline in body stores of protein, with or without fat depletion, or by a state of reduced functional capacity caused at least partly by inadequate nutrient intake relative to nutrient demand and/or which is improved by nutritional repletion. Approximately 40% of all patients with ESKD have protein energy wasting. The causes of protein energy wasting in ESKD are multi-factorial (see Table 8.1).

Protein energy wasting in ESKD is associated with:
• increased mortality and morbidity
• increased infection, poor wound healing, muscle wasting, fatigue and malaise.

Poor nutritional status prior to initiation of dialysis is associated with poorer outcomes on dialysis, increasing the odds ratio of mortality 2.5 times. Despite its limitations as an indicator of nutritional status, low serum albumin levels are independently associated with increased risk of death in HD, PD, and transplanted patients.

The decline in body protein stores and therefore in lean body mass, is mediated through metabolic processes present in ESKD:
• Metabolic acidosis stimulates degradation of protein and branched-chain amino acids via upregulation of branched-chain ketoacid dehydrogenase and the ubiquitin–proteasome proteolytic pathway.
• Pro inflammatory cytokines and insulin resistance may also activate proteolytic pathways.

Table 8.1 Factors causing protein energy wasting in ESKD

Factors increasing nutrient requirements	
Endocrine abnormalities	Hyperparathyroidism
Inflammation	Comorbid conditions, sepsis, increased cytokine and leptin activity
Dialysis treatment	Loss of nutrients through dialysis, e.g. amino acids in HD and PD
Factors decreasing nutritional intake	
Loss of kidney function and co-morbid conditions	Anorexia, nausea, fatigue, taste changes, anaemia, spontaneous reduction of energy intake with a GFR <25mL/min
Dialysis	Inadequate clearance of metabolic waste products through dialysis
Gastrointestinal disturbances	Phosphate binders, hypoalbuminaemia, antibiotics, polypharmacy, uraemic and diabetic gastroparesis
Psychosocial and socio-economic	Depression, anxiety, lack of social support, alcohol or drug abuse, poverty
Additional factors contributing to protein energy wasting in ESKD	
Metabolic and endocrine abnormalities	Metabolic acidosis, altered amino acid and lipid metabolism, insulin resistance
Dialysis treatment	Protein catabolism during HD

Assessment of nutritional status

Assessment of nutritional status involves quantifying the calorie intake and expenditure within an individual as well as their muscle and non-muscle (visceral) protein status. Multiple methods of assessments are required as individual markers of nutritional status are unable to capture the full spectrum of protein energy wasting and individual markers may reflect other underlying pathology. Nutritional assessment requires interpretation of a combination of dietary, clinical, and biochemical parameters.

Dietary intake

This should include current and past dietary intake, recent changes in food intake, and food preferences and aversions (including religious and cultural).

Appetite

Current appetite and recent changes to appetite and possible mechanisms, e.g. nausea, vomiting, gastrointestinal symptoms or tiredness.

Diet history

24–48h recall, food frequency, and general eating patterns and portions by careful prompting and use of food models/photographs.

Food diary

- Actual food and fluid intake are recorded for a minimum of 3 days by the patient.
- Include weekends and treatment (HD) days as these may reflect different eating patterns.
- Provide detailed instructions to enable accurate documentation of type of food, portion size, and relevant cooking methods.

The food diary is then used to determine macro- and micronutrient nutritional intake and estimate nutrient adequacy. This can help guide dietary modification and individualized menu planning.

Clinical assessment

Medical history

Past medical history of relevant illness or surgery
- Are energy requirements altered due to sepsis, need for wound healing, or gastrointestinal malabsorption?

Prescribed drugs
- Determine if nutritional intake compromised from side effects such as nausea or gastrointestinal disturbances.

Current medical condition
- Determine the nutritional requirements for the condition (e.g. stage of renal disease) and treatment (HD or PD).

Physical examination

Signs of nutritional deficiencies
- Determine whether current nutritional intake is meeting requirements by assessing appearance of skin, hair, lips, tongue, gums, and nails.

Signs of poor nutritional status
- Determine whether nutritional intake is meeting requirements by assessing signs of subcutaneous fat loss and/or muscle wasting.

Physical functioning
Declining or poor physical function can be due to suboptimal nutritional intake and subsequent loss of muscle mass.
- Review activities of daily living and the ease of basic physical activity (stair climbing or walking).
- Muscle strength can be determined using hand-grip dynamometry. Serial measurements are of more significance to highlight changes in muscle strength that can be indicative of changes in nutritional status.

Body weight
Dry weight (adjusted for fluid imbalance)
- Determine indication of nutritional status by assessing usual and current dry weight and changes over time.

Rate of weight loss
- Determine rate of weight loss and if intentional or unintentional. (See Table 8.2.)

Body mass index (weight (kg)/height (m)^2)
- A BMI of <18.5kg/m^2 is indicative of malnutrition. Nutritional intake may need to be adjusted if patient is obese (BMI >30kg/m^2) by adjusting requirements to their ideal body weight (based on BMI of 25) as opposed to actual body weight.

Body composition
Anthropometry
- Measures body composition (fat stores and muscle mass) using skinfold calipers and a tape measure.
- Triceps skinfold thickness provides an assessment of body fat. Mid upper arm circumference and triceps skinfold thickness are used to derive the mid upper arm muscle circumference, a measure of muscle mass. Values are compared with reference data tables to ascertain presence of malnutrition. These measurements require precise methodological techniques to enhance accuracy.
- *Serial measurements* are of more significance to highlight changes in muscle mass or fat.

Table 8.2 Classification of unintentional weight loss

Period	Significant weight loss	Severe weight loss
1 week	1–2%	>2%
1 month	5%	>5%
3 months	7.5%	>7.5%
6 months	10%	>10%

Other methods of body composition assessment
- Bioelectrical impedance (BIA), dual-energy X-ray absorptiometry (DEXA), and magnetic resonance imaging (MRI), but these are not routinely used in the clinical setting.

Social assessment
- Age, sex, social support and cultural background can influence nutritional risk factors and intake.
- Evaluation should include food preparation capabilities, food storage, available support, income, and education.
- Input from social services may be appropriate.
- Where communication is hampered by language, hearing or visual impairment, the following may be used to enable effective nutritional assessment and communicate appropriate advice: interpreting services, translated written and audio recorded information, food models, and pictures.
- Where food preparation is not undertaken by the patient, appropriate discussion with the whole family or carers is important.

Biochemistry

Biochemical markers that may indicate poor nutrient intake include reduced serum urea, albumin, potassium, and phosphate. In the long term, reductions in serum creatinine may reflect reduced muscle mass, and reduction in serum cholesterol may reflect inadequate energy intake.

Serum albumin
- Serum albumin requires careful interpretation: it can be influenced by fluid imbalance, by acute phase response (trauma, surgery, or infection), and protein loss through the urine and PD.
- The large body pool and long 14–20-day half-life renders albumin relatively insensitive to immediate changes in nutritional intake.
- Is a good predictor of mortality in ESKD. A single measurement at any point after initiation of dialysis is strongly associated with survival.
- Patients with serum albumin <25g/L have a risk ratio for dying 20 times higher than patients with serum albumin >40g/L.
- The association of albumin with outcome is likely to be due to the strong association between inflammation and mortality.

Serum pre-albumin
- Has a shorter half-life (2–3 days) and smaller body pool than albumin, and is more influenced by the acute phase response.
- It is less affected by liver disease and by hydration status.
- Levels elevated in progressive renal disease due to decreased degradation.
- Not a reliable indicator of nutritional status in ESKD.

Serum transferrin
- Serum levels are increased in iron deficiency, and reduced levels occur in uraemia per se, during an acute phase response, iron loading, and in patients with proteinuria.
- Not a good indicator of nutritional status in ESKD.

Serum creatinine
- Derived predominantly from creatinine catabolism in muscle and is produced at a constant rate when in energy and nitrogen balance.
- Varies according to residual renal function and muscle mass.
- Changes in serum creatinine over time may indicate changes in muscle mass, and should be confirmed using other parameters such as changes in body weight and/or body composition, and food intake.

Blood urea
- Derived from protein degradation.
- Influenced by diet, hydration, residual renal function, degree of anabolism, and the adequacy of dialysis.
- In ESKD, a low blood urea (<10 mmol/L) may indicate inadequate protein intake.
- In a steady state, protein catabolic rate (PCR) correlates well with dietary protein intake (DPI). However, in a catabolic state, urea generated by muscle breakdown far exceeds that derived from DPI. Conversely, anabolism may produce falsely low PCR values. PCR is usually normalized for actual body weight (nPCR). However, extremes in body weight will influence the interpretation of nPCR, with obese or underweight patients showing inappropriately distorted values unless metabolically active fat-free mass is considered and the body weight adjusted accordingly. Similarly the presence of oedema can cause errors, and oedema-free adjusted body weight should be used in such circumstances.

Potassium
- Potassium excretion is influenced by the degree of residual renal function, diarrhoea, anabolism, and the use of potassium-containing drugs or ACEIs/ARBs.
- Serum potassium below the normal range may indicate poor nutritional intake as potassium is found in a wide variety of foods.
- Low potassium may also result as part of the metabolic imbalances associated with re-feeding syndrome.

Phosphate
- Most patients with CKD and ESKD have raised serum phosphate and require phosphate binders.
- Low serum levels may indicate an overall poor nutritional intake due to wide distribution of phosphate in foods, in particular protein-rich foods.
- Low phosphate may also result as part of the metabolic imbalances associated with re-feeding syndrome.

Lipid profile
- Low total plasma cholesterol levels have been associated with increased mortality, possibly as an indicator of insufficient protein and energy intakes.

Subjective global assessment (SGA)

Eight clinical measures are used including dietary intake, co-morbid disease, gastrointestinal symptoms, physical examination, changes in body weight, and functional capabilities to produce a semi-quantitative nutritional assessment. An overall score of nutritional status is generated from a subjective weighting of all the clinical measures combined. The following provides the nutritional status associated with the 3- and the 7-point SGA scoring systems.

3-point SGA scoring system:
- A: well nourished
- B: moderately (or suspected of being) malnourished
- C: severely malnourished.

7-point SGA scoring system:
- 1–2: severely malnourished
- 3–5: mildly to moderately malnourished
- 6–7: well nourished.

Various SGA formats are in use. All rely on a subjective rating by the observer. (See Table 8.3.)

Table 8.3 Outline of SGA

Weight change	Current dry weight
	Change in dry weight in last 6 months
	Change in dry weight in last 2 weeks

Dietary intake	Meeting nutritional requirements:
	    Adequate
	    Inadequate
	    Poor

Gastrointestinal symptoms	None Diarrhoea Dysphagia Nausea Vomiting Anorexia
Functional impairment	Change in functional capacity
	Assess if related to nutritional intake
Disease and its relationship to nutritional requirements	None, high, or low metabolic stress
Muscle wasting	Biceps/triceps/quadriceps/deltoid, etc.
Subcutaneous fat loss	Eyes/perioral/palmar
Oedema	Hands/sacral/leg

Nutritional requirements in haemodialysis and peritoneal dialysis

- Appetite and food intake may gradually improve (but not always) when uraemic symptoms are alleviated through starting dialysis.
- Some patients may experience worsening nutritional status due to adverse effects of dialysis (PD or HD), e.g. loss of nutritional substrates such as protein through the dialysis process.
- Nutritional requirements for dialysis are shown in Table 8.4. Evidence from controlled trials is mostly lacking. Where possible, general healthy eating guidelines are recommended, e.g. 50% total energy from complex carbohydrates, high fibre (non-starch polysaccharide, NSP) and 30–35% energy from fat (predominantly poly- and monounsaturated fatty acid sources with low saturated fats). High soluble NSP intake is of particular importance in PD where uptake of dialysate glucose may increase the existing risk of hypertriglyceridaemia and poor glucose tolerance.
- There is significant evidence that nutritional interventions or supplementation (orally or by NG feeding) can improve markers of malnutrition, serum albumin, and hospitalization rates.
- Where intake is poor, relaxation of dietary restrictions (where appropriate) may be of help to achieve nutritional adequacy.

Table 8.4 Daily nutritional guidelines for patients on HD and PD

	HD	PD	Main food sources
Energy	30–35kcal/kg	30-35kcal/kg*	Cereals, bread, rice, pasta, potatoes, fats
Protein	1.1–1.4g/kg IBW	1.2g/kg IBW (1.5g/kg/IBW in peritonitis)	Meat, fish, eggs, pulses, milk (within allowance)
Potassium	0.8–1mmol/kg	Restriction only necessary if hyperkalaemic: 1mmol/kg	Fruit, vegetables, fruit juice, nuts, coffee, chocolate
Phosphate	<1000mg	<1200mg	Milk, yoghurt, cheese, offal, shellfish, fish with bones
Sodium	80–100mmol	80–100mmol	Table salt, smoked/cured foods, tinned and packet foods, ready meals
Fluid	500mL + previous day urine output	500mL + previous day urine output + ultrafiltration	Drinks, gravies, sauces, soups, jelly, yoghurts

IBW, ideal body weight. *Include calories absorbed through the dialysate fluid.

Strategies for achieving nutritional aims

Energy

PD

Use of higher dextrose concentration dialysate should be minimized especially in obese patients or those with diabetes or hypertriglyceridaemia. Icodextrin dialysate may be especially beneficial in these cases.

- Normal or overweight PD patients may require energy restriction to compensate for the additional calories absorbed from dialysate.
- Initial advice should concentrate on reducing excessive intake of fats and sugar (provide few nutrients other than energy).
- Excessive use of hypertonic (higher glucose) dialysate to control fluid balance will increase energy intake through additional calories absorbed from the dialysate. Fluid management and sodium restriction should then be emphasized.
- Long-term use of hypertonic solutions may cause damage to the peritoneal membrane, producing hyperpermeability and loss of peritoneal integrity, and weight gain.

HD

HD patients generally have more difficulty achieving recommended energy intakes. This group more frequently needs advice aimed at increasing their energy intake, using either energy-rich foods or prescribed energy supplements.

Protein

- The high protein requirements of dialysis are often difficult to achieve through diet alone, particularly in those with poor appetite, vegetarians, or during peritonitis in those on PD.
- Increasing intake of protein-rich foods and snacks, and use of prescribed protein supplements may be required.
- Combined energy and protein supplements may help, and occasionally intradialytic parenteral nutrition (IDPN) in those on HD (see ➲ Intradialytic nutrition, p. 409).

Potassium

- Potassium restriction is rarely needed in PD because of the continuous clearance.
- In HD, dietary potassium restriction may be required, but the level of restriction is partly dependent on residual renal function.
- Non-dietary causes of hyperkalaemia should be excluded. (See Table 8.5.)
- Limitation of potassium-rich food sources, including:
  - fruits: banana, rhubarb, avocado pear, dried fruit
  - vegetables: spinach, mushroom, beetroot, jacket, instant, or chipped potato (unboiled), crisps
  - drinks: fresh fruit juices, coffee, drinking chocolate, malted drinks, milky drinks
  - other: chocolate, evaporated and condensed milk, yeast extract, liquorice, salt substitutes, nuts, bran-based products.

Table 8.5 Non-dietary causes of hyperkalaemia

Metabolic factors	Acidosis, insulin insufficiency or resistance, hyperparathyroidism
Drugs	Potassium-containing drugs: Slow-K®, Sando-K® Affecting potassium excretion: ACEIs, ARBs, β-blockers, NSAIDs, K+-sparing diuretics
Cellular factors	Haemolysed blood sample, post-blood transfusion, infection, GI haemorrhage, crush injury, gangrene
Constipation	Reduced gut excretion
Dialysis	Inadequate dialysis, recirculation

- Advice on suitable cooking methods (as potassium is water soluble):
  - use large volumes of water for boiling vegetables and discard this cooking water
  - boil potatoes
  - parboil vegetables before adding them to stews, sauces, and soups
  - avoid the use of pressure cookers and microwave cooking (re-heating is permitted).
- Advice on portion size and quantities of fruit and vegetables.
- Review of protein intake: protein foods can also be rich in potassium, ensure protein intake is not excessive by diet history (cross-check against serum biochemistry and nPCR).
- Patients should have access to renal cookbooks for suitable recipes.

Phosphate
- Clearance of phosphate is not particularly effective with either PD or conventional HD.
- Daily dialysis and nocturnal dialysis achieve significantly better phosphate clearance, enabling some patients to relax their dietary restrictions and reduce (or cease) their intake of phosphate binders. Some patients may even require phosphate supplementation when dialysing daily.
- Management consists of dietary restriction of phosphate-rich foods, review of excessive protein portions and foods with added phosphate-containing additives (polyphosphates).
- Review of compliance, dosage, and timing of phosphate binders and vitamin D analogues is essential (see ⊃ Chapter 11).
- In general, all phosphate binders should be taken with or immediately after food, with the dose adjusted to protein portion and meal size.
- Hyperphosphataemia is often caused or exacerbated by patients eating away from home and neglecting to take their phosphate binders.

Phosphate-rich foods include:
- milk
- dairy products
- cheese
- chocolate
- dried fruit
- eggs
- fish (bony)
- shellfish and seafood
- nuts
- meat and poultry.

Special diets and eating patterns

It is common that individuals may follow different diets, eating patterns, or consume particular foods for personal or religious beliefs or cultural reasons.

Vegetarian or vegan diets

Generally provide less protein and may be higher in potassium and phosphate. Protein supplementation may be required. They may also contribute to vitamin B_{12} deficiency.

Fasting

Recommended energy and protein intakes are more difficult to achieve during fasting. Medications may be omitted inappropriately during a fast.

Cooking methods

Cooking methods for curries, stews, and stir-fries may conflict with potassium-lowering cooking techniques. Cooking utensils may contain iron, aluminium, or other trace elements, which can (rarely) accumulate.

Food items

May be rich in the following:
- potassium: spinach (sag), callaloo, karela, potato pakoras, plantain, yam, cassava, sweet potato, okra, banana, mango, paw-paw, nuts, coconut, sweetmeats, chevda
- phosphate: lassi, raita, Indian tea, nuts, sweetmeats, chapattis
- sodium: chevda, pickles, salt fish and pork, soy sauce, monosodium glutamate.

Rarely, some foods may be toxic in renal failure, e.g. star fruit (*Averrhoa carambola*; eaten especially in Asia) causes severe intoxication in patients with CKD, leading to intractable hiccoughs, agitation, muscle weakness, confusion, and fits. It can be fatal.

Supplemental vitamins and trace elements

Vitamins

- Vitamin deficiency can occur in ESKD due to dietary restriction, dialysate losses, and abnormal metabolism. Overt deficiency is rare.
- Most units prescribe a routine supplementary dose of the water-soluble vitamin B group, vitamin C, and folate, although good evidence for supplementation is lacking. Excessive dosing of vitamin C (>100mg/day) should be avoided since it is metabolized to oxalic acid which may accumulate in ESKD.
- Vitamin A is not routinely prescribed due to the risk of hypervitaminosis. However, vitamin E supplementation in ESKD may have antioxidant activity in relation to coronary heart disease prevention. (See Table 8.6.)

Trace elements

- Of the nine essential trace elements, deficiencies in zinc, copper, manganese, chromium, and selenium have been reported in CKD and ESKD, mostly due to dietary restriction (and drug interactions).
- Deficiency should be confirmed before starting supplementation which is not needed routinely.

For iron supplementation, see ➜ Chapter 10.

Table 8.6 Recommendations for vitamin requirements in HD

Vitamins	Recommended supplementation
Thiamine (B₁)	1.1–1.2mg
Riboflavin (B₂)	1.1–1.3mg
Pyridoxine (B₆)	10mg
Cobalamin (B₁₂)	2.4mcg
Niacin (B₃, nicotinamide, nicotinic acid)	14–16mg
Pantothenic acid (B₅)	5mg
Biotin (B₈)	30mcg
Folic acid	1mg
Ascorbic acid (C)	75–90mg
Vitamin E (alpha tocopherol)	400–800IU
Vitamin A (retinol)	700–900mcg intake (no supplement)

From European Best Practice Guideline on Nutrition 2007.

Use of nutritional supplementation

Oral nutritional supplements

- May be required if initial fortification of food remains insufficient to meet nutritional requirements or if it contributes to or exacerbates existing hyperphosphataemia or hyperkalaemia.
- Compliance with food supplements may be variable due to palatability, taste fatigue, and an unwillingness to use them as they contribute to the daily fluid restriction. (See Table 8.7.)

Nasogastric feeding

- May be used to supplement a poor intake, usually in the in-patient setting.
- Specifically formulated enteral feeds are available which are fluid restricted, electrolyte restricted, and nutrient-dense to assist meeting the nutritional requirements of dialysis patients.

Gastrostomy feeding

This is a more practical and longer term method of tube feeding compared to NG feeding, especially in HD patients. Increasing numbers of PD patients are also being fed this way, many units preferring to give a short period of peritoneal rest while the tube placement site heals.

Table 8.7 Nutritional products

Product	Examples of brands
Energy supplements	
Glucose powder	Vitajoule®, Caloreen®, Maxijul® Super Soluble Polycal®, Maxijul® Liquid
Glucose liquid	Calogen®, Duocal®, Liquigen®, Fresubin® 5 kcal
Liquid energy	shot, Pro-Cal® Shot
Protein powders	Renapro®, ProMod®, Maxipro®, Protifar®
Sip feeds	
Standard:	
milk based	Ensure Plus®, Fortisip®, Resource® Energy
non-milky	Ensure® Plus Juce, Fortijuce®, Resource® Fruit
High protein	Resource® Protein, Fresubin® Protein Energy Drink
Nutrient dense	Ensure® TwoCal, Fresubin® 2 kcal Drink
Low volume	Ensure® Compact, Fortisip® Compact
Low volume/electrolyte	Nepro HP®, Renilon® 7.5
High-protein desserts	Maxisorb®, Forticreme® Complete, Clinutren® Dessert, Fortisip® Fruit Dessert, Resource® Dessert Energy, Ensure® Plus Creme
Enteral tube feeds	
Nutrient dense	Osmolite® 1.5 kcal, Nutrison® Energy, Fresubin® Energy, Ensure® TwoCal
Low volume/electrolyte	Nepro HP®

Intradialytic nutrition

Intradialytic parenteral nutrition (IDPN)

- IDPN can be used to supplement energy and protein intake during each HD session.
- Provides nutrients without additional fluid (as the ultrafiltration (UF) volume is increased during the dialysis session).
- Short-term evaluation of IDPN suggests it is of benefit in some patients as it can reverse the acute catabolic state that occurs during dialysis and can lead to improvements in serum albumin, body weight, and dietary intake. However, no additional benefit in mortality was found in patients receiving IDPN together with oral nutritional supplements compared to nutritional supplements alone.
- Can provide up to 1100kcal and 50g protein per session although one can assume only 70% of this is absorbed and not lost through dialysis. This corresponds to daily additional 330kcal and 15g of protein. Metabolic side effects of IDPN (including hyperglycaemia and GI symptoms) require close monitoring.
- Patients may get more nutritional benefit from being encouraged to eat or take nutritional supplements during dialysis sessions (but occasionally this may exacerbate intradialytic hypotension).

Intraperitoneal amino acids

- Have been used in PD patients.
- Studies using 1.1% amino acid dialysate solutions to replace 1–2 of the usual daily glucose exchanges may show some improvement in nutritional status, especially in those patients with moderate to severe pre-existing malnutrition.
- Only leads to a small improvement in nutrition, and the exchange must be done at the same time as a meal to enhance amino acid uptake.

Carnitine and ESKD

Carnitine is trimethylated amino acid and an intermediary in fat metabolism, which is able to bind acyl groups. It transports long-chain fatty acids into mitochondria for cellular energy production by oxidation. It also acts as a scavenger of free acyl groups. Dietary sources include red meat, fish, and dairy products, but it is not an essential nutrient since it can be synthesized in liver, brain, and kidney, and is stored principally in muscle. Free and acyl carnitine both accumulate in renal failure, but the ratio of free to acyl form is markedly reduced which may impair its ability to bind acyl groups. Free carnitine is removed by HD so that the ratio is further reduced and a state of functional deficiency may exist. Rare genetic disorders of carnitine function exist, with clinical features including muscle weakness, cardiomyopathy, liver dysfunction, and increased infections. Some of these clinical problems are common in dialysis patients and it has been suggested that functional carnitine deficiency now called dialysis-related carnitine disorder (DCD), may be responsible at least in part.

Carnitine supplementation might therefore be expected to improve:
- anaemia, and erythropoietin responsiveness
- cardiomyopathy
- intradialytic hypotension
- hyperlipidaemia
- muscle weakness and fatigue.

Carnitine supplementation is not widely used due to the heterogeneity of the responses achieved in trials involving supplementation in dialysis patients. A systematic review and meta-analysis of studies involving levocarnitine supplementation in adults with ESKD on HD found no effect overall in improving haemoglobin, haematocrit levels, or reducing erythropoietin dose. This may be related to some people being 'responders' or 'non-responders' to treatment. Levocarnitine supplementation did lower serum low-density lipoprotein (LDL) but did not affect serum triglycerides, cholesterol, or high-density lipoprotein (HDL) levels. The effect of LDL lowering was significantly smaller than that achieved through statins. Levocarnitine did significantly lower levels of serum CRP but with no corresponding change in albumin levels. It is unclear whether this translates into improved morbidity and mortality.

When used, levocarnitine is usually given either as 100 mg IV or 20mg/kg IV after dialysis or 330 mg orally 2–3 times daily.

Fluid requirements in ESKD

Fluid management in ESKD is influenced by the degree of residual renal function and mode of dialysis. Patients with substantial urine output (>1L/day) do not usually require a strict fluid restriction. Patients with reduced urine output should restrict their fluid intake according to their dialysis modality (see Table 8.8).

Sodium intake should be restricted to a 'no added salt' diet which is equivalent to 80–100mmol sodium per day (equivalent to ~5–6g of salt per day).

Patients should be educated about salt as the major drive to thirst, as restricting sodium intake is likely to lead to better fluid control than attempting to restrict fluid intake per se.

PD fluid restriction
- Fluid loss by UF dependent on the dextrose concentration of dialysate (up to 2L/day). This is especially important to the anuric patient.
- The volume of UF, together with the volume of urine passed in previous 24 hours and 500mL (insensible losses) per day can determine the recommended fluid intake per day.

HD fluid restriction
Usually anuric and often requires a severe fluid restriction (volume of urine passed in previous 24 hours and 500mL daily to allow for insensible losses) and sodium restriction. Interdialytic fluid gain should be kept to ~1kg/day, or a maximum of 4% dry body weight (adjusted for metabolically active tissue in obesity).

Table 8.8 Strategies for achieving fluid restriction

No added salt intake	Little salt in cooking but no salt added at the table. Avoidance of high-salt foods—processed, cured, and smoked foods, soups, seasonings, stock cubes, yeast extracts. Avoid pre-prepared foods which contain large amounts of 'hidden' salt, e.g. ready meals
Reduced fluid intake	Use small-volume cups for drinks. Use of ice cubes and ice lollies. Taking tablets with food vs fluid (unless otherwise directed)
Increased awareness	Education of fluid content of certain foods—jelly, custard, soup, ice-cream, yoghurt, dhal. Measuring jug tally—fluid required throughout the day is extracted from a jug initially containing the desired daily volume (or a bottle of water frozen and kept in fridge to thaw slowly)
Thirst prevention techniques	Reduced salt intake. Use of sugar-free sweets or chewing gum. Use of fruit (within applicable potassium recommendations)
Regular mouth care	Use of mouth wash, lip salves, etc.

Nutrition in acute kidney injury

Assessment of nutritional requirements

Nutritional status in AKI is usually influenced by the underlying aetiology of disease, pre-existing malnutrition, degree of catabolism and pro-inflammatory response, and prolonged hospitalization. Increased plasma concentrations of catabolic hormones, including cortisol and catecholamines, are common. Severely catabolic patients usually require prompt nutritional support. The increased availability of dialysis and continuous filtration techniques means nutritional intake no longer need be compromised by controlling electrolyte and fluid balance. Assessment of nutritional status can be particularly difficult in patients with AKI.

Energy requirements

Non-septic patients have energy requirements similar to those of healthy individuals. In sepsis, the basal metabolic rate (BMR) may be increased by up to 30%. Provision of adequate energy is essential to prevent the breakdown of endogenous and ingested protein for gluconeogenesis. Energy requirements are determined from clinical circumstances, patient activity, and an estimate of BMR. (See Table 8.9.)

The additional requirements induced by a variety of clinical conditions (post-operative, infection, multiple long-bone fractures, burns) can be estimated from published nomograms. Bedbound and immobile patients have an increased energy requirement above BMR of 10%; bedbound but mobile patients require an extra 15–20%; and mobile patients require an additional 25% (precise value dependent on the extent of activity).

Protein requirements

Patients with AKI but no additional catabolic stress (e.g. sepsis) are usually able to maintain neutral or positive nitrogen balance. Catabolic patients may have a marked rise in blood urea nitrogen as nitrogen balance becomes negative. Urea nitrogen appearance can be measured to estimate total nitrogen balance.

Protein requirements can be estimated using weight and degree of catabolism and mode of dialysis, e.g. continuous renal replacement therapy (CRRT). (See Table 8.10.)

Table 8.9 Estimating basal metabolic rate

	Females (kcal/day)	Males (kcal/day)
18–30 years	13.1W+558	16.0W+545
30–60 years	9.74W+694	14.2W+593
60–70 years	10.2W+572	13.0W+567
70+ years	10.0W+577	13.7W+481

W, weight. (From Henry CJK. Basal metabolic rate studies in humans: measurement and development of new equations. *Public Health Nutr* 2005; 8(7A): 1133–52.)

Table 8.10 Estimation of protein requirements in AKI

	Protein g/kg/day
Conservative therapy, mild catabolism	0.6–0.8 (max 1.0) g/kg/day
Extracorporeal therapy, moderate catabolism	1.0–1.5 g/kg/day
CRRT, severe hypercatabolism	Maximum 1.7 g/kg/day

(From ESPEN Guidelines on Parenteral Nutrition: Adult Renal Failure. *Clin Nutr* 2009; 28: 401–14.)

Table 8.11 Amino acid (protein) losses during dialysis

	Estimated protein loss
HD	6–9g/session
PD	~10g/day
CRRT	9–12g/24h

Obese patients (BMI >30kg/m^2) have a lower proportion of metabolically active tissue, and the weight used in these calculations should be reduced to their ideal weight based on a BMI of 25kg/m^2.

Dialysis-dependent patients require additional protein to replace losses during dialysis. (See Table 8.11.)

Electrolyte and mineral requirements

- At different stages of AKI, supplementation or restriction can be necessary, often determined by the catabolic state of the patient and the modality of dialysis (e.g. intermittent or continuous).
- Conservatively managed patients usually require dietary restriction of potassium, sodium, and phosphate.
- Patients undergoing CRRT need a less restrictive diet, and many need full nutrition support. During CRRT many patients with AKI develop hypokalaemia, hypophosphataemia, and hypomagnesaemia requiring supplementation. These are important metabolic derangements, especially in ventilated patients, as electrolyte depletion can lead to increasing muscle weakness, alterations in acid–base balance, and further nephrotoxicity (especially tubular damage). Close daily monitoring is necessary. Patients can also have significant losses of selenium, chromium, copper, and zinc (in high-volume CVVHDF this can result in losses equivalent to twice the normal intake provided in parenteral feeding).

Routes for nutritional support in acute kidney injury

Wherever possible, patients should be fed orally. Non-dialysis-dependent patients may require potassium, phosphate, and fluid restrictions according to their serum biochemistry and fluid balance.

Oral nutritional support

If nutritional intake remains suboptimal after efforts to increase the nutrient density of the diet through fortification with calories and protein, oral nutritional supplements can be used to increase both energy and protein intake. The fluid and electrolyte content of these products should be considered, and, where possible, the most nutrient-dense brands selected.

Enteral tube feeding

Enteral tube feeding is recommended in AKI if the GI tract is functioning and nutritional requirements are unable to be met through oral means alone. Use of the enteral route helps maintain gut integrity and viability, and allows an additional route for the excretion of metabolic waste products, particularly potassium and phosphate.

In non-dialysed or haemodialysed patients, fluid- and electrolyte-restricted feeds may be appropriate. During CRRT, these feeds should no longer be necessary, and standard feeds may be better, with additional protein supplementation where necessary to overcome excessive dialysate protein losses.

Parenteral nutrition

Parenteral nutrition may be preferred in patients with impaired GI function, e.g. gastroparesis or bowel obstruction.

Energy requirements are best provided using a combination of both glucose and fat to prevent excess CO_2 production. Therefore the glucose oxidation rate should be within the range of 4–7mg/kg/min per day (including glucose derived from dialysate during CRRT). Provision of fat should be 0.8–1.2 (max 1.5) g/kg/day in AKI.

Routine use of low-electrolyte parenteral nutrition regimens in patients with AKI receiving dialysis (especially CRRT) may cause electrolyte depletion, and necessitate administration of additional potassium, phosphate, or magnesium, or the use of standard parenteral nutrition formulae. Close monitoring of serum biochemistry is paramount, especially at the onset of feeding.

Chapter 9

Special situations

Dialysis in the elderly

The median age of patients starting dialysis in the UK was 64.6 years in 2012, but this is highly dependent on race (66.1 years for white incident patients; 57.8 for non-white patients). The proportion of 'old' elderly is increasing; in the USA, there has been a 57% increase in the number of patients >80 years old starting dialysis. Although transplantation is now being offered to older patients, the majority will have too many co-morbidities to be suitable. It is therefore important that these patients are enabled to choose the dialysis modality best suited to their individual social circumstances. Although there are many reasons why older patients may prefer a home treatment, they are less likely to be started on PD; in the UK in 2009, 28% of incident patients <65 years were on PD at day 90 but only 14.5% of patients >65 years old.

Many working in the renal team think that older patients cannot cope with PD and they are therefore not given the opportunity to choose it. Many older patients can be trained to do their own PD, though this may take longer than with younger patients. Family members are often willing to help with all or part of the procedure and, increasingly, use of community nurses enables frail patients to be on PD in their own homes (see ➔ Assisted peritoneal dialysis, p. 420).

The North Thames Dialysis Study is the only prospective study looking at outcomes of patients ≥70 years old. The outcomes on HD and PD were similar and depended on age and co-morbidity. Overall mortality rate for both modalities was 25% per annum. A third of patients were not hospitalized over a 12-month period. Quality of life measured by SF-36 was also identical for both HD and PD. The striking feature of the patients studied was the high proportion on PD which reflected UK practice at the time of the actual study (late 1990s). Many of these patients would not be offered PD today in the UK, even though the results showed that outcome and quality of life were not different for patients on HD and PD.

Maximal non-dialytic conservative management is widely used in Europe but less in the USA, with support from multidisciplinary teams, in elderly patients usually with significant co-morbidities. In general, patients survive slightly less long than those started on dialysis (who 'lose' significant numbers of days to dialysis itself), but with significantly fewer hospitalization and interventions, higher quality of life, and death more likely to occur in the patient's place of choice (usually home). Starting dialysis in the frail elderly with co-morbidities is often associated with a worsening of quality of life (e.g. as measured by Satisfaction with Life scale).

Features of ageing

Older people on dialysis have the general features of ageing as well as kidney disease. Lifestyle and coping with dialysis can therefore be difficult whatever modality is chosen. The features to consider are:
- co-morbidities
- physical function
- cognitive function
- nutritional status
- depression

- social isolation
- vision
- hearing
- social support.

Physical function

Patients on dialysis of all ages have impaired physical function and lower levels of exercise than normal people of the same age. This is particularly marked in older patients with recent studies demonstrating that there is a marked deterioration in physical function resulting in increased dependence on social support within the first 6 months of starting dialysis. The level of physical function is also a predictor of survival on dialysis so that poor function is associated with worse survival. The term 'frailty' is used commonly, is not defined by chronological age per se, is increased in patients with CKD, and combines features including unintentional weight loss, slow walking speed, weakness, exhaustion, and low physical activity. Recognizing this can lead to attempts at rehabilitation. Falls are increased in older patients with ESKD, and associated with increased mortality.

Cognitive function

Cognitive dysfunction is remarkably often ignored and not recognized in older patients on dialysis. Given the burden of vascular risk, it is not surprising that cognitive problems are common when tested for. Cross-sectional studies show that cognitive impairment is more common in patients with CKD in general and in those on dialysis. Longitudinal studies are not available, though it would not be surprising for those to show faster deterioration in cognitive function with increasing age than normal. The BOLDE (Broadening Options for Long-term Dialysis in the Elderly) showed that a third of patients on PD and HD (all >65 years old) had impaired executive functioning, despite patients with clinical dementia being excluded from the study.

Depression

Depression is grossly under-recognized in patients on dialysis and particularly in the elderly: studies show that 20–30% patients with ESKD are depressed. Depression has been shown to predict survival in several studies with poorer survival in patients with higher depression scores. Treatment is not straightforward and there is in fact little data in patients with ESKD, although small studies have been reported on the efficacy of drug treatment and of cognitive behavioural therapy.

Choice of dialysis modality in the elderly

There are specific problems when considering dialysis in the elderly. (See Table 9.1.)

Table 9.1 Specific problems

	HD	PD
Advantages	Independent of patient ability	No need for vascular access Home treatment
	Less time on treatment	Less risk of hypotension
	Provides social support structure	Patient independence of hospital
		Ease of travel
		Better maintains residual renal function
		Can be done by family member or paid carer (assisted PD)
Disadvantages	↑ risk of hypotension	Not suitable in all patients
	↑ vascular access problems cause increased use of central catheters	↑ difficulty in learning—impaired vision, hearing, manual dexterity, cognitive function
	Patients often feel 'washed out' after HD session for many hours	
	Hours of treatment extended by reliance on hospital transport	Social isolation

Quality of life on HD versus PD

Only two studies have specifically compared quality of life of older patients on HD and PD:

- *North Thames Dialysis Study* showed no difference in the SF36 scores in patients >70 years old on HD and PD.
- *BOLDE (Broadening Options for Long-Term Dialysis in the Elderly)* showed no difference in adjusted SF12 and depression scores in patients >65 years old on HD and PD, though the Illness Intrusion Rating Scale was lower in patients on PD.

Further reading

Harris SAC et al. for the NTDS group. Dialysis modality and elderly people: Effect on clinical outcomes and quality of life *Perit Dial Int* 2002: 22; 463–70.

Brown EA et al. Broadening Options for Long-term Dialysis for the Elderly (BOLDE): Differences in quality of life on peritoneal dialysis compared to haemodialysis for older patients. *Nephrol Dial Transplant* 2010; 25: 3755–63.

Assisted peritoneal dialysis

Assisted PD (aPD), using community-based nurses or healthcare assistants, is being developed in many countries to enable patients to have PD at home even when they are unable to do it themselves and have no family support to help them.

French experience

In France, this has been standard treatment for older patients for many years. Of 11,744 French PD patients treated in the last decade (1995–2006), 56% were considered unable to perform their own treatment and needing assistance. This was provided by a community nurse for 86% of patients.

The availability of assistance has enabled PD in France to be predominantly a treatment of the elderly, with ~52% of patients on PD in January 2013 being >70 years of age. Non-disconnect CAPD with UV-flash is the predominant method used as this greatly shortens the time needed for the nurse visit—the nurse phones the patient or a relative to start the drain procedure so when s/he arrives they just have to remove the old bag and connect the new one, leaving the fluid to drain in and the patient to fold up the bag after their departure.

Assisted APD

In other European countries, APD is used as the PD modality for assisted patients. There are different models of how this is delivered:
- Community nurses visit twice a day:
  - Morning visit to disconnect patient from cycler machine, remove used bags, and set up machine with new bags for the evening.
  - Shorter evening visit to connect patient to cycler machine.
  - This model is being developed in some European countries (Sweden, Denmark, Netherlands, Belgium, France) and Canada.
  - Main disadvantage is cost of using nurses and providing two visits/ day.
- *In the UK*, the model of aPD that has been developed is to provide a daily visit from a healthcare assistant (individual with short basic training in healthcare):
  - Nursing qualification is not needed to perform PD (usually done by patients ± family support); salary of healthcare assistant is less than that of a nurse.
  - One visit a day only—assistant takes used bags off cycler machine and sets up machine with new bags; also checks blood pressure and weight of patient and can perform exit site dressings.
  - Patient (with or without family support) still has to do their own connection to and disconnection from the cycler machine. This obviously does limit the patient population suitable for aPD.

Training of assistants

In France, where there is the greatest experience, private community nurses receive only a half day of training from the PD unit at the initiation of treatment; the patient may then often train other nurse colleagues themselves. In Denmark, training is equally short—2.5h theoretical training and 2.5h from a PD nurse with the patient in their home. In the UK, using healthcare assistants, training is generally longer, with individuals spending 1–2 weeks in a PD unit or in a commercial PD training centre. In all programmes, the local PD team need to provide back-up and be available for advice for the PD assistant.

Future development of assisted PD in UK

The development of aPD enables frail patients with little or no family support to have their treatment at home and expands the proportion of patients able to have PD. It also enables some patients on PD who would have to transfer to HD for social reasons to remain on PD. Experience also suggests that some patients manage to learn how to do their own PD after some time with assistance; this enables patients to start PD acutely rather than having to start on HD if presenting as a 'crashlander'.

aPD is growing in the UK in most PD units, but its role remains to be fully established

- aPD is more expensive than standard PD; mostly this has been absorbed by individual renal units or funded by commissioners for limited number of patients. From April 2012, aPD has been reimbursed through the national tariff, though not at full cost.
- Cost mostly depends on source of assistants:
  - Most commonly, healthcare assistants are provided by a national healthcare agency who has formed a partnership with Baxter Healthcare (UK). Baxter provide the PD training, and the healthcare agency provides the infrastructure of transport for the assistants, holiday and sickness cover
  - Some PD units are employing and training their own assistants. This can sound attractive as costs are less, but it is also necessary to have the infrastructure to enable travel between patients, sickness and holiday cover. This model therefore only works in units with significant number of patients on aPD.
- More information is needed regarding comparison with HD for frail patients regarding costs (including transport), hospitalization, and most importantly, quality of life and physical function.

Managing diabetic patients on dialysis

Diabetes (mainly type 2) is an increasingly common cause of ESKD in all countries, accounting for almost 40% of dialysis patients in the USA and 20% in Europe. Patient survival is much worse than for non-diabetic patients, with a large proportion of patients dying within the first 3 months of dialysis. Major cause of death is cardiovascular disease. Outcome is better for transplanted patients, which should ideally be offered pre-emptively.

Many of the non-renal complications of diabetes will continue to progress after initiation of dialysis, including:

• coronary artery disease
• retinopathy
• cataracts
• cerebrovascular disease
• peripheral vascular disease
• peripheral neuropathy
• autonomic neuropathy
• sexual dysfunction
• depression.

The increasing prevalence of diabetic nephropathy among ESKD patients is primarily due to the increasing prevalence of type 2 diabetes in the general population. In comparison, the incidence of ESKD among those with type 1 diabetes may actually be decreasing with better management of blood pressure and blood glucose levels, and use of ACEIs/ARBs.

Diabetic patients on dialysis have more vascular-related co-morbidity than non-diabetics. (See Table 9.2.)

Initiation of dialysis

No controlled trials. Most units start at higher levels of GFR than for non-diabetic patients (10–15mL/min, and even up to 20mL/min, but with no evidence to support this) as uraemic symptoms may occur earlier, and renal function tends to deteriorate more rapidly in diabetic patients. Important also to avoid malnutrition. When determining when to start dialysis, rate of decline of renal function should be reviewed closely. With use of ACEIs and ARBs, suppression of proteinuria and good BP control can result in very slow rates of decline—such patients do not need to be rushed

Table 9.2 Frequency (%) of co-morbidities in diabetic compared with non-diabetic patients on dialysis (UK Renal Registry)

Co-morbidity	Non-diabetic	Diabetic
Ischaemic heart disease	18.6	32.6
Cerebrovascular disease	8.4	14.4
Peripheral vascular disease	8.3	23.6
Chronic obstructive airways disease	6.6	7.1
Malignancy	12.7	7.5

on to dialysis. Dialysis should, however, be started pre-emptively sooner in patients with documented rapid rate of decline in renal function—generally those with continuing heavy proteinuria and/or poor BP control.

Choice of modality

Discussion must take place on an individual basis. Advantages and disadvantages are similar to those of other dialysis patients.

Particular disadvantages of HD are vascular instability and increased cardiac risk, difficulty creating vascular access, increased complications from AVF (e.g. steal syndrome), increased hypotension on dialysis, and increased hypoglycaemia.

PD offers no cardiac instability or need for vascular access, but increased glucose loads, weight gain, and sometimes difficulty with diabetic control. Peritonitis rates are no higher than in non-diabetics. Visual disturbance may impair the ability to perform PD, but can usually be overcome.

Survival comparisons for PD and HD are difficult to assess because of patient selection. Most studies, after adjustment for co-morbid factors, have not found a statistically significant survival difference between HD and PD in diabetic patients, though observations vary for different patient groups, e.g. younger or older patients.

Younger patients with type 1 diabetes should be considered early for combined kidney–pancreas transplants (ideally pre-emptively), as well as isolated kidney transplantation and a subsequent pancreatic transplant (pancreas after kidney).

Problems for diabetic patients on dialysis

Gastroparesis
May significantly impair dietary intake. Diagnosed by gastroscopy, gastric emptying studies by scintigraphy, and radiolabelled breath tests. Volume depletion and electrolyte imbalance (hypokalaemia and metabolic alkalosis) can complicate severe bouts of vomiting. Managed initially using metoclopramide (starting with 5mg before meals), or (IV) erythromycin, and in difficult cases newer techniques such as injection of botulinum toxin into the pylorus.

Blood glucose control
HbA1C target for patients on dialysis has not been established. The suggested target is 7% (53mmol/mol) in the most recent KDIGO CKD guidelines (2012). There are several reasons why there is not so much emphasis on tight blood glucose control including:
- risk of severe hypoglycaemia with variable dietary intake related to dialysis sessions
- lack of symptoms with hyperglycaemia
- lack of evidence that other organ damage is affected by blood glucose levels
- potential inaccuracy in actual HbA1c measurement due to formation of carbamylated haemoglobin in presence of high urea concentrations.

Insulin delivery
Most patients carry on with SC injections. Doses may need to be increased in PD but reduced in HD. A common regimen in CAPD is short-acting insulin prior to each exchange, and once- or twice-daily long-acting insulin. Intraperitoneal insulin is no longer used because of the increased risk of peritonitis. Total daily insulin dose should be divided equally between the exchanges, with an additional dose added depending on the glucose concentration of the bag (usually an extra 2 units for 1.36%, 4 units for 2.27%, and 6 units for 3.86% bag). Patients should check their blood sugars 1h after each bag during the initiation of therapy to identify their insulin requirements. Patients on HD often require less insulin than prior to dialysis, because of reduced catabolism.

For all patients insulin requirements usually fall by 25–50% with advancing renal failure (GFR <50 mL/min) prior to initiation of dialysis.

Oral hypoglycaemic agents
Long-acting oral hypoglycaemic agents and metformin should not be used. Glipizide and tolbutamide are preferred *sulfonylureas*, both being hepatically metabolized. *Thiazolidinediones* are metabolized by the liver but carry a risk of oedema formation and worsening heart failure; whether this is worse in patients with ESKD is not clear, but they should be used with caution. *Alpha-glucosidase inhibitors*, e.g. acarbose, are not recommended because they and their metabolites are renally excreted and therefore accumulate in ESKD. *Insulin secretagogues*, e.g. repaglinide, stimulate the release of insulin,

and have a prolonged half-life in ESKD. Gliptins (dipeptidyl peptidase-4 inhibitors: include sitagliptin, vildagliptin, saxagliptin, linagliptin) can be used but may need dose modification. Exenatide (an injectable glucagon-like peptide) is contraindicated in ESKD.

Hypotension
More common in HD, and especially if patients have autonomic dysfunction. UF rate should be slow, Hb maintained with EPO, and sequential UF and dialysis, or sodium profiling may be helpful.

Vascular disease
All types—ischaemic heart disease, peripheral vascular disease, and cerebrovascular disease—are more common than in non-diabetic patients on dialysis. Peripheral vascular disease in particular is a predictor of poor survival. High-quality foot care is essential to minimize risk of amputation.

Retinopathy
Almost universal in diabetic dialysis patients. Needs regular formal review and laser therapy as necessary. BP and glucose control are preventative. Heparin should be avoided in HD at time of eye surgery or laser therapy, or after vitreal haemorrhage, but can be used safely if no overt bleeding.

Infections
More common (especially in grafts).

Vascular steal
Increased frequency in forearm AVF or AVGs.

Impotence
Extremely common, and may respond to sildenafil or vardenafil.

Surgery in dialysis patients

Surgery poses special problems for the dialysis patient, either general or specific to HD or PD. These result in increased mortality and morbidity, with longer hospital stays and a greater use of intensive care than for the general population. There are a number of reasons for this.

- Vascular co-morbidity—many patients have ischaemic heart disease and/or cardiac dysfunction, and calcified blood vessels which bleed more easily and are harder to suture.
- Difficulty in controlling fluid and electrolyte balance in peri-operative periods with particular risk of:
  - hyperkalaemia—may require post-operative dialysis
  - fluid overload
  - fluid depletion—in PD patients this can cause decline in residual renal function and therefore underdialysis
- Accumulation of anaesthetic and analgesic drugs
- Increased risk of bleeding
- Poor BP control.

General management

Dialysis patients need rigorous peri- and post-operative monitoring to prevent complications.

> **Pre- and Peri-operative monitoring of the dialysis patient**
> - Biochemistry: electrolytes especially potassium, liver function, urea, creatinine, calcium, phosphate
> - Anaemia status
> - Evidence of infection—WBC, CRP, temperature
> - Fluid and electrolyte management
> - BP control
> - Dialysis timing and dose
> - Nutrition
> - Cardiac status—ischaemic events, arrhythmias
> - Correction of bleeding problems
> - Glucose metabolism
> - IV access—avoidance of veins that may be required for arteriovenous access in future
> - Antibiotics—dosage, nephrotoxicity (important if residual renal function and especially on PD)
> - Pain control—appropriate and sufficient analgesia.

Management of specific problems

Hyperkalaemia

Occurs from release from damaged cells, absorption of altered blood, the potassium load from blood transfusion, hypotension, and decreased tissue perfusion, with production of lactic acid, and drugs (e.g. suxamethonium). Surgery, especially under general anaesthetic, should not be performed unless serum potassium is normal. Potassium should be rechecked within 2–4h of completion of surgery.

Anaemia

Although most anaesthetists prefer a normal Hb level, experienced 'renal' anaesthetists will usually accept a Hb level as low as 9g/dL. If surgery is planned, the Hb level should be optimized by adjusting the dose of EPO therapy rather than by transfusion.

Ischaemic heart disease

This is common and often clinically silent. ECG should always be performed pre-operatively. If the patient has IHD or other vascular disease, more detailed investigations such as echocardiography, thallium scanning, or coronary angiography may be needed before major surgery.

Bleeding

Impaired platelet function found in uraemia increases bleeding during surgery. Reduced in well dialysed patients or by use of:
- desmopressin 0.3mcg/kg (IV or SC; 3mcg/kg intranasally), acts within 1h, lasts 6–8h; do not use if history of IHD as may cause coronary vasoconstriction
- cryoprecipitate (10 units over 30min) acts within 1h, lasts 24–36h, risk of volume overload
- conjugated oestrogens 0.6mg/kg/day (IV) for 5days, but takes 1 week for peak effect, or 2.5–25mg oral conjugated oestrogens orally, or as transdermal patches 50–100mg/day.

Fluid overload

IV fluid both during and after surgery must be given with care, particularly if the patient is anuric.

Nutrition

Maintaining nutrition improves wound healing and reduces risk of infection and other complications. Many patients require nutritional supplements taken either orally or by nasogastric tube.

Haemodialysis

The specific problems related to HD are due to its intermittent nature and the use of heparin.

Timing of dialysis

HD can be planned round routine surgery, but acute surgery may have to be delayed if urgent HD is needed, e.g. to correct fluid overload or hyperkalaemia.

Use of heparin

Should be avoided completely or minimized if surgery is to take place as soon as dialysis is finished. If dialysis is needed soon after surgery, heparin-free dialysis should be performed.

Hypotension

Any drop of BP peri-operatively can cause fistula clotting.

Peritoneal dialysis

The specific problems related to PD are due to the presence of fluid within the abdominal cavity. Dialysate should be drained and the abdomen left empty prior to surgery, to avoid respiratory problems during anaesthesia. Hypotension or fluid depletion can cause a reduction in residual renal function and therefore underdialysis. It may therefore be necessary to increase the PD prescription. After abdominal surgery, depending on amount of residual renal function, temporary or permanent HD may be needed, and should be planned (especially need for access).

Myeloma and renal failure

Incidence of myeloma is about 40 new cases PMP per year, and 10% of patients will have severe AKI. Clinical features are caused by the B-cell clone itself, the secreted immunoglobulin (light chain nephrotoxicity, cryoglobulin), suppression of normal antibody production (immune paresis causing infections), or metabolic effects (hypercalcaemia). Renal failure itself is not an independent prognostic factor, but reflects increased tumour load. Renal failure pre-dates the diagnosis of myeloma in 50% of patients.

All patients with myeloma and AKI should be considered for RRT.

The most important cause of severe AKI is light chains precipitating in tubules as light chain casts. Hypercalcaemia increases cast formation. Dehydration, diuretics, NSAIDs, hypercalcaemia, and antibiotics may all exacerbate or precipitate renal failure by reducing GFR and increasing tubular light chain concentration, and as tubular toxins. (See Table 9.3.)

Clinical features

- Signs and symptoms of myeloma (bone pain, weight loss, weakness, infections).
- An acute precipitating event (infection, hypercalcaemia, dehydration, NSAIDs).
- Urinary light chains (>70% of patients).
- Proteinuria usually <1g/day (unless amyloidosis or immunoglobulin deposition disease).
- Large tumour mass (grade IIIB usually).
- Severe renal failure at presentation (>50% patients require immediate dialysis).
- Renal biopsy usually shows cast nephropathy and interstitial nephritis.

Table 9.3 Causes of renal dysfunction in myeloma

Renal disease	Precipitants	Electrolyte and fluid disturbances
Light chain proteinuria	Volume depletion	Hypercalcaemia
Light chain cast nephropathy	NSAIDs	Dehydration
Light or heavy chain deposition disease	Hypercalcaemia	Pseudohyponatraemia
Hypercalcaemic nephropathy	Radiocontrast media	Hyperviscosity
AL amyloidosis	Furosemide	Hyperuricaemia
Acute urate nephropathy	Septicaemia	Hyperkalaemia
Obstructive uropathy	Urinary tract infection	
Pyelonephritis		
Acute interstitial nephritis		
Cryoglobulinaemia		
ESKD		

Treatment of myeloma renal failure

- Remove precipitants.
- Volume repletion rapidly with normal saline (>3L/day required after rehydration).
- Treat infections.
- Correct hypercalcaemia, initially by rehydration. Steroids reduce serum calcium, and are usually used early as part of a chemotherapeutic regimen. If severe, consider bisphosphonates (pamidronate 60–90mg IV over 4–24h).
- Prevent hyperuricaemia with allopurinol (reduced dose).
- Maintain urine output >3L/day unless established oliguric renal failure.
- No evidence for benefit of alkalinization of urine.
- Furosemide may worsen light chain nephrotoxicity (increased tubular calcium concentration, dehydration).
- Plasma exchange (PE) has been used for patients with severe AKI. A single large RCT[1] in 97 patients could show no benefit of 5–7 PE sessions over 10 days in addition to chemotherapy in patients with AKI, although many were not dialysis requiring and not all had cast nephropathy. Retrospective studies have suggested patients in whom there is rapid reduction of light chains may have much better recovery of renal function whether by plasma exchange, modern chemotherapy, or high-flux dialysis. If PE is to be done, it should be performed daily for 5–7 days to produce maximum reduction in serum light chains and combined with chemotherapy.
- Preliminary data suggests intensive dialysis using a novel large pore protein permeable membrane (high cut-off dialysis) may clear light chains significantly better and improve the outcome of cast nephropathy. Trials are awaited.
- Chemotherapy should be begun early, and is justified in most patients. Renal failure is not a contraindication. Regimens have changed over the years as experience has increased with newer drugs and with increased use of autologous haematopoietic cell transplantation. Treatment plans should therefore be coordinated by specialist haematologists
- Commonly used first-line drug combinations for standard risk patients who are not candidates for transplantation but with renal failure are bortezomib; lenalidomide (or thalidomide) plus low-dose dexamethasone; or vincristine, doxorubicin, and dexamethasone. Where available, bortezomib is currently recommended as first-line therapy in patients with severe renal failure with trials showing a significant number of patients can recover renal function and stop dialysis.
- Toxicity from thalidomide (neuropathy, constipation, bradycardia especially) is more common in patients with kidney dysfunction. Thalidomide cannot be used in pregnant women.
- Similar treatment regimens are used in AL amyloidosis but without recovery of established renal failure.
- Younger patients who recover renal function may be considered for stem cell transplantation.

Dialysis

The outcome of patients with myeloma and renal failure is the same as for patients matched for tumour burden with normal renal function. Dialysis should be considered in all patients having chemotherapy, and should be begun early to avoid prolonged uraemia. Dialysis can be continued long term, or used as a short-term palliative therapy.

HD and PD have both been used. The major complication is infection—peritonitis and line-related sepsis. In patients who have presented acutely and are having plasma exchange, HD is preferable as the same line can be used for both procedures. Renal function can recover several months after treatment has begun and must be sought carefully. Mean time to recovery of renal function is 2 months.

Outcome

Overall survival of patients with renal failure and myeloma is ~17 months (mean). 20% of patients die within 1 month, and one-third survive 3–5 years. Response to chemotherapy is the best predictive factor for survival. About 50% of patients will recover renal function, usually between 30 and 70 days. Patients have recovered renal function from dialysis after bone marrow transplantation in both Europe and the USA (~20%), although mortality is high in this setting. Patients are increasingly recovering renal function with early use of bortezomib or lenalidomide chemotherapy and rapid reduction of serum free light chains (~40%).

Reference

1. Clark WF et al. Plasma exchange when myeloma presents as acute renal failure: a randomized, controlled trial. Ann Intern Med 2005; 143: 77–84.

Pain management in ESKD

50–60% of dialysis patients admit to pain when asked, often very severe, although many will not mention this to their doctors at clinic visits.

Pain is a major cause of depression in this group of patients.

Causes of pain

- Concurrent co-morbidity:
  - peripheral neuropathy
  - peripheral vascular disease
  - ischaemic heart disease
  - arthritis
  - immobility and bedsores
  - malignancy.
- Primary renal disease:
  - polycystic kidney disease (bleeding into cysts)
  - renal calculi.
- Complication of renal failure:
  - renal bone disease
  - gout and other crystal arthropathies
  - dialysis amyloid arthropathy
  - calciphylaxis
  - retroperitoneal haemorrhage from ruptured renal cyst.
- Infection:
  - septic arthritis
  - discitis and epidural abscess formation (as complication of *Staphylococcus aureus* septicaemia associated with central venous access)
  - peritonitis in PD patients.
- Dialysis-related pain:
  - AVF leading to 'steal syndrome'
  - cramps
  - headaches
  - abdominal pain related to PD
  - EPS with associated bowel obstruction.

Difficulty of pain management in renal patients

- Lack of awareness of pain in individual patients.
- Lack of training of nephrologists in pain management.
- Many causes and types of pain:
  - nociceptive:
    —sharp pain felt at site of tissue damage
    —usually responsive to opioids.
  - neuropathic:
    —shooting/stabbing pain occurring in area of abnormal sensation
    —poor response to opioids. Requires adjuvant, e.g. carbamazepine.
  - movement-related pain:
    —difficult to manage: no analgesia required at rest when no pain but often severe pain with movement requiring high levels of analgesia with consequent side effects.
- Pharmacokinetics of analgesics in renal patients:
  - accumulation of drug and/or active metabolite
  - changes in protein binding:
    —increased free drug in plasma
    —fluctuations in protein binding causing variable drug levels.
  - uraemia causing reduced metabolism in kidney.
- Difficulty in using NSAIDs:
  - decrease in renal blood flow causes reduction in GFR; this is particularly important in patients close to starting dialysis, or in PD patients with residual renal function
  - may increase bleeding risk in patients with uraemia because of effects on platelet function and GI mucosa
  - increase in renal sodium reabsorption can exacerbate hypertension and cause oedema
  - can cause severe hyperkalaemia in patients with ESKD, particularly in presence of diabetes with poor glycaemic control, multiple myeloma, and in patients given ACEIs, ARBs, and potassium-sparing diuretics.

Factors contributing to poor pain management

Clinician factors
- Failure to recognize problem
- Lack of training in pain management
- Failure to monitor effect of treatment and therefore adjust medications
- Fear of causing toxicity from opioids
- Fear of using strong opioids for non-cancer pain
- Complex pain management because more than one cause of pain.

Managing pain

Achieving pain control is not just a matter of handing out drugs. It is important to:

- establish the cause of the pain
- consider local treatment, e.g. steroid/local anaesthetic injection of joints
- explore what the pain means to that individual
- determine if there are any psychosocial issues
- treat any underlying depression
- set realistic goals for the patient.

Prescribing analgesics

Pain control is best achieved by using the WHO ladder (see www.who.int/cancer/palliative/painladder).

The WHO principles for managing pain are:

- by mouth—where the patient can swallow and absorb
- by the clock—if pain constant, medication must be given regularly
- by the ladder
- with as needed, prn, medication if pain breaks through
- for the individual
- attention to detail:
  - frequent assessment for efficacy and toxicity
  - dose adjustments according to assessment;
  - aggressive management of side effects.

Analgesic drugs

This list of analgesics by the WHO ladder (see www.who.int/cancer/palliative/painladder) is not comprehensive—rather it provides information about some of the commonly used analgesics and problems with their use in renal failure.

Step 1
Paracetamol
Metabolized by the liver; metabolites do accumulate in renal failure but accepted to be safe at normal doses.

Adjuvants
- NSAIDs—should be avoided if residual renal function, and increase in non-renal side effects in ESKD.
- Neuropathic agents (e.g. carbamazepine, gabapentin) often need to be started at low doses and titrated up.

Step 2: opioids for mild to moderate pain
Codeine
- Metabolized to codeine-6-glucuronide and morphine.
- Significant increase in half-life in renal failure.
- Accumulation of metabolites can cause vomiting, constipation, drowsiness, and confusion.
- Response idiosyncratic—can produce prolonged narcosis in some individuals with renal failure.
- Should be used with careful monitoring.
- Best to start use in a separate preparation from paracetamol.

Dihydrocodeine
- Little information about use in renal failure, so best avoided.
- Reports of CNS depression in patients with ESKD.

Dextropropoxyphene
Avoid—metabolized to norproxyphene, which is associated with CNS toxicity.

Tramadol
- Agonist at μ opioid receptor and inhibits noradrenaline (norepinephrine) and serotonin reuptake.
- May therefore have contributory role in neuropathic pain.
- Metabolized in liver to O-desmethyltramadol.
- 90% excreted by kidney; 30% unchanged.
- Dose adjustments are recommended in renal failure: 50mg bd–tds.
- Use normal release preparations.
- Watch for recognized side effects—confusion and sedation.

Step 3: opioids for moderate to severe pain

Morphine
- Metabolized in liver and excreted by kidney.
- Metabolites are more potent analgesics than morphine, but are responsible for much of the toxicity—drowsiness, respiratory depression, etc. in renal failure.
- Metabolites accumulate more than morphine itself in renal failure.
- Metabolites not cleared by dialysis.
- Chronic dosing with morphine is not recommended in renal failure.

Hydromorphone
- Semisynthetic morphine derivative.
- Orally 4–7 times as potent as morphine.
- Metabolites are not pharmacologically active.
- Useful alternative to morphine in renal patients.
- Used safely by some palliative care physicians at a dose of 1.3mg 4–6-hourly plus 1.3mg as needed if pain breaks through.

Oxycodone
- Semi-synthetic μ agonist with similar profile to morphine.
- 90% of drug is metabolized in liver, with active metabolites.
- Elimination half-life is significantly prolonged in advanced renal failure.
- Can cause sedation and CNS toxicity.

Buprenorphine
- Partial μ agonist/antagonist; sublingually 30–60 times as potent as oral morphine.
- Metabolized in liver; metabolites accumulate in renal failure but are pharmacologically inactive.
- Can be given sublingually and transdermally, though lack of evidence about long-term use in ESKD.

Fentanyl
- Potent synthetic μ receptor agonist 50–100 times as potent as morphine.
- 1000 times as lipophilic as morphine and therefore suitable for transdermal administration.
- IV administration: peak effect at 5min with a duration of 30–60min.
- SC administration: 10–15min to onset with duration of 60–120min.
- Poor oral availability.
- Metabolized in liver to norfentanyl which is inactive.
- <10% excreted unchanged in urine.

Use of fentanyl skin patch
- Not appropriate for uncontrolled pain.
- Effective analgesia not reached until 24h after patch applied.
- Continue normal release medications for first 12h.
- Normal-release strong opioid must be available for breakthrough pain.
- Maximum analgesia may not be reached until 72h so do not increase patch dose until time for patch change.
- A depot of fentanyl remains under the skin for 24h after patch removal.

Pain at the end of life

Most dying patients are frightened of pain. Pain control is therefore an important part of their management, and should not be avoided because of fear of using analgesics in ESKD. The goals of management are different from chronic pain management:

- Patients are often unable or are too weak to swallow.
- Use the WHO ladder (www.who.int/cancer/palliative/painladder)—paracetamol and NSAIDs can be given rectally.
- If pain is continuous, analgesics can be given by syringe driver:
  - in patients who have not previously been on opioids, start with fentanyl 150–300mcg/24h or alfentanil 0.5–1mg/24h
  - if the patient has previously been on strong opioids, calculate the previous 24h dose and convert to alfentanil.
- If pain is intermittent:
  - use strong opioids as needed, e.g. fentanyl 12.5–25mcg SC or alfentanil 0.1–0.2mg SC
  - change to syringe driver if patient unable to ask for pain relief, or if >2–3 doses/24h are needed.

Pregnancy in dialysis patients

Pregnancy is uncommon in women on any form of dialysis, and is usually unplanned. Maternal risks are high and fetal outcome poor, although has improved considerably in recent years. Only 42% of pre-menopausal women on dialysis have normal menstrual periods, and most women are anovulatory. The causes are not clear, but women on dialysis are hyperprolactinaemic, with low serum progesterone levels, and absent luteinizing hormone/follicle-stimulating hormone surges. The frequency of conception in dialysis patients is 0.3–1.4% per year. Pregnancy rates are greater in a woman on HD than CAPD.

Successful pregnancy is more likely in women with CKD prior to the need for dialysis, or in those who only start dialysis after conception. Women with moderate or severe CKD frequently have accelerated loss of renal function in pregnancy, poor BP control, and fetal growth retardation, but overall 90% of pregnancies succeed.

Outcome

Frequency of live births from pregnant dialysis patients has increased over the last decade and now 40–50% of pregnancies in dialysis patients will result in a surviving infant, compared with 75% of pregnancies in women starting dialysis after conception. During the first trimester, 40% abort; 20% of the remainder suffer spontaneous abortions during the second trimester; and ~10% of infants are stillborn. Up to 20% of live born infants will die neonatally, mostly from prematurity. Delivery before 32 weeks is common. Mean gestational age at delivery is 31 weeks. Maternal complications are frequent; hypertension in 80%, accelerated-phase hypertension in up to 10%, and polyhydramnios (urea causing an osmotic diuresis).

There is no difference in the outcome of pregnancy in women on CAPD or HD. Frequent obstetric monitoring is crucial. Second trimester abortions and neonatal death from prematurity are common, and may be preventable. The recent improved outcome is most probably from more intensive dialysis during pregnancy, in both HD and PD.

Diagnosis

Urine tests are unreliable even in patients passing urine, and pregnancy should be confirmed by serum β human chorionic gonadotropin (βHCG) testing. False-positive and false-negative results have both been reported.

Serum α-fetoprotein testing for Down syndrome is not reliable as levels are often elevated in patients with ESKD.

Managing pregnancy in dialysis patients

Management of dialysis during pregnancy

There is no indication to change the modality of dialysis in women who become pregnant on dialysis; however, there is increasing evidence for the benefits of significantly increasing the amount of dialysis, which may be difficult (or impossible) to achieve with PD. Choice of modality for women beginning dialysis during pregnancy is independent of the pregnancy itself, although HD may be preferred given the need for large amounts of dialysis. PD catheters can be placed even late in pregnancy. The value of intensive (daily) HD has not been proven, but a trend to better outcome is seen in women receiving >20h dialysis per week, and women with residual renal function have a better outcome (80% vs 40% infant survival with or without residual function). Intensive dialysis can be associated with hypokalaemia, hypercalcaemia, and alkalosis, but minimizes IDH. A target Kt/V of 2.5 has been suggested (no trials), and most women are now treated with dialysis for 4h, 6 days per week. Such intensive regimens aim also to maintain blood urea <16–17mmol/L (45–50mg/dL). Serum calcium and phosphate should be checked weekly, and some patients become hypophosphataemic. A major problem is determination of fluid overload since pregnant women will increase weight weekly with progression of the pregnancy, and accurate estimation of fluid balance is crucial to prevent both hypotension on dialysis and hypertension from volume overload. Volume status should be assessed carefully each week. Heparin can be used normally.

Women continuing CAPD will usually need reduced volumes and an increased number of exchanges late in pregnancy. Combining daytime CAPD exchanges with APD is often necessary. There are no data on the effect of PD regimens on pregnancy outcome. Peritonitis is rare.

Nutrition

Women need to increase their protein intake (~1.5g/kg/day), dietary potassium, water-soluble vitamins: folic acid (4mg/day), vitamin C (150mg/day), thiamine (3mg/day), niacin (20mg/day), B_6 (15mg/day), and calcium (2g/day as phosphate binders). Calcium-containing phosphate binders (if needed) are safe. There are no data on sevelamer or lanthanum use in pregnancy but neither are absorbed. Careful weekly assessment is vital to determine fluid status especially with planned weight gain of 0.3–0.5kg/week from pregnancy.

Management of hypertension in pregnancy

Hypertension is often caused by volume overload, and careful assessment and management of volume status are crucial. If antihypertensive agents are needed, methyldopa or labetalol are the drugs of first choice, especially during the first trimester. Hydralazine, nifedipine, and prazosin (and other α-blockers) are safe to use. β-Blockers are used but may cause fetal growth retardation. ACEIs and ARBs are contraindicated (oligohydramnios, pulmonary hypoplasia, neonatal anuria, or neonatal death). Exposure during the first trimester is probably safe (although there remains some controversy), and thus women with CKD trying to get pregnant may remain on them until pregnancy confirmed since the benefits on proteinuria for a possible prolonged time to pregnancy may be important. Patients can then switch to methyldopa or labetalol.

Pre-eclampsia is common and should be actively managed with prompt delivery.

Infections

CMV, herpes viruses, and toxoplasmosis may be more common in pregnant dialysis patients.

Anaemia

Worsening anaemia is almost universal. EPO requirements increase by 50–100%, and serum iron falls. EPO dose should be doubled from the onset of pregnancy in all women prior to a drop in Hb. IV iron is safe and useful. Women should be on increased folate supplementation (4mg/day) as folic acid is lost in dialysis.

Pregnancy after renal transplantation

Fertility rapidly returns to women after successful kidney transplantation, and pregnancy occurs in up to 12% of young women. All young women receiving a transplant should be advised to use contraception. Over 75% of pregnancies will result in a surviving infant (often premature), and >90% after the first trimester. There is an increased risk of graft loss and maternal morbidity in women with an elevated serum creatinine at conception.

Travelling and holidays

Patients on dialysis often want to travel for work, family reasons, and holidays. This is possible to many destinations, but does need organization and advance planning. There are also potential financial implications and health risks associated with many countries.

Patients on dialysis are at increased risk from the following:

- Heat: fluid balance will be affected in hot climates. Fluid losses are increased and patients can become dehydrated and hypotensive if they do not increase their fluid intake. Some patients, though, become fluid overloaded as they drink too much because of increased thirst.
- GI infections: these are more common when travelling, and can result in fluid depletion and hypotension, as well as electrolyte imbalance.
- Vaccinations: dialysis patients should not be given live vaccines (e.g. yellow fever) but can (and should) be given inactivated ones and antitoxins (e.g. typhoid).
- Malaria: most antimalarial drugs are renally excreted and need dose adjustment. The choice of antimalarial depends on the precise location visited, and is not predicated by ESKD.
- Drugs and supplies: patients should carry the drugs they need, a formal list of the drugs, syringes, and needles in case of problems at customs or security, and a summary of their medical information. EPO needs to be kept cold, should be kept in a cold box for travel, and placed into a fridge immediately on arrival at the destination.

Peritoneal dialysis

Travelling on PD is relatively easy. Supplies can be put in the back of a car, and most APD machines come in cases on wheels. PD companies have 'travel clubs' that arrange delivery of fluid locally round the world. This does take time to organize (from 1 month if travelling in Europe to 2–3 months if travelling further afield). The dialysis unit often absorbs the cost of this, as fluid is not required at home while the patient is away. There are some countries that do not have PD facilities and do not allow the import of fluid. Patients should therefore always check before organizing travel.

Specific problems and precautions:

- Some APD patients prefer to change to CAPD while travelling rather than take their machine.
- Some countries provide no back-up for APD machines if they go wrong so it is advisable for patients to use CAPD while there.
- As fluids come from local suppliers, the range of fluids available may be different from home, e.g. some countries just have high calcium (1.75mmol/L) dialysis fluid—most European patients are on 1.25mmol/L calcium dialysate, so should be advised to reduce calcium supplements.

- Patients should travel with a supply of antibiotics in case they develop peritonitis, as they could be some distance from a hospital with a renal unit. To avoid the need for blood levels and frequent dosing, a simplified regimen can be used, e.g. vancomycin (30mg/kg body weight) for 2 doses and ciprofloxacin 500mg bd for 2 weeks. Patients should be instructed to contact their home unit if they have to use the antibiotics.

It is also important to ensure return of the antibiotics after the holiday so they are not subsequently misused!

Haemodialysis

Travel requires significant advance planning. Patients need to identify a dialysis unit at their destination, make contact in advance to book dialysis slots, send a medical report in advance, including recent hepatitis (and often HIV) serology, as well as details of the dialysis regimen, and may need a supporting doctor's letter. Patients will usually have to pay for the dialysis, which may come as a shock to patients used to free provision. It may be possible to reduce the number of sessions to 2/week for a short period to reduce the cost, inconvenience, and disruption to the holiday. This is easier in patients with good pre-dialysis biochemistry and residual renal function. Patients on home HD especially when using newer technologies such as the NxStage® may find travelling easier, and in some countries (especially Australia) patients often travel in specially set-up vehicles.

Specific problems and precautions:
- Advance planning is crucial.
- Some patients take their dialysers with them.
- There is a risk of acquiring hepatitis viral infections if dialysing in a developing country, or one with a high prevalence. Patients should be warned of this risk, and will have more regular blood testing on their return for several months to detect seroconversion for hepatitis B or C. Infection with hepatitis C might jeopardize future transplantation.
- Patients especially dialysing with central venous lines are at increased risk from bacterial sepsis when dialysing in a temporary dialysis unit.

Plasmapheresis

Has been used to treat a large number of conditions, often without good evidence. Diseases for which PE has an important role should be treated aggressively, and PE performed intensively. (See Tables 9.4, 9.5, and 9.6)

Table 9.4 Conditions for which PE has an established role

Anti-GBM disease	Especially non-oliguric renal failure pre-dialysis and pulmonary haemorrhage
ANCA-associated vasculitis	Patients with severe renal failure (controlled trial data—MEPEX study) and/or pulmonary haemorrhage
Haemolytic uraemic syndrome (HUS)/ thrombocytopenic thrombotic purpura (TTP)	PE or infusion both beneficial
Type I and II cryoglobulinaemia	Patients improve symptomatically, vasculitic syndromes improve, variable effect on renal function
Hyperviscosity syndrome	Usually Waldenström's macroglobulinaemia

Table 9.5 Conditions for which PE may be useful

Recurrent nephrotic proteinuria (FSGS) post-transplantation	Reduction in proteinuria occasionally permanent, usually transient
Acute vascular allograft rejection	May help patients with resistant rejection
Highly sensitized transplant recipients	May help remove anti-HLA antibodies and allow successful transplantation
SLE	May be of use in the most severe disease or cerebral lupus. No benefit in moderate renal disease
Crescentic IgA glomerulonephritis	Possible short-term benefit
Guillain–Barré syndrome	But IVIG may be as good or better
Myasthenia gravis	In an acute crisis
Homozygous familial hypercholesterolaemia	Chronic treatment necessary

Table 9.6 Conditions with little or no evidence for benefit of PE

SLE	No benefit in mild/moderate renal disease
Primary glomerulonephritides	Except anti-GBM disease
Chronic transplant rejection	No benefit
Myeloma with cast nephropathy	No benefit in severe AKI after rehydration in a single large randomized trial

Techniques of plasmapheresis

Two major methods: centrifugal cell separators and membrane plasma filters. Both require IV access and large volumes of replacement fluids. The systems may not be equivalent (see Figs 9.1 and 9.2).

A single plasma volume exchange (50mL/kg) will lower plasma macromolecule levels by ~60%, and 5 exchanges over 5–10 days will clear 90% of the total body immunoglobulin. This regimen (5–7 exchanges over 1 week) produces maximum efficacy for removal of macromolecules such as immunoglobulin. Rebound in the plasma concentration of macromolecules occurs after PE due to resynthesis and redistribution, and PE should almost always be accompanied by some form of immunosuppression to prevent re-synthesis of immunoglobulins.

Cascade filtration (serial haemofilters with varying pore sizes to deplete larger MW components only), and cryofiltration (plasma passed through cold chamber after separation to precipitate cryoglobulins) are not routinely available.

Centrifugal devices

Withdraw plasma from a spinning bowl with either synchronous (Cobe Spectra system) or intermittent (Haemonetics system) return of blood cells to the patient. There is no upper limit to the MW of proteins removed by this method. Plasma, platelets, or WBCs can be isolated separately. Can be done through a single needle in an antecubital vein (intermittent system).

Membrane haemofiltration

Uses highly permeable membranes through which blood is pumped at ~100–150mL/min. Plasma readily passes through the membrane pores (0.2–0.5µm; MW cut-off ~2000kDa), while the cells are simultaneously returned to the patient. In general all immunoglobulin will cross the membrane (IgG more efficiently than IgM); however, some large immune complexes and some cryoglobulins may not be adequately cleared. Membrane filtration is faster.

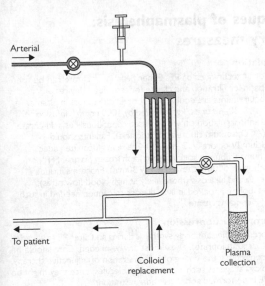

Fig. 9.1 Membrane plasma filtration.

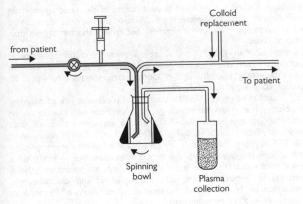

Fig. 9.2 Centrifugal cell separation.

Techniques of plasmapheresis: ancillary measures

Anticoagulation

Necessary for all techniques of PE. Either heparin or citrate can be used, generally heparin for filtration and citrate for centrifugal devices.

- Heparin requirements are double that for HD due to loss in plasma. Loading dose is 30–60 units/kg, followed by 1000 units/h infusion.
- For citrate anticoagulation citrate is infused continuously as acid-citrate dextrose (ACD; sodium citrate and citric acid). Patients should receive calcium IV or orally (2–4mL 10% calcium gluconate added to 500mL human albumin solution (not fresh frozen plasma, FFP), or calcium carbonate 500mg chewed every 30min). Problems include hypocalcaemia and alkalosis (more likely at high blood flow rates). Citrate metabolism impaired in liver disease so caution needed in such patients. FFP contains citrate.

Ancillary immunosuppression

Used to suppress further antibody synthesis during and after PE (e.g. cyclophosphamide or azathioprine), and almost always needed. Care should be taken when considering the timing of administration of adjunctive therapy, especially biological agents such as antibody molecules, since they might be removed if PE is performed soon after administration.

Replacement fluids

Crystalloids should not be used alone because of the need to maintain colloid oncotic pressure. Synthetic gelatin-based plasma expanders can be used as part of a replacement regimen, but have a shorter half-life than human albumin.

Human albumin (5%) remains the mainstay of fluid replacement. Reactions are rare, and it is virologically safe having been heat treated. The major disadvantages are the lack of clotting factors, leading to a post-PE depletion coagulopathy, and the cost.

FFP is also used (in addition to albumin) in patients at risk of bleeding (post-biopsy, pulmonary haemorrhage, etc.), or those with low fibrinogen levels. For patients with HUS/TTP, plasma replacement rather than removal may be critical for recovery, and full exchanges for FFP are usual. In HUS/TTP, cryoprecipitate-poor FFP (plasma from which the cryoprecipitate has been removed) offers theoretical advantages over whole plasma (depletion of von Willebrand factor multimers that are potent endothelial activators). FFP replaces clotting factors, complement, and non-pathogenic immunoglobulin, but almost all the serious complications of PE occur in patients receiving FFP including anaphylaxis.

Complications of plasmapheresis

Occur in <10% of exchanges, most being trivial (leg cramps, dizziness, nausea, urticaria, citrate-induced paraesthesiae). In patients receiving albumin replacement (not FFP), complications occur in <2% of exchanges. Serious complications—hypotension, chest pain, anaphylaxis—are rare, but significantly more common with use of FFP.

- Complications of vascular access—haematoma, bleeding, local infection, line sepsis, venous thrombosis.
- Ethylene oxide hypersensitivity (from plasma filter or sterile disposable centrifugal bowl).
- Citrate (in FFP or used as an anticoagulant) induced hypocalcaemia is averted by infusing 10–20mL 10% calcium gluconate during PE.
- Alkalosis can be caused by metabolism of citrate to bicarbonate and the failure to excrete it adequately.
- Dilutional hypokalaemia is avoided by adding potassium to replacement fluids.
- Risk of bleeding is increased due to depletion of coagulation factors. Prothrombin time is increased by 30%, and PTT by 100% after a single plasma volume exchange. FFP should be used in patients at risk of bleeding. PE should be avoided if possible for 24–48h after a renal biopsy, and FFP used for 48–72h.
- Platelet consumption is more common after centrifugal PE. PE should be withheld if platelet count <80×10⁹/L (except in TTP/HUS).
- No increased risk of infection.

Specific indications for plasmapheresis

Anti-GBM disease
PE removes anti-GBM antibodies effectively. The introduction of PE was associated with dramatically improved patient survival. Only one controlled trial has been performed, which showed benefit of PE (non-significant). PE rapidly reverses pulmonary haemorrhage. Patients presenting as dialysis dependent or with creatinine >600µmol/L have less benefit (unless pulmonary haemorrhage), but may still recover function. There are no controlled trials of IV methylprednisolone vs PE. PE should be performed daily for at least 14 days and continued until anti-GBM antibody is undetectable (may be >14 days). FFP should be added to replacement fluids in pulmonary haemorrhage. Avoid fluid overload (can precipitate pulmonary haemorrhage).

Pauci-immune crescentic RPGN (ANCA associated)
The MEPEX prospective RCT of PE vs IV methylprednisolone (in addition to conventional immunosuppression) in >140 patients with ANCA-associated RPGN and severe renal failure has shown significant short-term benefits of PE in recovery of renal function (~75% vs 50%). Three previous small controlled trials of PE in focal necrotizing GN had been performed. Two showed benefit in patients with creatinine >600µmol/L or requiring dialysis. From uncontrolled data, 85% of dialysis-dependent patients treated with PE recover renal function, compared with 40% of those receiving immunosuppressive drugs alone. PE is performed daily for 7–10 days. May need to be repeated. Monitor ANCA titres.

Other crescentic nephritides
No controlled trials. May be beneficial in patients with a rapidly progressive clinical course and histological evidence of acute crescentic glomerular damage.

HUS/TTP
Full exchanges for FFP offer benefit. RCTs in adult TTP have shown unequivocal advantage of PE over plasma infusion (78% vs 50% 6-month survival); however, patients received 3× more plasma during PE than with simple plasma infusion. PE should be continued until platelet counts >100, lactate dehydrogenase normal, and minimal ongoing haemolysis. May be better to use cryo-poor FFP as replacement. Some evidence that exchanges for 50% FFP and 50% albumin may provide similar efficacy to full exchange for FFP alone. No good trial data in pure HUS for benefit of PE.

SLE
No benefit in mild or moderately severe SLE (RCTs). May be useful in patients with most severe disease, with pulmonary haemorrhage, cerebral lupus, or severe lupus unresponsive to conventional drugs, or patients in whom cytotoxic therapy has been withdrawn because of bone marrow suppression or other toxicity.

Cryoglobulinaemia, myeloma, and paraproteinaemia

No controlled trials in cryoglobulinaemia. In type I cryoglobulinaemia, symptoms are closely related to the presence of the cryo-immunoglobulin, and treatment with PE is efficacious. In type II cryoglobulinaemia, PE removes circulating immune complexes effectively, but recurrence common. Particularly useful if ongoing vascular occlusion or active renal disease. Chronic treatment often required (1 session per week/fortnight). Warm replacement fluids.

Utility of PE in myeloma probably low (see ➔ Myeloma and renal failure, p. 430). A large prospective RCT in patients with myeloma and AKI demonstrated no benefit of PE over chemotherapy alone (after rehydration). Patients did not all, however, have a renal biopsy, and patients with cast nephropathy as the predominant pathology may benefit. More recent data suggests any treatment which rapidly reduces free light chains may allow renal recovery, and newer chemotherapeutic drugs can achieve this (e.g. bortezomib and lenalidomide) as well as PE or high cut-off dialysis. If using PE, patients should be treated daily for 5–7 days.

Transplantation

No benefit in chronic rejection. Used in severe vascular rejection, but no controlled trials vs antibody therapy (antilymphocyte globulin/OKT3). Can remove anti-HLA antibodies in sensitized recipients pre-transplant and allow successful engraftment, and anti-ABO blood group antibodies to allow ABO-incompatible transplantation. Needs to be continued for several days. Highly effective in recurrent FSGS (with nephrotic syndrome) post-transplantation, although effect may be transient (see ➔ Indications for immunoadsorption, p. 455).

Immunoadsorption techniques

Immunoadsorption (IA) selectively removes immunoglobulin molecules from plasma. Compared with PE, immunoglobulins are eliminated in large quantities and with high specificity, replacement blood products (human albumin, FFP) are not required, and there is no depletion of circulating clotting factors and complement.

Techniques

• Most commonly using protein A columns. Protein A binds IgG with high affinity and specificity (via the Fc domain), and small quantities of IgA and IgM. Columns can be re-used many times, but are costly.
• Phenylalanine- or tryptophan-coated columns: relatively low selectivity and efficiency, cheap, but cannot be re-used.
• Antihuman IgG antibody-coated columns: highly specific for human immunoglobulins, very effective, but very costly.

The latter two systems are not widely available. In all systems, blood is circulated extracorporeally through a fibre haemofilter, and the filtered plasma is pumped through short columns containing Sepharose® beads coated with immunosorbent. Unbound plasma is returned to the patient. Protein A columns are regenerated by stripping off the bound IgG with acid.

Patients requiring HD can have simultaneous sequential IA and HD, but this requires skilled nursing.

Patients receiving IA need concurrent immunosuppression with steroids and cyclophosphamide, mycophenolate, or azathioprine to minimize further antibody synthesis.

Complications

Side effects are rare. IV access is required, volume overload, and anaphylactic reactions to protein A (a staphylococcal product) can occur during treatment. Coagulopathy and metabolic derangement do not occur.

Indications for immunoadsorption

Few controlled clinical trials have been performed. Evidence for benefit is based on uncontrolled trials or small series.

- IA has been used successfully to treat anti-GBM disease and ANCA-associated vasculitis with severe renal failure either in place of PE or in patients with ongoing pulmonary haemorrhage or resistant renal disease. A single controlled trial in vasculitis showed no difference in outcome compared with PE.
- Patients with moderately severe SLE have been treated with phenylalanine and anti-IgG columns, with marked improvements in organ dysfunction, and disease scores improving for at least 6 months.
- IA can remove anti-HLA antibodies in sensitized dialysis patients awaiting renal transplantation. Treatment can be continued either intermittently for several months while awaiting a donor kidney, or intensively for 6–12h immediately prior to transplantation. Panel-reactive antibodies can become undetectable with continued treatment, and allow a negative cross-match between recipient and donor. Treatment is continued for several days after transplantation to allow accommodation of the graft, but can be stopped after ~1 week. In many patients the subsequent return of cytotoxic antibodies does not cause rejection.
- IA has been used to treat recurrence of FSGS in renal allografts. FSGS commonly recurs in patients after transplantation as nephrotic syndrome, and predisposes to graft loss. PE and IA have both been successfully used to remove an uncharacterized circulating factor from the serum of these patients. In most cases the response is temporary, and IA or PE need to be continued intermittently for prolonged periods. However, some patients never relapse after a short course of IA, and are cured.
- IA has been used to treat patients with myasthenia gravis, immune thrombocytopenia, Guillain–Barré syndrome, idiopathic dilated cardiomyopathy, Grave's disease, and a number of other immune-mediated diseases. The number of patients treated is small.

Chapter 10

Complications of ESKD: anaemia

Causes of anaemia

Anaemia is universal in ESKD, primarily due to a relative lack of EPO. Plasma EPO levels are within the 'normal' range (6–30mU/mL), but not increased to the levels seen in other severe anaemias (>100mU/mL), due to the failure of diseased renal tissue to respond to the anaemic hypoxic stimulus. Anaemia usually develops as the GFR falls below 35mL/min, and worsens with declining GFR. Other causes of anaemia in renal failure include:

- shortened red blood cell survival
- uraemic and cytokine inhibition of erythropoiesis (especially infections and inflammatory conditions)
- iron deficiency
- hypothyroidism
- active blood loss (including HD circuits, GI bleeding)
- haemolysis
- haemoglobinopathies
- aluminium overload
- hyperparathyroid osteitis fibrosa
- folic acid or vitamin B_{12} deficiency
- elevated circulating hepcidin.

Anaemia in ESKD is not a trivial problem. There is a strong association between Hb and risk of death in ESKD.

Benefits of treating anaemia

Major improvements have been demonstrated in:
- morbidity and mortality
- quality of life
- exercise capacity
- cognitive function
- sexual function
- immune responsiveness
- nutrition
- sleep patterns
- cardiac status (reduced LVH and dilatation, improved cardiac output, reduced angina).

Recent trials have, however, demonstrated increased mortality, stroke and cardiovascular events in pre-dialysis patients treated with EPO to Hb levels >11g/dL which may be more a consequence of higher doses of EPO (see ➲ Target haemoglobin, p. 466), but which has engendered some concerns over targets when treating anaemia in CKD.

Assessment of anaemia and haemolysis

Investigating anaemia in ESKD

Should be performed when Hb <11.0g/dL. Initially:

- red blood cell indices
- blood film
- WBCs and platelets
- reticulocyte count
- serum iron and total iron binding capacity
- transferrin saturation (TSAT)
- serum ferritin (and CRP)
- stool occult blood.

These tests will exclude causes for anaemia other than renal failure itself, especially haemolysis, haematinic deficiency, bone marrow suppression, or infiltration.

Haemolysis

Can be caused by:

- contaminants in the dialysate (chloramines—an oxidant—copper, nitrates)
- hypo-osmolar or overheated dialysate
- re-use sterilants (formaldehyde inducing antibodies)
- blood pump trauma to red blood cells
- high flows through narrow IV catheters or needles
- drug induced (penicillin, cephalosporin, quinidine, methyldopa)
- causes of microangiopathic haemolytic anaemia or autoimmune haemolysis.

Management of anaemia

Erythropoietic stimulating agents (ESAs) and IV iron are the mainstays of management of the anaemia of renal failure. There are currently five forms of ESAs—all are recombinant forms of either native human EPO or with modifications to improve pharmacokinetics or activity, or EPO receptor activators. All ESAs increase Hb effectively in renal anaemia.

EPO is a 165-amino acid secreted glycoprotein. Recombinant EPO (epo-etin) is available in four forms: alfa, beta, theta and zeta. Each is administered 1–3 times/week by SC or IV injection (see ➔ Erythropoietin: administration, p. 462).

The other two ESAs in clinical use are darbepoetin alfa and methoxy polyethylene glycol-epoetin beta.

Darbepoetin alfa is a 'longer acting' erythropoietic molecule with a half-life ~3-fold longer than recombinant EPO, achieved by adding two extra N-linked carbohydrate side chains to the EPO molecule. As a result, darbepoetin alfa needs less frequent dosing, usually only once a week or once every 2 weeks, and sometimes only once a month in stable patients.

Methoxy polyethylene glycol-epoetin beta is a continuous erythropoietin receptor activator with extended half-life which enables once-monthly dosing of patients.

ESAs have been shown to have a beneficial effect in most patients with anaemia of CKD, improving quality of life, exercise capacity, and cognitive function, and reducing LVH and cardiac dilatation. They are beneficial in patients on HD or PD, or in those with CKD prior to dialysis. Their use has removed anaemia as a major cause of morbidity in ESKD, and reduced the need for blood transfusions. Almost 90% of dialysis patients receive ESAs in the USA, slightly fewer in Europe. Response to ESAs varies between individuals, and particularly depends on the dose and route administered, adequacy of iron stores, and concurrent inflammation. Ideally ESAs should be begun when the Hb falls below 10.0g/dL, before LVH begins to develop, although there are no long-term trials available comparing timing of initiation. Economic constraints may prevent early use.

Indications and preparation for use

- All dialysis patients with symptoms attributable to anaemia or a Hb <10.0g/dL (but precise level controversial, and no good evidence for absolute starting level of Hb).
- Pre-dialysis patients with ESKD and symptomatic anaemia (and maybe with a Hb <10.0g/dL).
- Treat iron deficiency first.
- Ensure adequate iron stores.
- Ensure good BP control.

Use in pre-dialysis patients

ESAs are safe and effective in pre-dialysis patients with ESKD, although not without concerns. Their use has not been associated with increased rate of loss of residual renal function. Early use may help prevent cardiac dysfunction associated with anaemia. Recent RCTs of ESAs in patients with CKD not yet on dialysis have shown:

- no improvement in mortality with higher Hb levels
- variable improvement in quality of life
- high-risk groups:
  - increased risk of stroke
  - worse prognosis if pre-existing malignancy
- poorer outcome with high doses of ESA.

Erythropoietin: administration

EPO α and β are available as vials containing 1–10,000 units/mL, as larger volume multidose vials, as pre-filled syringes with 1–10,000 units per syringe, and in the form of a multidose injecting 'pen'. EPO is relatively unstable at room temperature and must be kept in a fridge at 4°C. Stability varies somewhat between the main preparations. Multidose vials in particular should not be left warm for very long, and pen injectors (containing multidose cartridges) should be carried only for short periods with cooled inserts. Other ESAs also need injection, and have variable needs for cold storage and come as pre-filled syringes or vials.

Route of administration

SC administration of EPO α and β has historically been shown to allow a 35% (15–50%) reduction in dosing for a given Hb response (compared with the IV route). More recently, however, only a small increase in dose has been needed in patients transferring from the SC to IV routes. The SC route had been the preferred route, until the advent of pure red cell aplasia (PRCA). Patients should be taught to self-administer where possible. The injection site should be changed at each injection. Some patients report stinging with injection, probably induced by the citrate buffer in some preparations. The presence of benzyl alcohol (as a preservative) in other EPO preparations acts as a local anaesthetic and minimizes stinging. For darbepoetin alfa there is no dose differential between SC and IV routes. For convenience, many patients on HD are given EPO IV.

Patients can generally be dosed once a week or fortnight with EPO α and β now, although the original licensed indication suggested dosing 2 or 3 times per week; darbepoetin alfa is given once per week to once per fortnight, and methoxy polyethylene glycol-epoetin beta is given once a month.

Recombinant human erythropoietins (epoetin alfa, beta, theta, and zeta)

Note: it is essential to specify which epoetin is to be prescribed. This is particularly important with the increasing number of biosimilar products emerging around the world—the active substance of a biosimilar medicine is similar, but not identical, to the biological reference medicine.

Darbepoetin alfa

Comes in a range of colour-coded pre-filled syringes or as a prefilled disposable injection device ((*Aranesp®SureClick*), both ranging from 10 to 500mcg. 1mcg darbepoetin alfa is equivalent to 200IU EPO. There is no difference between the IV and the SC doses (unlike EPO). Treatment should start initially at a dose of 450ng/kg once weekly; maintenance dose can be given weekly, fortnightly, or monthly. The less frequent dosage regimens are useful for community treatment (pre-dialysis or PD patients), particularly for patients who require a nurse to give the injection.

Methoxy polyethylene glycol-epoetin beta

Comes in a range of pre-filled syringes, ranging from 50 to 250mcg. Initial dose is 1.2mcg/kg once every 4 weeks, by SC or IV injection, or 600 ng/kg once every 2 weeks. Maintenance dose is given every 2–4 weeks. The sole advantage of this drug is the extended dosing regimen making it convenient for community-based patients needing nurse assistance for injections.

Erythropoietin

Initiating therapy

- Patients must have adequate iron stores prior to starting ESAs. Serum ferritin should be >200mcg/L and TSAT >20%. Oral iron is poorly tolerated and ineffective in HD patients, and IV iron infusions are preferred.
- Iron stores can be depleted rapidly once erythropoiesis is induced. Ferritin levels therefore need to be closely monitored and further iron replacement given as needed.
- BP should be well controlled. Severe hypertension and fits were a complication of starting EPO when it was first introduced, but are rarely seen with current dosage regimens, with slower rises in Hb levels.
- Starting doses of ESAs for patients on PD or not yet on dialysis are about 30% lower than for patients on HD.
- Starting dose of EPO α and β should be 80–120 units/kg/week (typically 6000 units/week) either once per week or in two or three divided doses. IV doses need to be increased by 30–50% (average 9000 units/week).
- Starting dose of darbepoetin alfa is 0.45mcg/kg weekly either SC or IV once per week.
- Starting dose of methoxy polyethylene glycol-epoetin beta is 600ng/kg once every 2 weeks either SC or IV.

Titrating dose

- Target Hb should be reached in 3–4 months (increase in Hb of ~1g/dL per month).
- Hb should be monitored every 2–4 weeks after initiating therapy or after a change in dose.
- If Hb rises too fast, temporarily withhold ESA. Hb should fall ~1g/dL per month. Reinstate at a dose ~25% below previous dose.
- Decrease dose by between 25% and 50% if Hb increases >2g/dL in a 4-week period.
- *Increase* dose by ~25% if increase in Hb <1g/dL over 4 weeks and iron stores are adequate.
- Frequency of administration depends on type of ESA:
  - EPO α and β are usually given once per week, but can be given once per fortnight if Hb level is maintained using a relatively low dose.
  - Darbepoetin alfa can be given weekly and fortnightly—and in some patients even monthly if only a low dose is required
  - Methoxy polyethylene glycol-epoetin beta can be given monthly after Hb has stabilized.
- Patients using longer-acting ESA and being treated at home (i.e. pre-dialysis or on PD) can change dose by altering interval between injections, e.g. from weekly to 2-weekly if dose needs to be reduced, or 2-weekly to weekly if dose needs to be increased. This avoids having to supply new vials for a different dose—and wasting existing home supplies.
- Longer dosage intervals, e.g. fortnightly or monthly, are particularly useful for patients who need assistance from a nurse to receive their injection.

Maintenance therapy

- Hb level should be monitored monthly in HD patients and 2-monthly in pre-dialysis or PD patients.
- If Hb remains at target level, drug dose can be kept unchanged, although dose frequency can be reduced (keeping total dose unchanged). Some patients can be maintained on 2-weekly EPO, or monthly darbepoetin alfa.
- Iron status is crucial to maintaining adequate Hb levels. Ferritin and TSAT status should be checked monthly in HD patients and 2-monthly in pre-dialysis and PD patients. Regular IV iron is needed by many patients.
- Maintenance dose of ESAs is often 75% of the final dose used during the initial phases of treatment.
- Increased doses may be required during intercurrent illnesses to maintain Hb, but there are no data on the best management strategy. Post-transplantation it may take a month for the graft to resume secretion of EPO.
- If given IV, EPO should be infused towards the end of dialysis. AN69® in particular can adsorb large amounts of EPO.

Side effects

- Hypertension is the most common complication (20–50% patients):
  - associated with rate of rise in Hb, absolute level of Hb achieved, vasoconstriction induced by treatment, arterial remodelling, and enhanced responsiveness to noradrenaline
  - hypertensive encephalopathy was seen during the early days of EPO and was associated with a rapid rise in Hb and BP
  - severe hypertension is not seen with slow controlled rise of Hb.
- Hypertension should be managed by fluid removal and appropriate drug treatment.
- EPO and darbepoetin alfa should not be withheld unless evidence of accelerated hypertension.
- Pain at injection site occurs in a few patients using darbepoetin alfa SC; it is much less common with EPO β.
- Trials have suggested an increased risk of cardiovascular events and stroke in patients with CKD, but this may be an effect of high doses of EPO and remains controversial.

Pure red cell aplasia

This is rare but devastating.
- Caused by formation of antibodies to EPO.
- Very rare.
- Historic cluster in patients treated with Eprex® (European brand of EPO A), in total affecting ~250 patients worldwide. Thought to be due to change in the immunogenicity of the EPO molecule brought about by removing human albumin from solvent and replacing with polysorbate which reacted with compounds leached from the uncoated rubber stoppers.
- Mostly occurs with SC route of administration, because of increased immunogenicity of proteins when injected SC.

- Diagnosis should be suspected if Hb falls (usually abruptly) despite increasing dose of EPO—and reticulocyte count is <1% (or $<10 \times 10^9$/L), with normal platelet and white cell counts.
- Diagnosis confirmed by finding anti-EPO antibodies in serum, and bone marrow features of PRCA.
- If diagnosed, EPO should be stopped. Various immunosuppression strategies have been used as treatment with some success; Hb will rise, but often reintroduction of EPO (any brand) will re-stimulate production of antibodies. Kidney transplantation can be curative.

Target haemoglobin

- Target Hb remains controversial and are regulated by NICE (UK) and the FDA (USA), with several other bodies also producing guidelines.
- Randomized controlled studies on which guidelines are based have all been performed in predialysis patients.
- Increasing evidence that there is little benefit of maintaining Hb >12g/dL in predialysis patients.
- Some evidence of potential risk with increased morbidity and mortality in predialysis patients on ESAs with Hb maintained at level >12g/dL.
- Surprisingly, quality of life measurements in predialysis patients on ESAs have not been shown to be directly related to Hb level.
- Current UK Renal Association Hb target is 11.0–12.0g/dL, and KDIGO Hb target <11.5g/dL.
- Patients with angina may get fewer symptoms at higher Hb levels.
- Fears about increased vascular access thrombosis with higher Hb levels have not been proven.
- Hb levels in a dialysis population on EPO follow a normal distribution. Therefore, in order to achieve 80% of patients having a Hb within a target range, a dialysis unit must aim for a higher Hb level overall.

Higher values of Hb have been associated with better cognitive function, better quality of life, further improvement in exercise capacity, and in some patients prevention of progressive left ventricular dilatation. However, the several trials randomizing patients to more normal Hcts, with or without heart disease, have either been stopped early because of a trend to increased mortality in the normal Hct group, or at completion showed similar results.

Failure to respond (resistance)

Most common cause is iron deficiency, often induced by the rise in Hb. Other causes include:
- inadequate dosing
- concurrent infection/inflammation
- compliance
- hyperparathyroidism
- bone marrow fibrosis
- occult malignancy
- aluminium
- malnutrition
- inadequate dialysis

- haemoglobinopathies
- other haematinic deficiency
- other bone marrow disorders, e.g. myelodysplasia
- PRCA
- blood loss
- haemolysis
- ACEIs
- carnitine deficiency.

True resistance (to 500–900 units EPO/kg/week or 1.5mcg/week darbepoetin alfa in iron-replete patients) is rare. Relative resistance is quite common.

Adequate doses of EPO should induce an increase in reticulocytes in the blood.

Iron store should be maintained (ferritin 400–800ng/mL) with regular iron. Increasing evidence that regular IV iron reduces requirements for EPO.

Iron metabolism

Iron deficiency

Commonly associated with the anaemia of CKD, so achieving and maintaining adequate iron stores are an essential part of anaemia management. There are numerous reasons for this:

- Decreased iron absorption through GI tract
- Reduced intake of iron—dietary restrictions, loss of taste for iron-rich foods
- Low-grade GI bleeding
- Frequent blood tests
- Blood left in dialyser circuit on HD
- Erythropoietic agents stimulate bone marrow to supraphysiological rates of red blood cell production so normal amount of circulating iron can be insufficient
- Reticuloendothelial blockade—occurs in setting of acute or chronic inflammation or infection:
  - Correlates with high CRP
  - Ferritin is an acute-phase protein and so is also elevated
  - Iron gets trapped in reticuloendothelial system and is not released to transferrin
  - Results in low TSAT despite a normal or elevated ferritin.

Hepcidin

Hepcidin is a relatively newly described peptide that is crucial for iron absorption and mobilization:

- Synthesized in the liver in response to level of iron stores—high iron stores result in increased synthesis.
- Feeds back to GI tract to reduce iron absorption.
- Inhibits release of iron from the reticuloendothelial system to circulating transferrin.
- Hepcidin therefore protects against iron overload.
- Interestingly, haemochromatosis has turned out to be genetic defect causing low hepcidin activity, resulting in iron overload.
- Hepcidin is an acute-phase reactant so levels increase in presence of inflammation and infection—this results in reduced iron absorption and release of iron from the reticuloendothelial system causing the low TSAT and high serum ferritin described earlier in this topic.
- Serum hepcidin levels appear to correlate directly with serum ferritin in healthy subjects, are highest in inflammatory states, and lowest in iron deficiency anaemia.
- No standardized assay, so hepcidin not yet ready as a clinical test.

Assessing iron status

Serum ferritin and transferrin saturation

There are various problems with measuring iron status and therefore diagnosing iron deficiency in patients with CKD and those on dialysis:

- Ferritin is an acute-phase protein so can be elevated in an iron-deficient patient who is in an inflammatory state.
- Ferritin is generally lower in women.
- Transferrin may also be elevated in inflammatory state—this results in lower TSAT if circulating iron is constant.
- Decreased transferrin synthesis with malnutrition—results in raised TSAT if circulating iron is constant.
- Significant diurnal fluctuation (up to 70%) in TSAT—will result in different levels depending on whether patient is dialysed on morning or evening shift.
- Reticuloendothelial blockade discussed above ➔ Iron metabolism, p. 468 will result in low TSAT and high ferritin—often found in patients on dialysis.

Reticulocyte Hb content

- Measure of amount of Hb in reticulocytes.
- Reflects amount of iron available to bone marrow for incorporation into new red cells.
- Test is widely available on multichannel haematology analysers.
- Studies have shown it to be less variable than TSAT or ferritin.
- Cut-off of reticulocyte Hb content of <32pg has been suggested.

Percentage of hypochromic red cells

- Based on concentration of Hb in red blood cells.
- Takes into account absolute amount of Hb as well as size of cell.
- Red cells tend to expand when stored so can only be done on fresh samples.

Soluble transferrin receptor

- Bone marrow erythroblast membrane transferrin receptor increases in setting of iron deficiency.
- Some erythroblasts enter the circulation and are therefore detectable.
- Total erythroblast mass, and therefore also soluble transferrin receptor, will be increased by use of erythropoietic agent.
- Elevated level therefore can be due to treatment with EPO or due to iron deficiency—makes test difficult to interpret.
- Test not widely available.

Iron supplements: oral iron

All dialysis patients should receive iron unless they have documented excessive iron stores (ferritin >800ng/mL or TSAT >50%). In pre-dialysis patients, iron supplements (oral and/or IV) should be given to achieve ferritin >200ng/mL or TSAT >20%, if Hb <11g/dL, before starting treatment with erythropoietic agents. Approximately 1000mg iron is needed in the first 3 months of EPO treatment to sustain the increase in Hb, and then ~25–100mg/month.

Oral iron

- Oral iron should be first-line treatment and IV iron only used if patients are intolerant of oral iron or remain absolutely or functionally iron deficient despite oral iron.
- Many patients, however, suffer GI side effects (proportional to the dose of iron taken).
- 200mg elemental iron needed a day.
- Ferrous sulfate 325mg tablet provides 65mg elemental iron; other iron formulations are more expensive and provide less elemental iron.
- Compliance is poor.
- May cause constipation in PD patients (to be avoided).
- Absorbed best from duodenum and proximal jejunum. More expensive enteric-coated or sustained-release capsules release iron further down the GI tract and are therefore counterproductive.
- Timing of taking iron tablets important particularly when considering potential interactions with other drugs:
  - Should not be given with food as absorption impaired.
  - Should be given 2h before or 4h after antacids.
  - Absorption impaired by quinolones, e.g. ciprofloxacin.
  - Should not be taken at same time as oral phosphate binders.

Intravenous iron

- Efficacious in all studies in increasing Hb, increasing ferritin and TSAT index, and reducing EPO requirements.
- Needed in most HD patients as iron loss from GI bleeding and blood loss in dialysis lines exceeds ability of gut to absorb oral iron.
- Potential concerns about iron overload, infection, and cardiac dysfunction have not been realized.
- Iron should be withheld if ferritin >800ng/mL to avoid iron overload.
- Increased risk of infection probably not of great significance, but IV iron should not be given while infection present because of theoretical risk that neutrophil function may be adversely affected.
- Macrocytosis developing during the use of IV iron may reflect the development of folate deficiency.
- Needs to be given with care to avoid adverse reactions:
  - Free iron reaction:
    —symptoms include hypotension, nausea, vomiting, sweating, back pain, pruritus, and a sudden feeling of being unwell
    —owing to either the effect of iron overload or the result of infusing IV iron too rapidly
    —can be treated if necessary with IV hydrocortisone and chlorphenamine.
  - Anaphylaxis:
    —symptoms include laryngeal oedema, erythema, urticaria, palpitations, collapse, loss of consciousness
    —risk very low, but all nurses giving IV iron should be trained in resuscitation, and adrenaline (epinephrine), chlorphenamine, hydrocortisone, and resuscitation equipment should be immediately available.

Preparations of intravenous iron

There are various preparations available:
- Iron dextran
- Iron sucrose
- Ferric carboxymaltose
- Iron isomaltoside 1000
- Ferumoxytol.

Intravenous iron and hypersensitivity reactions

In August 2013, the UK Medicines and Healthcare Products Regulatory Agency issued a warning about serious hypersensitivity reactions with IV iron.

- Life-threatening and fatal anaphylactic reactions reported. These reactions can occur even in patients who have previously tolerated IV iron and when the test dose has been negative.
- IV iron should therefore only be given by appropriately trained staff and in locations where patients can be monitored for signs of hypersensitivity for up to 30min after administration and where resuscitation facilities are available.
- In the event of a hypersensitivity reaction, the IV infusion should be stopped at once and appropriate management started.
- Risk of hypersensitivity is increased in patients with known allergies, history of severe asthma, eczema or other atopic allergy.
- During pregnancy, IV iron should be avoided during the first trimester and only given during the second and third if benefit is considered to outweigh the potential risks for mother and fetus.

Intravenous iron preparations

Iron sucrose

- A complex of ferric hydroxide with sucrose containing 2% (20mg/mL) of iron.
- Efficacious with a very low incidence of adverse reactions, and no deaths due to anaphylaxis.
- Supplied as 100mg/5mL single-dose vial.
- Usual dosing:
  - 100mg at end of HD on 10 successive dialysis sessions if ferritin <200ng/mL, then weekly while ferritin <600ng/mL
  - 200mg can be given every 1–3 months in PD or pre-dialysis patients as an IV infusion.
- Can be given as IV infusion or as slow IV injection (at 20mg/min).
- Administration protocols:
  - 100–200mg undiluted over 5–10min (20mg/min) is recommended
  - 100mg undiluted over 2min has been reported as being safe
  - 100mg in 100mL normal saline over 15min.
- Changes in TSAT and ferritin levels can be measured 48h after IV administration.

Sodium ferric gluconate complex in sucrose

- Increasingly used.
- Non-dialysable; free of dextran polysaccharides.
- Fewer life-threatening and fatal adverse reactions than iron dextran and may be safe in patients who are allergic to or are intolerant of iron dextran.
- Mild reactions not uncommon.
- Usually given as 62.5–125mg IV infusions undiluted over 5–10min (12.5mg/min) during consecutive dialysis sessions until 1g administered, then weekly (while ferritin <600ng/mL). As with iron sucrose.
- Can be given as larger doses to PD and pre-dialysis patients (300mg 1–3-monthly, over 90min) to avoid frequent hospital admissions, or 125mg in 100mL normal saline over 60min.

Ferumoxytol

- A complex of iron oxide with polyglucose sorbitol-carboxymethylether containing 3% (30 mg/mL) of iron.
- Appears to be safe when given as a single dose of up to 510mg iron.
- Can be administered at a rapid rate—up to 30mg/sec.
- For treatment of iron deficiency, manufacturers recommend single dose of 510mg followed by further dose of 510mg within 3–8 days.

Iron dextran

- A complex of ferric hydroxide with dextran containing 5% (50 mg/mL) of iron.
- Risk of anaphylactic reactions (0.6–1.5%), but probably less commonly than previously reported.
- Can lead to generation of antidextran antibodies (extremely infrequently).
- Because of risk of anaphylaxis, test dose needed for first administration (20mg diluted in 50mL saline over 30min).
- Other adverse effects include itching (1.5%), dyspnoea and wheeze (1.5%), arthralgia, myalgia, fever, headache (often delayed by 24–48h).
- Dose on each dialysis session initially to treat iron deficiency (usually 20–100mg, for 10–20 sessions), and then intermittently (usually weekly, fortnightly, or monthly) to maintain iron stores (~50–100mg). Alternatively, 250mg over half an hour monthly. Give at end of dialysis by slow injection or infusion.
- In PD or pre-dialysis patients, 500mg can be diluted into 250mL saline and given over 30–60min.
- Total dose iron infusions of specially fractionated iron (III) dextran (20mg/kg iron over 4–6h) may avoid the need for repeated infusions.
- Not commonly used in view of adverse reactions.

Iron isomaltoside 1000

- A complex of ferric iron and isomaltosides containing 10% (100 mg/mL) of iron.
- Can be given as a single dose to replace iron.
- Does not contain dextrans so low rate of anaphylaxis.

High ferritin and low transferrin saturation index

As discussed earlier, patients in an inflammatory state related to co-morbidities and/or infection frequently have an elevated ferritin level in the presence of a low TSAT. It is difficult to establish whether such patients are functionally iron deficient and would therefore benefit from further IV iron. Some authorities suggest that there should be an upper limit of serum ferritin level (500–800ng/mL) above which further IV iron should not be given because of the risk of iron overload.

There has been one RCT examining use of IV ferric gluconate compared with no iron in a group of patients with low Hb, low TSAT and high ferritin resulted in:

• treatment group—rise in Hb, TSAT, and ferritin
• control group—fall in ferritin and reticulocyte Hb content.

This was a short-term study (6 weeks) and therefore does not address the issue of long-term safety of IV iron in this situation or whether there is an upper limit of serum ferritin above which IV iron should not be given.

Because of these various concerns, use of non-iron adjuvants should also be considered for this group of patients.

Non-iron adjuvants to erythropoietin therapy

Various non-iron pharmacologic agents have been evaluated as adjuvants to EPO treatment. Although these are sometimes recommended in patients not responding to EPO treatment, they have mostly not been studied in patients with EPO resistance. The agents include L-carnitine, ascorbic acid, androgens, pentoxifylline, and statins.

Levocarnitine

(See also ➋ Carnitine and ESKD, p. 410.) Important in energy metabolism—required for transport of long-chain fatty acids into mitochondria. Reported that levocarnitine increases formation of colony forming-unit-erythroid colonies in bone marrow cell cultures, though not known whether this is clinically important. Also alters red blood cell phospholipid membrane, thereby affecting red blood cell deformability, resulting in increased red cell survival.

Efficacy
- Anecdotal reports, small case series and uncontrolled studies suggesting that IV or oral levocarnitine increases Hb levels and/or reduces EPO requirements in patients on HD.
- Conflicting data from RCTs.
- None of studies conducted in patients with EPO resistance.
- Bioavailability of oral carnitine is low and there is some concern about breakdown products formed in GI tract—use of IV carnitine is therefore preferred.
- K/DOQI guidelines suggest empiric trial of oral or IV levocarnitine in selected patients for 4 months.

Ascorbic acid

Ascorbic acid increases release of iron from ferritin and the reticulo-endothelial system, enhances iron utilization during Hb synthesis, and is an antioxidant.

Efficacy
- Some encouraging uncontrolled observations in EPO-resistant HD patients with around half of patients achieving a 25% reduction in EPO dose when given ascorbic acid IV.
- Conflicting results from RCTs, with some showing around half of patients responding and some showing no effect.
- Oral vitamin C has not been shown to be of benefit as adjunct to EPO therapy.
- K/DOQI guidelines in 2006 suggest insufficient evidence to recommend ascorbic acid as an adjuvant to EPO therapy.
- European Best Practice guidelines suggest that correction of impaired vitamin C status can reduce EPO resistance or functional iron deficiency, but does not recommend routine use.
- If used, treatment should be limited to a 2–6-month course of IV ascorbic acid at dose of 300mg at each HD treatment.

Safety issues
- Secondary oxalosis remains a concern—very high levels of plasma oxalate can occur with regular use of high-dose IV ascorbic acid.
- Possible harmful pro-oxidant effects, either directly or through mobilization of iron.

Androgens

Increase endogenous EPO production, sensitivity of erythroid progenitors to EPO, and red blood cell survival. Were previously used regularly for treatment of anaemia before the use of EPO. A few studies have considered possible role for androgens in combination with EPO.

Efficacy
- Giving IM nandrolone daily to patients on EPO does cause a greater rise in Hb—demonstrated in several uncontrolled studies, but all are small and have relatively short follow-up.
- Both K/DOQI and European Best Practices guidelines conclude that the role for androgens is limited and that side effects prevent their use in most patients.

Disadvantages
- Need to be given by IM injection.
- Side effects include acne, virilization, abnormal liver function tests, risk of hepatocellular carcinoma.

Pentoxifylline

Has anti-inflammatory properties. One small, open-label, uncontrolled study suggested that pentoxifylline 400mg daily for 4 months in patients with EPO resistance resulted in higher Hb levels. Larger studies are needed before routine use can be recommended.

Statins

Have anti-inflammatory and antioxidant properties. One retrospective study suggested that Hb level rose and EPO dose requirements fell by 25% when statin treatment was started. Further prospective studies are needed. Recommendations for their use as an adjuvant to EPO treatment cannot be made, but statins are used widely in patients with CKD and on dialysis.

Complications of ESKD: bone mineral disorders

Renal bone disease

All patients with ESKD will have renal bone disease by the time they require dialysis, though of varying severity. Dialysis is not a cure but merely a prolongation of the state of renal failure. Renal bone disease is therefore not improved by starting dialysis, and may instead progress.

Contributing factors to renal bone disease

- Acidosis
- Hyperparathyroidism
- Low vitamin D levels
- Suppressed parathyroid activity (after treatment)
- Aluminium accumulation (now rare)
- Osteoporosis in elderly patients
- Osteopenia caused by steroids used to treat initial disease or for transplantation.

Types of renal bone disease

- High turnover:
  - hyperparathyroidism.
- Low turnover:
  - treated hyperparathyroidism
  - osteomalacia (due to vitamin D deficiency)
  - aluminium deposition.

Hyperparathyroidism and hyperphosphataemia

Causes of hyperparathyroidism

Hyperparathyroidism is the key to renal bone disease. The primary cause is the failure of the kidney to synthesize 1,25 dihydroxyvitamin D_3 (calcitriol), the active metabolite of vitamin D. This leads to:

- reduced intestinal calcium absorption → hypocalcaemia → ↑ PTH synthesis
- reduced inhibition of PTH synthesis by 1,25 vitamin D_3
- parathyroid cell proliferation
- increased PTH action on skeleton, releasing calcium and phosphate, thereby restoring plasma calcium levels towards normal
- phosphate retention
- ↑ phosphate → ↓ serum calcium level → ↑ PTH secretion
- reduces formation of 1,25 vitamin D_3 by enzymatic inhibition (more important in early renal failure)
- directly reduces sensitivity of parathyroid gland to hypercalcaemia, i.e. raised plasma calcium level causes less inhibition of PTH synthesis.

Hyperphosphataemia

Phosphate levels are an independent predictor of survival on dialysis and start rising when GFR falls below 30mL/min/1.73m^2. Factors determining phosphate levels include:

- level of residual renal function
- dietary intake of phosphate
- degree of secondary hyperparathyroidism
- use of vitamin D metabolites
- dialysis adequacy and time on dialysis per se
- dose of phosphate binders (and compliance with their use).

Fibroblast growth factor 23

Over the last few years, Fibroblast growth factor 23 (FGF23), in addition to PTH, has emerged as an important regulator of plasma phosphate levels. FGF23 is an endocrine hormone secreted by osteocytes and osteoblasts; it binds to FGF receptors in the kidney and parathyroid gland.

Physiological role
- Stimulate phosphaturia
- Reduce systemic levels of 1,25 vitamin D
- Inhibit PTH secretion.

Regulation of FG23 secretion in 'normal' individuals
- With high phosphate intake FGF23 secretion rises and:
  - lowers 1,25 vitamin D levels thereby reducing gut phosphate absorption
  - induces greater urinary phosphate excretion.
- With low phosphate intake FGF23 secretion falls and:
  - higher levels of 1,25 vitamin D enable increased gut phosphate absorption
  - reduces urinary phosphate excretion.
- Negative feedback loop between FGF23 and 1,25 vitamin D:
  - 1,25 vitamin D stimulates FGF23 secretion
  - FGF23 lowers 1,25 vitamin D levels.
- Negative feedback loop between FGF23 and PTH:
  - FGF23 inhibits PTH secretion
  - PTH stimulates FGF23 secretion
- High serum calcium stimulates FGF23 secretion.

FGF23 in CKD
FGF23 levels rise with falling levels of GFR. Levels may be >1000 times normal in patients on dialysis and decline rapidly after transplantation.
- High FGF23 levels are associated with adverse outcomes in CKD:
  - Some studies suggest an independent association with increased mortality and cardiovascular events.
  - Risk factor for CKD progression.
- Emerging as most sensitive screening test for development of bone mineral disorders.

Hyperparathyroid bone disease

Symptoms do not develop until an advanced stage of renal bone disease. The early stages can be detected biochemically. There are clinical implications to all stages.

Symptoms

Related to calcium phosphate metabolism
- Pruritus (calcium phosphate deposition under the skin)
- Soft tissue calcification leading to tender lumps under skin
- Calcification of tendons leading to acute joint problems
- Symptoms of hypercalcaemia if present (i.e. nausea, vomiting, confusion).

Related to bone pathology
- Joint pains—usually mild and widespread
- Aches in bones
- Fractures—particularly of pelvis with vitamin D deficiency (osteomalacia).

Related to raised PTH level
- Mild depression.

Clinical implications

Hyperphosphataemia
- Soft tissue and vascular calcification. Calcification of coronary arteries contributes to ischaemic heart disease and acute coronary syndrome (ACS). Calcification of larger vessels increases vascular stiffness, which contributes to LVH.
- Increasing evidence of reduced survival on dialysis.

Severe or tertiary hyperparathyroidism
- Hypercalcaemia
- Hyperphosphataemia more difficult to control
- Resistance to EPO therapy.

Radiological changes

Only with advanced renal bone disease. X-rays less important as a diagnostic or monitoring tool than measurement of plasma PTH levels. Principal changes are:
- subperiostial bone resorption (best seen on the distal and middle phalanges of hands and feet)—correlates with PTH and alkaline phosphatase levels
- erosion of distal end of clavicles in severe cases
- areas of osteosclerosis, particularly in the spine, leading to the characteristic 'rugger jersey' appearance seen on lateral X-rays of the thoracic spine
- solitary cysts or 'brown tumours' particularly in jaw, pelvis, or ribs—only with very severe hyperparathyroidism.

Bone histology

Bone biopsies can be obtained from the iliac bone by a trephine or drill technique. This is rarely performed in clinical practice and is mainly a research tool. Demonstrates characteristic features.

Biochemical abnormalities

These will depend on the severity and duration of hyperparathyroidism. PTH level is the key to diagnosing the severity of the bone disease. Any significant degree of renal impairment is inevitably associated with secondary hyperparathyroidism. Tertiary hyperparathyroidism occurs when the parathyroid gland no longer responds to the normal feedback mechanisms resulting in hypercalcaemia either spontaneously or with minimal treatment. (See Table 11.1.)

Table 11.1 Biochemical features of renal osteodystrophy (secondary hyperparathyroidism) and tertiary hyperparathyroidism (HPT)

	Calcium	Phosphate	Alkaline phosphatase	PTH
Secondary HPT				
Mild	↔ or ↓	↔ or ↑	↔	↑
Moderate	↓	↑	↔	↑↑
Severe	↓↓	↑↑	↑ or ↑↑	↑↑↑
Tertiary HPT	↔ or ↑	↑↑	↔ or ↑	↑↑↑

Parathyroid hormone assays

- Serial measurements of PTH are useful in assessing degree of secondary hyperparathyroidism, and response to treatment, though with some limitations:
  - PTH levels <2× normal range associated with low turnover bone on bone biopsy
  - high PTH levels are not always associated with other markers of severe bone disease, e.g. raised alkaline phosphatase levels, X-ray changes.
- Abundant bone histology data correlate PTH levels to histological findings.
- Conventional PTH assays (first-generation immunometric techniques) detect biologically active PTH(1–84) and also PTH fragments, which accumulate in renal failure.
- Secondnd-generation immunometric PTH assays are now available though not yet in general clinical use:
  - assay detects only biologically active PTH(1–84) and not fragments;
  - possible to calculate level of PTH fragments by subtracting second-generation PTH level from first-generation test—and then possible to calculate ratio of PTH(1–84)/PTH(fragments)
  - very few data so far correlating new assay PTH levels to bone histology
  - biological relevance of PTH(1–84)/PTH(fragments) not yet fully established, although known that some PTH fragments have inhibitory action on osteoblasts and bone remodelling. A ratio <1 has been correlated with low turnover bone, suggesting accumulation of inhibitory fragments relative to biologically active PTH.
- Oversuppression of PTH is important since increasing evidence suggests low PTH levels and low bone turnover are associated with deposition of calcium in vasculature, and increased vascular and soft tissue calcification.

Low turnover bone disease

Clinical features
There are three main causes (see Tables 11.2, 11.3, and 11.4). In order of importance these are:
- treated hyperparathyroidism—results in 'adynamic bone disease'
- vitamin D deficiency (osteomalacia)
- aluminium deposition (now very rare as aluminium salts rarely used as phosphate binders, and water for dialysate is treated to lower aluminium levels).

Table 11.2 Adynamic renal bone disease

Symptoms	Clinical implications
None	No evidence of increased risk of fractures
	Resulting osteopenia may increase risk of steroid-induced osteoporosis after transplantation
	Increased risk of hypercalcaemia when using calcium compounds as phosphate binders
	Possible increased risk of vascular and soft tissue calcification

Table 11.3 Osteomalacia

Symptoms	Clinical implications
Bone pains	Fractures (can be spontaneous)
Proximal myopathy associated with vitamin D deficiency	

Table 11.4 Aluminium bone disease

Symptoms	Clinical implications
Severe and diffuse bone pains	High risk of spontaneous fractures
Muscle weakness	Risk of aluminium encephalopathy or 'dialysis dementia'
	Resistance to EPO therapy

Radiological changes

Adynamic bone disease
- X-rays may be normal.
- Osteopenia often difficult to detect on standard X-rays.

Osteomalacia
- X-rays may be normal.
- Spontaneous fractures or pseudofractures (particularly in pelvis—'Looser zones') are occasionally seen.

Aluminium bone disease
- X-rays may be normal.
- Spontaneous fractures may be seen.

Histology

As with hyperparathyroid bone disease, bone biopsy is a research rather than a clinical tool. PTH has proved to be a good predictor of bone histology, as shown in Table 11.5.

Osteomalacia can be diagnosed by finding a low 1,25 dihydroxy vitamin D level, so again a bone biopsy is not required. The diagnosis of aluminium bone disease should probably be confirmed by histology. However, the diagnosis is so rare, and bone biopsies so rarely performed, that the patient should be referred to a specialized centre for expert advice.

Biochemical features

These will depend on the cause. (See Table 11.6.)

Table 11.5 Bone histology

Bone turnover state	PTH level (normal: 10–50pg/mL)
Low turnover	<120pg/mL
Normal turnover	100–200pg/mL
High turnover	>400pg/mL

Table 11.6 Causes of low turnover bone disease

Cause	Calcium	Phosphate	Alkaline phosphatase	Aluminium	25-OH vitamin D	PTH
Treated hyperpara-thyroidism	↔	↔ or ↑	↔	↔	↔	↓, ↔, or ↑
Osteomalacia	↓	↓, ↔, or ↑	↑ or ↑↑	↔	↓	↑ or ↑↑
Aluminium toxicity	↔ or ↑	↔ or ↑	↔	↑	↔	↔ or ↑

Medical management of renal bone disease

The aim of management is to prevent the development of severe hyper-parathyroid bone disease with the complications of tissue calcification, severe hyperphosphataemia, and, in particular, hypercalcaemia (i.e. tertiary hyperparathyroidism). This should be regarded as a therapeutic failure as parathyroidectomy is then needed. Management should be started as soon as any evidence of disturbance of calcium phosphate metabolism is detected, whatever the level of renal function. Patients who present late with more severe renal failure are at special risk of developing severe hyperparathyroidism.

Objectives of management

- Calcium and phosphate blood levels in the normal range.
- Ensure bone metabolism is as near normal as possible.
- Maintain PTH blood levels within a 'safe range' thereby avoiding high or low levels (probably 150–250pg/mL).
- Prevent the development of parathyroid hyperplasia.

This is done by:
- maintenance of normal phosphate levels
- use of active metabolites of vitamin D
- selection of appropriate dialysate calcium concentration to prevent hypercalcaemia.

Maintenance of normal phosphate levels

Failure of the kidney to excrete phosphate, inadequate removal of phosphate by dialysis, and excessive dietary intake all contribute to the hyperphosphataemia seen in renal failure. All need to be addressed, as well as the increased phosphate release from 'high turnover' bone disease induced by increased PTH secretion, by the following:
• Dietary phosphate restriction.
• Ensuring dialysis adequacy (but adequate small molecule clearance and volume control do not necessarily mean adequate phosphate clearance. Often only improved by daily or nocturnal dialysis).
• Use of *phosphate binders*—taken with each meal to reduce intestinal phosphate absorption. Large quantities are needed and many patients find them unpalatable—compliance is a major problem. Currently available phosphate binders are:
  • calcium carbonate
  • calcium acetate
  • aluminium hydroxide
  • magnesium carbonate very rarely used (causes diarrhoea)
  • sevelamer hydrochloride and carbonate
  • lanthanum carbonate.
• The use of *calcium salts* is often limited by the development of hypercalcaemia, though this is less of a problem with calcium acetate (less calcium is absorbed). Even without the development of hypercalcaemia, there is increasing evidence that they may contribute to soft tissue and vascular calcification.
• Aluminium hydroxide should no longer be used as a first-line phosphate binder because of the potential risk of aluminium absorption, except in those patients whose phosphate levels cannot be controlled by other binders, or as a short-term measure while awaiting parathyroidectomy. Plasma aluminium levels must be monitored regularly (every month initially and then 3-monthly); treatment should be stopped if aluminium levels move into the toxic range.
• *Sevelamer hydrochloride* is a non-calcium-, non-aluminium-containing polymeric phosphate binder:
  • Comes as 800mg tablets which are swallowed at start of meal. Sevelamer is a relatively weak phosphate binder and the starting dose should be 2 tablets (1.6g) tds
  • Average dose is 8 tablets a day—it is therefore not surprising that compliance is often poor.
  • Main side effects relate to GI intolerance—abdominal discomfort and bloating.
  • Main advantage is absence of calcium and therefore achieving lower calcium–phosphate (Ca–P) product.
  • Good evidence that sevelamer attenuates progression of cardio-vascular calcification.

- Polymeric nature of sevelamer has other beneficial effects: lowering of low-density lipoprotein (LDL), reduced inflammation, lower plasma urate, and lower oxidative stress. These may account for survival benefit of sevelamer compared with calcium-based phosphate binders seen in some trials.
- Main limitations for use of sevelamer in clinical practice are the number of tablets and its cost, which is several-fold greater than calcium-based phosphate binders.

- *Sevelamer carbonate* has the same phosphate binding properties as sevelamer hydrochloride but causes less acidosis. It is also available as a powder which may aid compliance for some patients.
- *Lanthanum carbonate* is the newest non-calcaemic phosphate binder.
  - It appears to be a highly effective phosphate binder associated with a lower risk of hypercalcaemia and systemic calcium accumulation than calcium-based phosphate binders.
  - It is a tasteless chewable table taken with each meal, most patients need a single tablet on each occasion (500mg, 750mg, or 1g).
  - Intestinal absorption of lanthanum is miniscule (~0.00005%) and, in contrast to aluminium, lanthanum is eliminated primarily through the biliary system and the gut wall, rather than through the kidney, thereby minimizing systemic accumulation.
  - There remains concern that long-term use may result in lanthanum accumulation in the bone, though evidence for this has not been found in any clinical study; however, these are limited to <3–5 years. This concern is going to be more important for younger patients than older ones with shorter life expectancy.
  - Use of lanthanum carbonate as a phosphate binder is going to be limited by the above concerns and its cost.

Features of phosphate binders

Comparison of phosphate binders: evidence reviewed by **UK NICE (March 2013)**

- All phosphate binders (see Table 11.7) effective in lowering serum phosphate compared to placebo.
- No binder emerges as the most effective.
- Non-calcium-based binders were associated with lower serum calcium levels.
- Sevelamer hydrochloride was better than calcium-based binders in controlling coronary calcification scores.
  - When the effectiveness of calcium-based binders considered separately, sevelamer hydrochloride was only better than calcium carbonate; there was no statistically significant difference in coronary calcification scores between sevelamer hydrochloride and calcium acetate.
- Fewer GI side effects with lanthanum carbonate compared to sevelamer hydrochloride.
- Some evidence that patient survival may be slightly longer in patients using sevelamer hydrochloride.
- A cost–utility model was built based on effectiveness data from meta-analyses comparing various phosphate binders.
- While the use of non-calcium-based binders may be associated with some extension of quality-adjusted life expectation compared with conventional calcium phosphate binders, this gain is insufficient to justify the additional costs of the proprietary binders (around £90,000 per QALY gained).

Table 11.7 Phosphate binders: features

	Dose	Advantages	Disadvantages	Effectiveness /cost
Calcium carbonate	1–3 tablets with meals	Corrects hypocalcaemia	Hypercalcaemia Constipation	++/cheap
Calcium acetate	1–3 tablets with meals	Corrects hypocalcaemia	Hypercalcaemia	++/cheap
Aluminium hydroxide	1–2 capsules with meals	Less hypercalcaemia. Lower Ca–P product	Aluminium toxicity. Need to monitor aluminium levels. Constipation	+++/cheap
Sevelamer hydrochloride or carbonate	1–3 800mg tablets with meals or 0.8–2.4g of carbonate as power	Lower plasma cholesterol. Lower plasma calcium. Lower Ca–P product may result in less coronary artery calcification	GI side effects	++/ expensive
Lanthanum carbonate	500mg–1g tablets with meals	Less hypercalcaemia. Lower Ca–P product.	Long-term effects of lanthanum in bone not known Short-term studies show no toxicity. Mild GI upsets	++/ expensive

Vitamin D

Vitamin D metabolism

There is mounting evidence that vitamin D and its metabolites have systemic effects beyond their actions on the skeleton. An overview of vitamin D metabolism is shown in Fig. 11.1.

Vitamin D therapy in renal bone disease

Vitamin D analogues currently used therapeutically include:

- Calcitriol
- Alfacalcidol (not available in the USA, but used in the UK)
- Paricalcitol
- Doxercalciferol (not available in the UK, but used in the USA).

Calcitriol and alfacalcidol

As the key to the development of secondary hyperparathyroidism is the failure of the kidney to synthesize 1,25 dihydroxycholecalciferol, it is logical that this should be used in its management. There are two main forms currently used: *calcitriol*, the physiological metabolite; and *alfacalcidol* (1-α-hydroxycholecalciferol), a synthetic equivalent. The actions of both are the same:

- increased intestinal calcium and phosphorus absorption
- increased calcium mobilization (and thereby phosphate release) from bone
- reduced synthesis of PTH
- reduced rate of cell growth within the parathyroid gland.

Dose (generally 0.25–1.0mcg orally daily) should be tailored to maintain normal plasma calcium, and PTH in a safe range (2–4 normal range).

- The major side effects are hypercalcaemia and hyperphosphataemia.
- Probably less hypercalcaemia if dose given at night.
- Dose needs to be adjusted according to calcium and phosphate levels.
- Should not be started if plasma phosphate is poorly controlled.
- Pulsed therapy (1–3mcg 2-3 times per week) provides better suppression of PTH with lower risk of hypercalcaemia than daily therapy.
- Pulsed oral therapy probably as effective as IV treatment and cheaper, though IV administration while on HD can be useful if compliance is thought to be a problem. Pulsed oral therapy can also be administered on dialysis if compliance a concern.

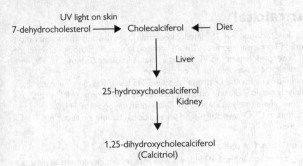

Fig. 11.1 Overview of vitamin D metabolism.

Paricalcitol

Paricalcitol, 19-nor-1-α,25-dihydroxyvitamin D2, is the only 'third-generation' vitamin D receptor agonist (VDRA) licensed in the UK, although doxercalciferol (a second-generation VDRA) is available in other countries.

- Paricalcitol is available for IV or oral use.
- Initial dosing for the IV preparation is PTH level/8 given after each dialysis session. Dosing often needs reducing over time as PTH falls. When given orally in stage 5 CKD, the starting dose is PTH/7.
- Studies in CKD have suggested an additional benefit on reducing proteinuria.

Indications for use

- Suggested to suppress PTH level with less severe increments in plasma calcium, by selectively stimulating parathyroid vitamin D receptors rather than GI tract receptors responsible for calcium absorption.
- Only one prospective randomized trial has been done comparing paricalcitol and calcitriol. This showed that paricalcitol reduced PTH more rapidly and to a greater extent than calcitriol with fewer sustained episodes of hypercalcaemia and less elevated calcium–phosphate product, though these remained significant side effects. Most treated patients achieved target PTH levels.
- Retrospective analysis of large patient databases of patients dialysing in the USA, and in the DOPPS studies, have shown the following:
  - Overall mortality significantly lower in paricalcitol-treated patients, with similar cardiovascular mortality in all patients
  - Lower levels of calcium and phosphate and greater degrees of PTH suppression in paricalcitol groups, though data on calcium and non-calcium phosphate binder use was not available
  - This study was not randomized and there were significant differences in baseline characteristics such as age, race, and length of time on dialysis between the 2 groups. The results, therefore, cannot be used as an indication for widespread use of paricalcitol, but are interesting.
- As paricalcitol is more costly than other VDRAs, its use should be targeted to patients with resistant symptomatic hyperparathyroidism who cannot have (or do not want) a parathyroidectomy (as an alternative to cinacalcet), patients with hyperparathyroidism who develop rising calcium levels or elevated Ca–P product using calcitriol or alfacalcidol, and patients who are intolerant of cinacalcet.

Systemic effects of vitamin D

Role of 1,25-OH vitamin D

Systemic effects of vitamin D

There is increasing awareness that vitamin D and its metabolites may have important systemic effects. Distribution of vitamin D-dependent genes points to a number of physiological functions of 1,25-dihydroxycholecalciferol:

- 'Classical' roles—regulation of plasma calcium and phosphate levels by actions on intestine, bone, parathyroid, and kidney.
- 'Non-classical' roles—actions on cell differentiation and antiproliferative effects in a number of cell types including immune system, skin, breast.
  - These actions have led to claims that vitamin D is involved in the pathogenesis of a wide range of conditions including psoriasis, some cancers, multiple sclerosis, BP regulation, and many others.
- Supporting such observations are fairly convincing retrospective data that mortality is reduced in HD patients on vitamin D therapy compared with those who were not.
- This suggests that simply correcting calcium–phosphate balance using other medications (calcimimetics, phosphate binders), could mask underlying circulating calcitriol deficiency leaving non-classical effects untreated.

Role of 25-OH vitamin D

Blood 25-OH vitamin D levels may be a better health indicator than calcitriol levels. Data are now emerging that conversion to calcitriol occurs in many sites outside the kidney, suggesting additional roles for vitamin D outside its classical functions on calcium/phosphate metabolism.

Vitamin D (cholecalciferol) deficiency is common in CKD patients. Measurement of levels in non-dialysed CKD populations have shown that >80% have low levels, with nephrotic patients having the lowest levels; there was no relationship to GFR. The clinical implications of this and the effects of correcting the vitamin D deficiency are not known. In the general population, secondary hyperparathyroidism associated with low vitamin D levels is associated with bone loss, and oral vitamin D supplementation in a dose of between 700 and 800IU/day reduces the risk of hip and non-vertebral fractures by ~25% in older populations.

Clinical consequences of vitamin D deficiency in the general population include:

- non-specific musculoskeletal pain; prevalence of vitamin D deficiency in patients with non-specific musculoskeletal pain can be ~90%
- bone disease—osteomalacia, osteoporosis
- secondary hyperparathyroidism causing bone loss.

Physiological doses of vitamin D attenuate bone loss and decrease fracture rate in older men and women. There is also a reduction in the risk of falls in the elderly, possibly through improvement in muscle strength.

For patients on dialysis it is now generally recommended that:

- Vitamin D status should be assessed 6-monthly by measuring 25-hydroxycholecalciferol levels
- Vitamin D deficiency is defined as levels <25nmol/L (10ng/mL)
- The Renal Association guidelines suggest supplementation if levels are <70–80nmol/L
- Not clear how this supplementation should be achieved. There are arguments for the general population whether this should be achieved by encouraging more exposure to sun or by food supplementation
- New controlled-release formulations of vitamin D may be necessary to eradicate vitamin D insufficiency
- Currently, supplementation should be with colecalciferol 800U/day either as calcium with ergocalciferol, or calcium carbonate D_3 (which gives a larger dose of calcium)
- Doses of up to 800U of ergocalciferol will not elevate 1,25 dihydroxycalciferol levels so will not cause hypercalcaemia, and are therefore safe in patients with CKD or on dialysis.

Calcimimetics

- A class of drugs that suppress PTH secretion by increasing the sensitivity of the parathyroid gland calcium-sensing receptors; this is the principal factor regulating parathyroid gland hyperplasia and PTH secretion.
- Can be given in conjunction with vitamin D analogues as both work on different targets.
- Use of calcimimetics should result in lowering of PTH without rise in plasma calcium or phosphate; indeed hypocalcaemia may occur.

Cinacalcet

- Cinacalcet is only calcimimetic currently available.
- It is given orally once a day, starting at 30mg and then titrated every 2–4 weeks to a maximum of 180mg once daily to achieve a target level of PTH of 2–4 times the normal range.
- Main side effects are nausea and vomiting, which are more common with higher doses; giving the drug at night or dividing the drug into 2 doses daily can reduce this side effect. Some patients have to stop the drug.
- Cinacalcet should not be started if the plasma calcium is below normal as it can reduce the calcium level further.
- Using cinacalcet is expensive, particularly at higher doses.
- Trials have shown improvement in mean levels of PTH, calcium, phosphorus, and Ca–P product, usually for all four measures.
- Target mean PTH levels are reached in 40% of patients randomized to cinacalcet; ~60% patients on cinacalcet will have a reduction in PTH of at least 30%.
- The EVOLVE study[1] is the largest RCT determining outcomes of treatment with cinacalcet:
  - 3883 patients with moderate-to-severe hyperparathyroidism randomized and followed for up to 64 months.
  - Cinacalcet did not significantly reduce the risk of death or major cardiovascular events in patients with moderate-to-severe secondary hyperparathyroidism who were undergoing dialysis.
  - Hypocalcaemia and GI adverse events were significantly more frequent in patients receiving cinacalcet.
  - Parathyroidectomy rate was halved in the cinacalcet group (7% compared to 14% in control group).
  - There was no difference in fracture rates (12% and 13% in cinacalcet and control groups respectively).
- Isolated case reports of regression of parathyroid hyperplasia and 'cure' (PTH levels return to near normal) and no relapse after cinacalcet is withdrawn, though follow-up periods are short
- UK NICE guidance on the use of cinacalcet is summarized below. The interpretation of this guidance depends on contraindications to parathyroidectomy. Furthermore, the use of cinacalcet avoids the development of low turnover bone syndrome after a total parathyroidectomy (see ➲ Parathyroid hormone control, p. 507; Paracalcitol, p. 500).

NICE guidance (January 2007)

- 'Cinacalcet is not recommended for routine treatment of secondary hyperparathyroidism in patients with ESRD on maintenance dialysis therapy.
- Cinacalcet is recommended for treatment of refractory secondary hyperparathyroidism in patients with ESRD (including those with calciphylaxis) only in those:
  - *who have 'very uncontrolled' plasma levels of PTH (>85 pmol/l) that are refractory to standard therapy, and a normal or high adjusted serum calcium level AND*
  - *in whom surgical parathyroidectomy is contraindicated, in that the risks of surgery are considered to outweigh the benefits*
- Response to treatment should be monitored regularly and treatment should be continued only if a reduction in the plasma levels of intact PTH of 30% or more is seen within 4 months of treatment, including dose escalation as appropriate.'

Review of guidance (July 2013)

- In the absence of clinical trials showing any benefit of cinacalcet on survival or quality of life, the decision was made not to change the above guidance.
- Cinacalcet should therefore continue to be used only where patients are at very high risk of adverse events from standard medical and surgical treatment and have poor quality of life. The incremental cost-effectiveness ratio was then likely to be reduced to the extent that cinacalcet could be considered a cost-effective use of NHS resources.

Reference

1. The EVOLVE Trial Investigators. Effect of cinacalcet on cardiovascular disease in patients undergoing dialysis. *N Engl J Med* 2012; 367: 2482–94.

Treatment of renal bone disease

Aims of treatment
The new drugs are considerably more expensive than standard treatment with alfacalcidol/calcitriol and calcium-based phosphate binders. Guidelines should therefore be followed for their use.

Phosphate control: NICE guidelines
UK NICE published guidelines for phosphate control in patients with CKD 4 and 5 in March 2013.

Dietary control
- All patients should have regular review by a dietician.
- Advice on dietary phosphate management should be tailored to individual learning needs and preferences.

Phosphate binders
- For adults, calcium acetate is the first-line phosphate binder.
- Consider calcium carbonate if calcium acetate is not tolerated or patients find it unpalatable.
- For patients with stage 4 or 5 CKD who are not on dialysis, consider switching to a non-calcium based binder if:
  - patient does not tolerate calcium-based binder
  - if hypercalcaemia develops or serum PTH level is low.
- For patients on dialysis, consider adding in or switching to a non-calcium based binder if:
  - persistent hyperphosphataemia despite adherence to the maximum recommended or tolerated dose of calcium-based binder
  - serum calcium goes above upper limit of normal
  - serum PTH level is low.

Box 11.1 UK Renal Association 2010 guidelines

Calcium (adjusted for albumin)
- Maintain within normal reference range for laboratory used.

Phosphate
- CKD 3b–5 (not on dialysis): maintain at 0.9–1.5mmol/L.
- Dialysis: maintain at 1.1–1.7mmol/L; measure before a 'short gap' dialysis in HD patients.

Parathyroid hormone
- CKD 3b–5 (not on dialysis): start treatment if serum PTH level rising and persistently greater than upper range of reference level for assay.
- Dialysis: target range for PTH measured using an intact PTH assay should be between 2 and 9 times the upper limit of normal for the assay used.

General comments regarding management of hyperphosphataemia

- Consider reducing dose of calcitriol/alfacalcidol if being used.
- Review dialysis adequacy:
  - In HD, phosphate removal is determined by time so better removal is achieved with longer hours/dialysis session or more frequent short hour dialysis.
  - In PD, phosphate removal is mostly determined by residual kidney function and is much more difficult if patient is anuric.
- Remember that the most common causes of continuing poor phosphate control are poor compliance with or timing of phosphate binders and diet.
- *Do not* keep increasing the dose and/or adding in newer and expensive phosphate binders before checking compliance.
- Refer and/or discuss with dieticians; they are good at assessing compliance with phosphate binders as well as diet.

Parathyroid hormone control

- Raised PTH levels can be detected early in CKD and is not uncommon in stage 4. PTH levels should be measured:
  - yearly when GFR 30–45mL/min
  - 6-monthly if PTH >7mmol/L or in stage 4 CKD
  - 3-monthly if PTH >12mmol/L or stage 5 CKD or on dialysis.
- Aim for appropriate targets, e.g. UK Renal Association guidelines (see Box 11.1).
- At lower levels of elevated PTH, ensure that phosphate is controlled and plasma calcium is in normal range.
- If Ca <2.15mmol/L, use calcium carbonate if stage 3 or 4 CKD, and on HD consider increasing dialysate Ca concentration and check 25-OH vitamin D.
- First-line drug treatment is alfacalcidol or calcitriol:
  - Monitor calcium and phosphate monthly and PTH levels 3-monthly.
  - Use calcium carbonate/acetate to control phosphate as long as plasma Ca <2.5mmol/L and Ca–P product <4.2mmol^2/L^2.
  - Titrate dose of alfacalcidol/calcitriol according to Ca and P level as well as PTH.
  - Remember to reduce dose once PTH is back into target zone and stop if PTH falls below target. This is essential to avoid hypoparathyroidism and low turnover bone problems.
- *Parathyroidectomy* should be considered in patients with persistent severe hyperparathyroidism (PTH >60pmol/L) with one or more of the following: raised alkaline phosphatase, hypercalcaemia, or high Ca–P product on standard treatment, bone symptoms, unless contraindications to surgery or likely planned living donor transplant in near future.

- *Cinacalcet or paricalcitol* should only be used in persistent severe hyperparathyroidism (as described on ➲ Calcimimetics, p. 504) when:
  - patient has had a failed parathyroidectomy attempt and continues to be severely hyperparathyroid with symptoms
  - patient unable to tolerate (or refuses) surgery
  - likely planned living donor transplant in near future.
- Use of cinacalcet:
  - Recheck PTH level before starting—you can be surprised and patient has responded to treatment.
  - Starting dose is 30mg od.
  - Continue with existing phosphate binders and vitamin D supplements.
  - Check Ca and PTH level at 2 weeks.
  - If PTH has fallen <30%, increase dose by 30mg increments up to 90mg/day (and very rarely up to 180mg/day).
  - Monthly PTH and Ca levels for first 6 months of treatment.
  - Hypocalcaemia has been reported so calcium supplements may be needed, and alfacalcidol/calcitriol probably needed in all.
  - As calcium levels fall, remember to add or change to calcium carbonate/acetate for phosphate control.
- Use of paricalcitol:
  - Now available as IV and oral preparations.
  - Indications similar to cinacalcet, and may be especially useful if plasma Ca <2.4mmol/L.
  - If cinacalcet not tolerated (usually nausea or hypocalcaemia) or failed to suppress PTH.
  - Stop any oral vitamin D supplements.
  - Start at a dose of PTH level/8 IV with each dialysis. Oral dosing is 1mcg daily or 2mcg three times/week if PTH <500pg/mL; 2mcg daily or 4mcg three times/week if PTH >500pg/mL.
  - Monitor PTH and Ca monthly and adjust dose accordingly.
  - Maximum dose 40mcg/dialysis IV; dose often needs reducing as PTH suppressed.
  - If no response after 4months, paricalcitol should be stopped.

Parathyroidectomy

Indications

- Spontaneous hypercalcaemia in the presence of an elevated PTH level, i.e. tertiary hyperparathyroidism.
- Inability to suppress severe secondary hyperparathyroidism without producing hypercalcaemia when using therapeutic doses of calcitriol (0.5mcg orally daily or 1mcg IV three times a week) or alfacalcidol (1mcg orally daily or 2mcg IV/orally three times a week). There is usually evidence of bone destruction with a raised alkaline phosphatase level. PTH levels are invariably high—>500pg/mL (55pmol/L). Phosphate levels are also very high, frequently >3mmol/L, as the use of calcium-based phosphate binders has to be limited or stopped as they will worsen hypercalcaemia.
- Calciphylaxis, raised Ca–P product, or intractable pruritus despite dietary phosphate restriction, phosphate binders, and vitamin D analogues.

Surgical techniques

- Subtotal parathyroidectomy (removing 7/8 of total parathyroid tissue)—carries risk of redevelopment of parathyroid hyperplasia of remaining tissue and need for repeat parathyroidectomy, with technical difficulties of repeated surgery on the neck.
- Total parathyroidectomy with autotransplantation of small amount of parathyroid tissue into forearm—theoretically attractive as tissue in arm easily accessible, but refractory recurrent hyperparathyroidism can still develop.
- Total parathyroidectomy with subsequent maintenance of plasma calcium using calcitriol or alfacalcidol and calcium supplements— increases risk of development of aplastic bone disease with its unknown long-term sequelae.
- Surgery may involve open neck exploration or minimally invasive surgery.

Management

- Pre-operative localization of parathyroid glands.
- Parathyroid glands are usually in the neck, but can also be found in the submandibular region or in the mediastinum.
- The glands are large (pea- to walnut-sized) so no localization techniques are needed before the first parathyroidectomy. Even experienced surgeons, however, may not find all four glands.
- Patients who have had a subtotal parathyroidectomy are at risk of needing repeat surgery as severe hyperparathyroidism will almost invariably recur.
- Pre-operative localization of the glands is needed for second operations, using radioisotope scanning (technetium, sestamibi or thyroid–parathyroid subtraction scans), US, CT, or MRI of the neck and mediastinum.

Peri-operative management
- Calcitriol (0.5mcg/day) or alfacalcidol (1mcg/day) for 1–3 days pre-operatively can reduce the degree of hypocalcaemia after surgery (sometimes significantly higher doses needed if patients already taking vitamin D analogues).
- Plasma calcium (and potassium, as with any surgery) should be checked 2–4h after surgery, and then once to twice daily for the next 2–3 days. Calcium levels can fall precipitately; however, if insufficient parathyroid tissue has been removed, calcium levels will fall only slightly, if at all.
- Some surgeons measure PTH levels peri-operatively to ensure total PTH gland removal.

Post-operative management
- Calcitriol (or alfacalcidol) should have been begun pre-operatively. They should continue, and calcium supplements should be started as soon as the calcium level falls below the normal range. These should be given orally even immediately post-operatively. IV calcium is only needed if the patient develops tetany (very rare).
- Plasma calcium should always be measured before dialysis. Dialysate calcium is all ionized so calcium levels will rise during dialysis if the patient is hypocalcaemic, or fall after dialysis if ionized plasma calcium level is higher than that of dialysate (as when plasma calcium levels are normal or high).
- Patients can be discharged 3–4 days after surgery, but calcium levels need to be checked weekly or more frequently for 2–3 months until they are stable.
- Bone is often very 'hungry' for calcium immediately after parathyroidectomy, and very high doses of calcitriol or alfacalcidol (up to 2mcg/day) and calcium supplements (up to 6g calcium carbonate/day) are needed.
- As soon as serum calcium starts rising, calcium and vitamin D doses should rapidly be reduced as the patient can become hypercalcaemic within a few days once bone is 'filled'.
- Alkaline phosphatase levels often rise during this period—this represents bone healing and is not a cause of concern.

Calciphylaxis

- A syndrome of vascular calcification and skin necrosis occurring rarely in patients with ESKD:
  - Most common in patients on HD
  - Occasionally seen after recent transplant.
- Pathogenesis poorly understood, though abnormalities in mineral metabolism that predispose to vascular and soft tissue calcification are clearly involved.
- Associated with hypercalcaemia, hyperphosphataemia, hyperparathyroidism, vitamin D treatment, and IV iron, but precise cause unknown.
- Occurs in 1–4% of patients with ESKD.
- High mortality (60–80%); mostly sepsis from infected necrotic skin.
- Characterized by areas of ischaemic necrosis that usually develop in the dermis, subcutaneous fat, and less often in muscle.
- Lesions very painful, usually on legs, develop suddenly and progress rapidly. Start as erythematous papules, then necrotic or even bullous.
- More common proximally on thighs, buttocks, and lower abdomen, but not uncommon distally.
- Vascular calcification a constant feature, but distal pulses usually present.
- Rarely associated with hypercoagulable state (including protein C and S deficiency).
- No specific diagnostic tests, although a high PTH and Ca–P product are suggestive.
- Diagnosis can be confirmed by skin biopsy showing arterial occlusion and calcification in absence of vasculitic changes, but healing can be a problem.
- Differential diagnosis includes cholesterol emboli, cellulitis, and vasculitis.

Treatment

- As this is a rare condition, there are no randomized trials, and evidence for any particular treatment is entirely anecdotal
- Treat aggravating factors (stop parenteral iron, vitamin D analogues).
- Normalize serum calcium and phosphate, increase dialysis times, low calcium dialysate.
- Non-calcaemic phosphate binders, e.g. sevelamer or lanthanum carbonate, are preferable to avoid risk of further calcification.
- Consider parathyroidectomy or use of cinacalcet, though role of urgent parathyroidectomy has not been proven.
- Aggressive wound care and debridement.
- Antibiotics as necessary.
- Hyperbaric oxygen may be of benefit (usually if can demonstrate tissue hypoxia).
- Sodium thiosulfate increasingly used (20mmol IV, slowly over 24h for 15–30 days, or 25g IV after every dialysis).
- Response to therapy is assessed by physical examination.

Complications of ESKD: cardiovascular disease

Cardiovascular disease

Cardiovascular disease accounts for 50–60% of deaths in patients with ESKD and is considerably more common in patients on dialysis than in the age-matched general population. The figure most commonly quoted is that a 40-year-old man on dialysis has a 100-fold greater risk of a cardiovascular death than a 40-year-old man with normal renal function. Patients with early renal disease are also at increased risk; most die from cardiovascular causes before developing ESKD, and many will have cardiovascular disease by the time they start dialysis. Interventions to reduce the incidence need to be begun early.

Clinical features of dialysis-related cardiovascular disease

Cardiovascular disease in dialysis patients is different from that found in the general population.
- Classical MI is found in only 8–12% patients at autopsy.
- Atherosclerosis is widespread but there is considerably more vascular calcification in dialysis patients.
- Coronary artery and valvular calcification are common.
- LVH is common.
- Primary cardiac muscle dysfunction is common, e.g. heart failure, cardiomyopathy.
- Sudden death is common.

Cardiovascular risk factors in dialysis patients

Include those that are the same as for the general population, and those that are unique for renal failure. (See Table 12.1.)

Table 12.1   Cardiovascular disease risk factors

General risk factors	Risk factors with increased prevalence in renal failure	Risk factors unique to renal failure
Age	Hypertension	Anaemia
Male sex	Diabetes	Hyperparathyroidism
Smoking	Physical inactivity	Uraemia
Family history	LVH	Hyperphosphataemia
Thrombogenic factors	Cholesterol	Malnutrition
Obesity	Lipoprotein (a)	AVFs
	Homocysteine	Volume overload
	Inflammatory state	

Cardiovascular risk factor intervention in dialysis patients

Cardiovascular risk factor intervention in dialysis patients

There have been few RCTs specific to patients with CKD. Most advice is therefore based on trials in the general population, and on epidemiological data from dialysis patients. Some guidelines are shown in Table 12.2.

Cholesterol-lowering trials

Analysis of both diabetic and non-diabetic patients with reduced GFR enrolled in conventional lipid-lowering trials has shown that statin therapy reduced cardiovascular events by 20% over 5 years for every 1mmol/L reduction in LDL cholesterol, but with no effect on overall mortality. More recently, studies specifically in patients with kidney disease have reported results:

- The *SHARP* (Study of Heart And Renal Protection) is the largest RCT with >9000 pre-dialysis and dialysis patients with and without vascular disease (patients with classical myocardial ischaemia were excluded). Patients were randomized to a fixed combination of simvastatin 20mg and ezetimibe 10mg daily or to placebo. Follow-up was for 5 years. The results confirmed a reduction in myocardial infarction by 20% over 5 years for every 1mmol/L reduction in LDL cholesterol (as in the general population), but with no effect on mortality.
- The *4D Study* (the German Diabetes and Dialysis Study) randomized diabetic patients on dialysis and with known vascular disease to atorvastatin or placebo. There was no difference in cardiovascular events between the two groups, though the study was underpowered to look specifically at MI.

Reverse causality

Epidemiological observations have shown that there is a U-shaped relationship of outcomes to many risk factors in comparison with the straight-line relationship found in the general population. For example, mortality is increased in patients with both low and high plasma cholesterol levels, and with low and high systolic BP. This is most probably due to the heterogeneous nature of a dialysis population with a group of patients with multiple co-morbidities, poor cardiac function, low BP, and poor nutrition, with low plasma cholesterol.

Table 12.2 Guidelines for treatment

Risk factor	Target level and treatment
Smoking	Stop
Hypertension	<140/90mm Hg predialysis
Diabetes	HbA1c <55mmol/mol
Thrombogenic factors	Aspirin 75mg daily unless contraindication
Obesity	Appropriate dietary advice
Physical inactivity	Encourage exercise
LVH	BP control, treat anaemia
Cholesterol	<5.0mmol/L
Lipoprotein (a)	No treatment available
Homocysteine	Folic acid—no evidence of benefit
Anaemia	Aim for Hb 10.5–12.0g/dL
Hyperphosphataemia	<1.7mmol/L
Uraemia	Appropriate adequacy of dialysis
Malnutrition	Improve nutrition as much as possible

Management of ischaemic heart disease

Some special problems occur investigating and treating ischaemic heart disease (IHD) in dialysis patients.

Investigations

Coronary angiography is often the only reliable means of diagnosing or screening for IHD (e.g. pre-transplant assessment). Many patients cannot complete an exercise ECG because of anaemia, 'unfitness', or peripheral vascular disease.

Medical management

- Use of antiangina drugs is sometimes limited by hypotension, particularly during HD.
- Anaemia treatment should be optimized with a Hb level of 10.5–12.0g/dL. Higher levels have been associated with increased mortality.
- HD should be as 'gentle' as possible to avoid sudden hypotension precipitating angina. BVM may be helpful.
- Patients can receive ACEIs, statins, β-blockers, control of diabetes, and should be advised to stop smoking.

Surgical management of ischaemic heart disease

- Both coronary angioplasty and coronary artery bypass grafting (CABG) can be completed successfully in dialysis patients.
- Patients should be well dialysed prior to angioplasty to avoid the risk of fluid overload. >500mL of fluid (as contrast) may be given during angioplasty.
- Haemofiltration can often be performed within the bypass circuit during CABG.
- Continuous haemofiltration may be used post-operatively if immediate dialysis is required, or the patient is in ICU.
- Most patients can be safely dialysed 48h post-CABG if not hypotensive or haemodynamically unstable.
- Early PD may hinder withdrawal of ventilatory support, but can usually be recommenced within 48h.
- The risks of CABG are greater than in non-dialysis patients due to increased incidence of other vascular disease (cerebral and/or peripheral).
- Prolonged hypotension during the procedure may cause a decline in residual renal function; this is particularly important in PD patients who may subsequently become underdialysed. Contrast load during angioplasty may have the same effect.
- Mortality from coronary artery bypass surgery in dialysis patients is ~3-fold higher than in the general population—one large survey found a mortality rate of 11%.
- As there is a very high risk of cardiovascular death without intervention, CABG may nevertheless be life-saving in dialysis patients.

Acute coronary syndrome

Aggressive management of ACS in the general population improves survival. The same is true for patients with renal disease, though there are some important differences:

• No firm data that ACS is more common in patients with renal failure, but they do have significantly worse outcomes.
• Symptoms are frequently absent in renal patients.
• Silent ischaemia makes true incidence of ACS in renal disease difficult to estimate.
• Restenosis rate after angioplasty is higher.
• Coronary artery disease is common in dialysis patients, but acute MI is a relatively rare cause of death.

Diagnosis

• High index of suspicion needed because of lack of symptoms—ACS should be considered in all patients with episodes of hypotension. unexplained by fluid status, or fluid overload with no change in weight.
• ECG—can often be difficult to interpret because of LVH, bundle branch block, effect of hyperkalaemia.
• Troponin levels can be difficult to interpret—elevated troponin levels (T > I) are often found in HD patients without evidence of acute coronary disease, but not usually very high.

Coronary investigations

• Treadmill exercise tests often impossible to perform in patients on dialysis:
  • Patients often become exhausted before reaching maximal heart rate.
  • May have peripheral vascular disease.
• Coronary angiography can pose special problems:
  • Nephrotoxicity of contrast material can precipitate pre-dialysis patients on to dialysis although this is rare, and minimized by avoiding contrast load of a ventriculogram.
  • Contrast material is hypertonic, causing expansion of blood volume, which can lead to left ventricular failure.
  • Acute decline in residual renal function in patients on PD can cause symptomatic uraemia. If residual renal function is known to be critical for dialysis adequacy, then extra PD should be performed for 2–3 days after, e.g. increasing the number of CAPD exchanges from 3 to 4, or 4 to 5; if on APD, the volume of fluid cycled overnight can be increased, or an extra hour spent on the machine at night.
• HD should be avoided for 24h after angiography (which should be scheduled, if possible, for a non-dialysis day). If dialysis is needed, heparin should be avoided.

Cardiac management

• Little trial evidence as patients with renal disease excluded from most studies.
• Uraemia associated with prolongation of bleeding time and abnormal platelet aggregation, so increased risk of bleeding from antithrombotic agents.

- Dialysis patients with acute MI have high cardiac mortality and poor long-term survival; they are also less likely to be treated with thrombolytic drugs because of risk of bleeding. Angioplasty or urgent CABG may be preferred. There is no reason to avoid treating dialysis patients with acute MI urgently.
- Aspirin and clopidogrel should be given as with non-renal patients; risk of bleeding should be assessed for each individual patient, but is higher than in non-dialysis patients.
- LMWH superior to unfractionated heparin (UFH) but higher risk of bleeding in patients with renal failure; patients with GFR <30mL/min have been excluded from studies. Doses need reducing in renal failure. Until data are available, it may be safer to use UFH.
- Platelet glycoprotein IIb/IIIa inhibitors vary in mechanisms of clearance. Dose of tirofiban and eptifibatide, but not abciximab, needs to be adjusted for renal failure.
- Thrombolytics, according to local guidelines, should be considered when cardiac criteria indicate their use.
- Contraindications to thrombolysis are more common in renal patients, such as:
  - insertion of catheter (CVC, PD) within 14 days
  - recent renal (native or transplant) biopsy
  - active peptic ulceration
  - uraemic pericarditis
  - uncontrolled hypertension (>220/110mmHg).

Renal management

- ACS in renal patients can be related to anaemia; and oxygenation of myocardium and chest pain improve if patient is no longer anaemic.
- If Hb <11g/dL, patient should be transfused with careful monitoring of fluid status and plasma potassium:
  - Pre-dialysis patients will mostly need additional diuretics with careful monitoring of renal function.
  - PD patients should use hypertonic dialysate to cover transfusion, e.g. a 2.27% glucose exchange substituted for a 1.36%.
  - HD patients should receive blood during a dialysis session, unless the patient is clinically volume depleted and the blood needed as an emergency.
- Patients will continue to need dialysis, and fluid status should be optimized. Both volume depletion and volume overload will compromise myocardial perfusion.
- CAPD and APD regimens can usually continue unchanged, though alterations to glucose concentrations may be needed.
- HD can be difficult immediately after ACS, and unless patient needs urgent UF or is severely hyperkalaemic, dialysis should be avoided for at least 24h until patient is stable.
- HD should be more 'gentle' immediately after ACS, e.g. shorter, with reduced UF (depending on fluid status), to avoid electrolyte shifts that could precipitate arrhythmias and hypotension.

Hypertension

- Hypertension is probably the most important complication of renal disease.
- Hypertension complicates most types of renal disease.
- It is also the most important factor contributing to the rate of progression of renal damage whatever the original cause.
- Untreated or poorly controlled hypertension can directly damage the kidneys, causing hypertensive nephropathy.
- RVD and peripheral vascular disease are more common in patients with hypertension.
- Hypertension, both on its own and by causing LVH, plays a major role in the increased risk of cardiovascular death in patients with renal failure.

Aetiology of hypertension

- Extracellular fluid volume expansion (major cause)
- Increased sympathetic activity
- Renin–angiotensin–aldosterone system stimulation
- Increased body weight
- Calcified arterial tree (contributing to systolic hypertension).

Management of hypertension

The aims are to:
- slow the rate of deterioration of renal function
- reduce the degree of LVH
- reduce the prevalence of cardiovascular disease
- reduce the rate of cardiovascular death
- reduce prevalence of renal disease in the general population.

Targets for BP control

In patients with CKD (pre-dialysis) see ➡ Management of renal failure: blood pressure control, p. 36). There have been no trials establishing the optimal level of BP control in patients on dialysis, and guidelines extrapolate from trials in other high risk patients (e.g. diabetics). UK Renal Association guidelines suggest a goal of <130/80mmHg in both HD (post-dialysis) and PD patients. This target is unrealistic, however, for the growing number of older patients on dialysis. As in the general population, older patients do not tolerate low systolic BP and a more realistic target would be a systolic of 140–150mm Hg.

BP control in patients on haemodialysis

Achieving BP targets in patients on HD is difficult:

- Hypertension is multifactorial.
- Volume overload is a major problem.
- Timing of measurement of BP is controversial (pre- or post-dialysis).
- Compliance with salt and fluid intake and polypharmacy are major issues.

BP measurement

- BP falls during dialysis because of UF, and rises gradually before the next session because of salt and water retention.
- In practice, pre-dialysis BP level is used to determine level of control.
- Patients, however, may be anxious before dialysis and many do not take their antihypertensive drugs on the day of dialysis to avoid IDH. The overall level of BP may therefore be overestimated by pre-dialysis readings.
- Pre-dialysis BP may also be >20/10mmHg higher when measured on arrival in the dialysis unit (even after rest), than that measured over the previous 6h by ambulatory BP monitoring (ABPM).
- Post-dialysis BP may give an estimate of hypertension not due to volume overload, assuming adequate volume control during dialysis.
- Interdialytic measurement, or ABPM, are probably more meaningful but not easy to achieve in practice.

Management of BP on haemodialysis

- It is possible to achieve excellent BP control without the use of any drugs by normalizing extracellular fluid volume and maintaining 'dry weight' with UF on dialysis.
- Salt (especially) and fluid intake between dialyses must be low.
- This is the experience of the few units (e.g. Tassin, France), which still practise long HD (8h three times a week) and aggressive salt management. The risk of hypotension during dialysis is much reduced as the UF rate is lower (the same amount of fluid removed but over a longer period). Patients achieve true dry weight, and >90% need no drugs for hypertension. Mortality is significantly reduced.
- Most units cannot offer long dialysis because of resource implications, and most patients prefer shorter hours of dialysis, hence BP control is usually achieved by reducing post-dialysis weight as low as possible, and by using antihypertensive drugs.
- It is still possible to control BP by getting patients to their true dry weight, but often takes several months of gentle reductions in weight, strict control of salt intake, and avoidance of antihypertensive drugs during the process.
- IDH associated with rapid UF worsens the problem by necessitating use of saline, and preventing the achievement of dry weight. BP can be controlled if antihypertensive drugs are weaned as dry weight is reduced progressively.
- Patients undertaking daily short dialysis, and especially nocturnal dialysis, usually have good BP control with minimal use of drugs.

Achieving BP control on haemodialysis

Aim to bring patients to their dry weight, even if no other clinical features of fluid overload (other than hypertension):

- Bring weight down slowly over several dialyses, e.g. 0.5–1kg/week. There can be a delay of several weeks between control of fluid overload and reduction in BP.
- Minimize symptomatic hypotensive episodes so patients will tolerate weight reduction, and ideally use as long hours as possible. UF profiling should be standard and sodium profiling avoided because of the risk of sodium loading. Low temperature dialysis may help. HDF often better tolerated.
- Minimize use of antihypertensive drugs as these contribute to risk of hypotension on dialysis.
- As most modern antihypertensive drugs are active for >24h, stopping them on day of dialysis probably has little effect on risk of hypotension during dialysis, but reduces their efficacy.
- Encourage patients to restrict weight gains between dialyses to <2kg by limiting salt and water intake. Salt reduction is more important as this drives thirst.
- Educate patients about the importance of BP control.

Use of antihypertensive drugs

- Doses should be kept low to avoid hypotension on dialysis.
- If BP rises, response should be to lower post-dialysis weight and not increase drug therapy.
- β-blockers are useful as they block sympathetic overactivity contributing to renal hypertension. They may contribute to hypotension on dialysis as they block the baroreceptor response, so short-acting agents should be stopped on dialysis days in patients with frequent hypotensive episodes.
- Calcium antagonists can be useful, but prevent reflex arteriolar vasoconstriction, which is important in preventing IDH.
- α-blockers do not increase risk of hypotension.
- ACEIs and ARBs can cause dramatic hypotension with volume depletion. Anaphylactic reactions can also occur when ACEIs are used in patients dialysing on polyacrylonitrile (PAN) membranes. These drugs should be used with great care and when BP control cannot be achieved by any other means, but are effective. Both are increasingly used in patients with left ventricular dysfunction on HD (with no evidence of benefit in this group).
- For patients with pre-dialysis hypotension:
  - BP check whether patient is truly volume depleted, i.e. beneath their target weight; if they are, give fluids.
  - Stop or reduce antihypertensive drugs and allow patient to remain at this new 'dry weight'.
- If hypotension occurs in the absence of fluid depletion or drug therapy, the most likely cause is poor cardiac function—echocardiography should be performed.

BP control in patients on peritoneal dialysis

This is less of a problem than on HD.

- Only half of the patients on PD have hypertension.
- Extracellular fluid volume expansion is the predominant cause as in HD.
- There is no problem of interdialytic weight gains or dialytic hypotensive episodes affecting BP.
- BP control is easier in patients with residual renal function as continued urine output makes it easier to control fluid intake and achieve 'dry weight'.

Management of BP on PD

- Aim for the patient's 'dry weight' using UF and restriction of fluid intake.
- Any antihypertensive drug can safely be used.
- ACEIs and/or ARBs have been shown in small RCTs to preserve residual renal function.
- ACEIs and ARBs are not particularly effective in patients who are fluid overloaded (RAS will be suppressed).
- If patient becomes hypotensive, cut back on drug therapy rather than allowing their weight to rise.
- If BP rises, initially bring down the patient's weight by increasing UF or encouraging fluid restriction, and by ensuring that the patient is restricting their salt intake. Loss of residual renal function is also a cause.

Cerebrovascular disease

Cerebral and peripheral vascular diseases are important causes of morbidity and mortality in patients with renal failure.

Cerebrovascular disease

- Patients with CKD are at increased risk of stroke.
- There is some evidence that stroke is more common in patients on HD than on PD.
- Increased stroke rate on HD is partly due to episodes of hypotension on dialysis and the increased risk of haemorrhage related to anticoagulation on dialysis.
- Patients at most risk are those with poorly controlled hypertension, diabetes, the elderly, smokers, and those with other vascular disease.
- As in the general population, a CT scan should be done as soon as possible, particularly because of the increased risk of cerebral haemorrhage.
- Extrapolating from studies in the general population, aspirin should probably be given to all patients with renal disease (unless there is a contraindication) to reduce the incidence of stroke (but no primary trial data). There are greater potential risks of bleeding from aspirin in view of the platelet and endothelial dysfunction of uraemia.
- Thrombolysis is usually contraindicated in patients on haemodialysis as in many centres, use of heparin in the previous 48h is a contraindication to the use of thrombolytic agents.
- Heparin use on dialysis should be limited or avoided in both cerebral haemorrhage (risk of re-bleeding) and in infarction (risk of bleeding into infarct).
- No decision on the long-term outcome should be made immediately, as the prognosis is very variable.
- Important long-term sequelae of stroke in a patient on dialysis include social independence, ability to continue performing PD, and nutritional status.

Peripheral vascular disease

This is one of the worst predictors of outcome and survival on dialysis:
- Most patients with peripheral vascular disease also have other vascular disease, so are at high risk of IHD and/or cerebrovascular disease.
- Vascular access for HD is often difficult to achieve.
- Limits chances of transplantation as anastomosis on to the iliac artery may be technically difficult or may cause critical limb ischaemia.
- Arteries are usually heavily calcified. This makes non-invasive investigations, such as Doppler studies and ankle–brachial pressure ratio, inaccurate as the arteries cannsot be compressed. The diagnosis is therefore often made late when critical ischaemia has already occurred.
- The arterial disease is predominantly distal, making bypass surgery technically difficult.
- There is a high rate of amputations. Survival after amputation is poor. Nutritional support is very important.

Patients with RVD or diabetes are most at risk of developing peripheral vascular disease. All patients on dialysis are, however, at risk, particularly if they are smokers. The key investigation is arteriography as non-invasive tests are not always accurate. It is essential that patients not yet on dialysis, and those on PD with significant residual renal function, be well hydrated prior to arteriography, to avoid development of contrast-induced nephropathy, but avoiding pulmonary oedema! Patients with diabetes are at particular risk. Acetylcysteine orally (600mg bd, starting before contrast exposure) may reduce the risk. Management of surgery in these patients is the same as with any other surgery. However, the patient's 'dry weight' must be reduced after limb amputation or they will become fluid overloaded.

Complications of ESKD: infection

Infection risk in dialysis patients

Infections are the second most common cause of death in ESKD (up to 30% of all ESKD deaths; mostly from septicaemia and pneumonia). Patients with ESKD or CKD are relatively immunosuppressed, have an increased incidence of diabetes, and hence may develop more severe or occult infections, and require a higher index of suspicion by the clinician. Lymphocyte, monocyte, macrophage, and neutrophil function may be impaired in uraemia, bacterial clearance is reduced, dialysis membranes may be immunomodulatory, and malnutrition and blood transfusions impair immune responses.

Infections are usually due to common pathogens (staphylococci, streptococci, *Escherichia coli*) and not opportunistic organisms. Vascular access-related infections are the most common cause of morbidity and mortality. Bacteraemia occurs in up to 20% of patients, and can be complicated by osteomyelitis, cerebral abscesses, endocarditis, and septic arthritis in up to 30% of cases.

Viral infections may be transmitted nosocomially and must be screened and detected.

Nephrotoxic drug use should be minimized, and antibiotic dosing made appropriate to the level of renal function and modality of dialysis, as under- and overtreatment are both common.

See also:
- Management of access (catheter) infections (p. 132)
- Exit site infections (p. 318)
- Peritonitis (p. 323).

Non-access-related infections in dialysis patients

Respiratory infections
- Upper respiratory tract infections not increased in ESKD—treatment unchanged.
- Pneumonia more difficult to diagnose in ESKD because of fluid overload or pulmonary oedema—treat early.
- Gram-negative pneumonia increased in hospitalized patients.

Nervous system
- Meningitis not increased in ESKD.
- Mucormycosis more common in patients treated with desferrioxamine for aluminium overload.

Gastrointestinal system
- *Helicobacter pylori* infection probably not increased in ESKD. Treatment should be as for patients without kidney disease.
- Gastroenteritis more commonly leads to problems with intravascular volume in both HD and PD.
- Diverticulitis can lead to peritonitis in PD.
- *Clostridium difficile* colitis is more common in dialysis patients (up to 5 times), because of increased exposure to antibiotics. Can be more severe.
- Hepatitis is an important cause of morbidity and mortality. Hepatitis B and C incidence has fallen in dialysis patients in most countries.

Urinary tract infection
Difficult to diagnose in anuric patients. Pyuria not a sensitive marker of infection in ESKD.

Cellulitis and osteomyelitis
Important causes of morbidity in dialysis patients. Patients have vascular disease, diabetes, and repeated needle sticks and percutaneous assaults. Can spread rapidly.

Tuberculosis

- Increased incidence (6- to 50-fold) in dialysis patients. 100-fold increase has been reported in dialysis patients in West London, UK, over the local population.
- Often extrapulmonary disease. Fever, malaise, and weight loss are the most common symptoms.
- Patients with ESKD often anergic to cutaneous testing (up to 40% of patients), making diagnosis difficult. Diagnosis is often delayed. ELISPOT or other interferon release assays may be useful in diagnosing TB in dialysis patients, but not yet confirmed in formal studies.
- Therapeutic trial of treatment may be necessary in patients with undiagnosed fever or illness in whom the index of suspicion is high, including EPO resistance of undetermined cause.
- Drug dosing can cause problems. In general give drugs after dialysis.
- Infectious patients require appropriate management (isolation) within dialysis units until non-infectious.

Resistant organisms: MRSA

Resistant bacteria are an increasing problem in hospitalized patients. Infection control policies, handwashing, identification of infection rather than colonization, and collaboration with local microbiologists are crucial in their control. Ideal management of colonized patients within dialysis units (e.g. treatment in separate rooms) is often compromised by lack of resources (especially space).

MRSA

Meticillin-resistant *Staphylococcus aureus* is mostly a nosocomial pathogen affecting hospitalized patients. MRSA is endemic in many hospitals. Most dialysis units have colonized patients. May be found as a colonizing bacterium, or as a cause of bacteraemia or overt infections. Nasal carriage common. Up to 40% of all staphylococcal infections may be caused by MRSA.

Risk factors for colonization include previous antibiotic therapy, treatment on an ICU, or proximity to a colonized or infected patient. Healthcare staff are also carriers. Transmission is by skin contact, from hands or instruments. Up to 60% of colonized patients will develop overt infection. Risk factors for infection include invasive procedures, recent hospitalization, and recent surgery. MRSA infections cause increased morbidity, length of stay, and costs, but mortality rates are the same as for sensitive staphylococcal infections. MRSA bacteraemia is usually associated with vascular access. MRSA peritonitis is often more severe than sensitive strains.

MRSA prevention and treatment

- Hand washing with antimicrobial soaps or gels between patients provides the major route for preventing nosocomial spread; staff should wear gloves and gowns for close contact.
- Isolation within outpatient dialysis units not universally performed as the risk of spread is deemed minimal in clothed patients (no evidence).
- The value of eradication of carriage of MRSA is unclear. Current regimens include topical mupirocin to the nose three times a day for 3–5 days, and bathing with antimicrobial soaps. There is increasing evidence that mupirocin does reduce *S. aureus* sepsis rates, and can also be applied to permacath and PD catheter exit sites.
- Treatment should be restricted to patients with infection (not simply colonization), and be based on local antibiotic sensitivities.
- Pathogenic foci must be removed or drained (e.g. intravascular lines, drains, purulent collections).
- Vancomycin remains the drug of choice (but use should be restricted as much as possible), but only for truly meticillin-resistant bacteria. Teicoplanin is an alternative, and MRSA is occasionally sensitive to gentamicin. In patients intolerant/allergic to vancomycin, co-trimoxazole, ciprofloxacin, clindamycin, and minocycline have been used (but are all less effective than vancomycin). Rifampicin should not be used as a single agent as resistance reliably emerges.
- Linezolid (oral or IV) is an alternative. Its dose does not need to be adjusted for renal failure, but it should be given after a HD session as it is removed during dialysis. Linezolid has numerous side effects; thrombocytopenia is found in 1/3 of patients, and associated with optic and peripheral neuropathy, particularly after prolonged use.

Resistant organisms: VISA, VRSA, VRE, and others

VISA/GISA/VRSA

Vancomycin (glycopeptide) intermediate S. aureus (VISA/GISA), a strain of MRSA with reduced sensitivity to vancomycin, was first reported in 1996. Only a few cases to date, all of whom had received prolonged courses of vancomycin prior to the isolation of VISA. Patients must be treated under more careful isolation, with minimal contact with healthcare staff, other patients, etc. Treatment should be based on *in vitro* sensitivity studies. A couple of cases of vancomycin-resistant S. aureus (VRSA) have also been reported in dialysis patients, sensitive to linezolid, chloramphenicol, minocycline, and quinupristin–dalfopristin.

Vancomycin use should be minimized to prevent the more widespread emergence of vancomycin-resistant bacteria.

VRE

Enterococci are group D streptococci found in normal gut and skin flora—the most common is *Enterococcus faecalis*. Vancomycin and multidrug-resistant strains are common, and can transfer resistance to other organisms. VRE is primarily a nosocomial pathogen, becoming endemic in many hospitals. It is no more common in dialysis units than other hospital settings. Transmission is by direct or indirect hand contact. Major risk factor is previous antibiotic use (especially vancomycin and cephalosporins) and ICU care during hospitalization. Most common site of infections are urinary tract and blood. Not an intrinsically virulent organism, and mortality associated with underlying debility of the patient.

Prevention and treatment

Careful use of vancomycin in general, infection control (especially hand washing), and patient isolation. There is no way to eliminate colonization. If necessary, treatment should be based on *in vitro* sensitivity and local knowledge of susceptibility, but may include ampicillin, teicoplanin, gentamicin, ciprofloxacin, rifampicin, imipenem, chloramphenicol, linezolid, or quinupristin.

Others

Multidrug-resistant Klebsiella

Can cause outbreaks of infections (urine, blood). Dialysis patients not more at risk.

Multidrug-resistant tuberculosis

Increasingly common, especially in patients from sub-Saharan Africa, and in those with HIV. Treatment requires close collaboration with infectious disease specialists, knowledge of local susceptibilities, and *in vitro* sensitivity data.

Viral infections: HBV

HBV was highly prevalent 20+ years ago in HD patients, but has now been minimized in most developed countries by implementation of universal precautions, screening of blood products for HBsAg, vaccination of dialysis patients (or ideally patients with CKD prior to dialysis), isolation of HBsAg-positive patients, and use of dedicated machines for infected patients.

Acute HBV infection is usually asymptomatic, manifesting only as a rise in serum transaminases. Chronic carriage is common in infected dialysis patients, and increased in those with high serum ferritin levels.

All patients should be screened regularly (3-monthly) for HBsAg, and serum transaminases monitored (often monthly). Especially important in patients returning from holiday having had dialysis in countries with a higher prevalence of HBV (increase screening to 2-weekly or monthly with or without polymerase chain reaction-based techniques).

Treatment

Rapidly changing, but includes interferon alfa, lamivudine, famciclovir, adefovir, and tenofovir. Treatment for chronic carriage often less efficacious in dialysis patients. Patients must be isolated for dialysis.

Vaccination

All staff and patients (unless HBsAg positive) should be vaccinated, and the response assessed by measurement of anti-HBsAg antibodies. Dose should be doubled in patients to maximize efficacy (3–4 doses of 40mcg). Seroconversion more likely in patients vaccinated prior to need for dialysis.

Viral infections: HCV

Prevalence rates in dialysis patients vary round the world from 0% to 73% (0.4–15% in the USA). Symptomatic acute illness is rare, but infection may cause a rise in serum transaminases. Transmission is by blood products and shared needles, and much less commonly sexually. Increasing evidence for horizontal spread (patient to patient) within dialysis units by environmental blood contamination. Being dialysed next to an HCV-infected patient significantly increases the risk of HCV acquisition in some studies. No evidence for transmission by re-use of machines.

Diagnosis

By detection of antibodies (third-generation assays have high sensitivity and specificity) or viral RNA in serum by polymerase chain reaction. Antibody response may take several months to develop after infection, and is blunted in dialysis patients. Patients should be screened every 3 months (more frequently on return from holiday dialysis in high-risk countries).

Treatment

Interferon, PEG interferon, and ribavirin less successful in dialysis patients, but sometimes used, especially prior to attempted transplantation (~40% response rate). Side effects and serious adverse effects are common. Ribavirin needs careful dose reduction to avoid haemolytic anaemia, which is a common complication.

New drugs are now available and increasingly recommended including boceprevir, telaprevir, sofosbuvir, and simeprevir (HCV protease inhibitors). If available, these new agents in conjunction with PEG interferon and/or ribavirin are the treatment of choice and can offer complete eradication of HCV. This is especially useful in patients with preserved liver function suitable for subsequent kidney transplantation.

Patients with HCV are not usually isolated but separate machines are used. Universal precautions should be rigorously applied.

Vaccination

Not currently available.

Viral infections: other viruses

Hepatitis E

A self-limiting, enterically transmitted viral hepatitis especially common in Asia, Africa, Central America, and the Middle East. Not increased in dialysis patients. Prevalence 3% in Italy in dialysis patients, and no association with HCV or HBV.

HGV/GBV-C

HGV/GBV-C is a Flaviviridae RNA virus, initially described as putative agents of non-A–E hepatitis. (GBV-A and GBV-B are Tamarin monkey viruses rather than human pathogens.) They differ substantially from other hepatitis viruses. Detection requires polymerase chain reaction of serum virus RNA combined with serological response to a putative coat protein. The virus is transmitted parenterally, and has been found in 1–2% of normal blood donors in the USA, 0.9% in Japan, 3.6% in Australia, and 14% in West Africa. Serological prevalence may be higher (i.e. patients without viraemia). Prevalence in HD patients has been reported at between 3% and 57% (17% in the USA). Patient-to-patient transmission probably occurs, without evidence of associated symptoms or disease. Clearance of GBV-C/HGV is rare in HD patients, and many do not mount an antibody response to the envelope protein. Co-infection with HCV is common.

The pathogenicity of GBV-C/HGV remains in doubt, as infected blood donors have normal transaminases, experimentally infected primates frequently do not develop hepatitis, and viral DNA is not concentrated in the liver. In some patients there is an association between non-A–E hepatitis and GBV-C/HGV detection, but overall there is no clear relationship between infection and liver disease.

TT virus

Non-A–G predominantly blood transmitted hepatitis virus. Pathogenicity unclear. TT virus DNA found in up to 50% of Japanese and Spanish HD patients, 68% of Danish HD patients, 20% in Korea, 40% in Turkey, and 20% in Germany. No increase in prevalence over control populations in Korea, Japan, or Turkey. Most patients do not have abnormal liver function tests, but there is an association with a lower Hb level. Does not increase incidence of liver disease in HCV-co-infected patients.

Viral infections: HIV

Incidence and prevalence of HIV in dialysis patients varies hugely; up to 39% in some cities in the USA. In most countries the prevalence of HIV sero-positivity is <1% (0.13% in Italy, 1.5% in the USA). Survival of HIV-infected patients has increased hugely over the last 15 years in patients on dialysis, especially with the use of HAART (highly active antiretroviral therapy). One-year survival increased from 49% in 1991 to 74% in 2000 and is now nearly identical to non-HIV infected patients. Deaths are due predominantly to infections rather than cardiovascular disease, however, with increasingly long-term survival of patients with HIV, cardiovascular disease is emerging as a major cause of morbidity and mortality. Long-term survival is associated with CD4 T-cell count at the start of dialysis.

Dialysis modality

- Either PD or HD can be used. No difference in patient survival. Routine factors should determine choice of dialysis modality. Patients can be transplanted if no opportunistic infections, HIV virus fully suppressed and patients have normal CD4 counts.
- Anaemia is more common in HIV-infected patients and multifactorial. Parvovirus B19 is more common in HIV-infected patients and should be looked for in patients with unresponsive or new-onset anaemia.
- Low risk of transmission via HD, so routine isolation or dedicated machine use not necessary.
- Care should be taken during access needling, and disposal of sharps, but standard infection control procedures are sufficient.
- Standard disinfection is sufficient for machines.
- HIV can be isolated from PD fluids, but safe to flush PD fluids down toilet and disinfect after with viricidal agent (e.g. 10% household bleach).
- Staff exposed to blood from an HIV-positive patient (needlestick injury) should receive currently recommended post-exposure prophylaxis.

Drug treatment of HIV on dialysis

- Nucleoside reverse transcriptase inhibitors (NRTIs) mostly renally excreted and dialysed, so need 30–50% dose reduction and dosing after dialysis (except abacavir).
- Non-nucleoside reverse transcriptase inhibitors (NNTRIs) and protease inhibitors do not need dose reduction in ESKD.
- Protease inhibitors especially major cause for drug interactions through cytochrome P450 inhibition.
- See **➔** Chapter 18 for precise dosing.

Chapter 14

Symptoms related to ESKD

Introduction

Patients with ESKD have multiple symptoms related to co-morbidities and complications of renal disease. Many will be graded as moderate–severe in questionnaires and yet patients often do not tell physicians about them when seen in routine clinic appointments. This may be because patients are not given the opportunity to talk about them as the nephrologist is more interested in achieving various adequacy and biochemical targets.

Fatigue/tiredness, pruritus, and constipation occur in more than half of dialysis patients, and >40% experience anorexia, pain, and sleep disturbance. Quality of life can be profoundly affected by such symptoms. It is time-consuming to enquire about and manage symptoms, but this is an essential part of caring for the patient on dialysis. Patients also may acquire symptoms from drug side effects especially when renal function is deteriorating near end stage, e.g. drowsiness, confusion, and constipation from opioids, hypoglycaemia from insulin, and bradycardia from atenolol. Physicians and nurses looking after renal patients should explicitly enquire after potential drug-related symptoms. (See Table 14.1.)

Table 14.1 Common symptoms in ESKD

Very common (>50% patients)	Fatigue/lack of energy
	Pruritus
	Dry skin
	Bone or joint pain
	Dry mouth
Common (30–50% patients)	Sleep problems
	Sexual problems
	Numbness or tingling in feet
	Muscle cramps
	Dizziness
	Leg oedema
Moderately common (20–30% patients)	Nausea
	Shortness of breath
	Anxiety/depression
	Feeling irritable
	Muscle soreness
	Restless legs
	Cough
	Constipation
	Decreased appetite
Less common (10–20% patients)	Vomiting
	Diarrhoea
	Difficulty concentrating
	Headache
	Chest pain

Symptom evaluation

Although there are increasing numbers of publications demonstrating the high symptom burden and associated distress in patients with ESKD, it is also well reported that the renal healthcare team usually underestimate patients' symptoms and that patients do not always report them unless specifically asked. Currently symptom score tools have mostly been used in research studies, but are also beginning to be used clinically. The advantages of using such tools include:

• identifying symptoms that need immediate treatment
• changing model of care to a patient-centred model focusing on symptoms and quality of life
• enabling discussions about palliative care and prognosis when high symptom scores are reported
• evaluating response to any specific symptom treatment.

Various symptom scores have been evolved for research purposes. The most commonly used are POS (renal) and KDQOL-SF.

Palliative care Outcome Scale – renal (POS-renal)

Adapted from the Palliative care Outcome Scale (POS). Contains 17 questions which are rated in terms of impact to patient over the last week from 0 (not at all) to 4 (overwhelming). Symptoms assessed include pain, shortness of breath, weakness or lack of energy, nausea, vomiting, poor appetite, constipation, mouth problems, drowsiness, poor mobility, itching, difficulty sleeping, restless legs or difficulty keeping legs still, anxiety, depression, changes in skin, and diarrhoea with a space for any other symptoms. Takes patients <10min to complete.

Kidney Dialysis Quality of Life – Short Form (KDQOL-SF)

Focuses on symptoms, effects on daily life, burden of disease, cognitive function, work status, sexual function, quality of social interaction, and sleep. Symptoms assessed include general well-being, limit to activity, physical activity, depression and emotional problems, pain, anxiety, confusion, cramps, itch, dry skin, shortness of breath, dizziness, lack of appetite, numbness, nausea, sexual activity, and sleep. Although this is the 'short form', there are over 37 questions often with multiple parts and takes 20–30min to complete.

Fatigue/lack of energy

This common symptom complex is experienced by:
- over two-thirds of patients before the onset of dialysis
- a similar proportion after starting RRT
- one-third of conservatively managed patients.
- Poor sleep, discussed on ➔ Sleep disorders, p. 550, is associated with daytime somnolence and reduced quality of life.
- 45% of 507 dialysis patients rated drowsiness moderate or severe.
- Muscle weakness itself will contribute to fatigue and reduced mobility and activity.
- This may lead to further reduction in activity and hence further muscle weakness, with the potential for a spiral downwards of function if not actively managed.

Contributory factors
- Inadequate dialysis
- Hypotension—can be caused by fluid depletion, poor cardiac function
- Anaemia
- Biochemical abnormalities particularly hyper- or hypokalaemia, hypomagnesaemia, hyper- or hypocalcaemia, hyponatraemia, and hypophosphataemia
- Severe hyperparathyroidism
- Poor nutritional state
- Poor quality sleep
- Depression
- Renal bone disorders leading to reduced activity because of pain
- Pain
- Co-morbidities
- Medications, e.g. β-blockers.

Impact of fatigue and weakness
This symptom complex has a major impact on quality of life and can lead to a vicious circle of being unable to work or perform many daily activities, leading to loss of self-esteem with the potential for depression and psychological distress with a worsening feeling of tiredness and weakness.

Post-dialysis fatigue
Some patient experience severe fatigue immediately post-dialysis. Surveys suggest that the average time to recovery after dialysis is 6–7h, but it can be significantly longer. This can be caused by the fluid shifts and possible hypotension related to dialysis. There is an expectation among patients that they will feel better when dialysis starts; for the frail and elderly the reverse may happen and they actually feel worse.

Management

General non-drug measures

- Appropriate changes to dialysis regimen to ensure good adequacy
- Address nutritional problems—may need supplements
- Assess sleep pattern
- Physiotherapy and rehabilitation programmes are associated with improved exercise tolerance and reduced fatigue
- Address social issues—may need support with some activities or help with caring for another family member, e.g. children, elderly spouse.

Specific and drug measures

- Optimal anaemia management
- Screen for and manage depression if present
- Appropriate treatment of associated co-morbidities
- Discontinue drugs that may be implicated, e.g. β-blockers
- Pain control—will improve sleep pattern
- Levocarnitine IV after HD has been used with some (poor quality) evidence for benefit.

Pruritus and dry skin

Pruritus is one of the most common and distressing symptoms of ESKD, occurring in 20–90% patients in various studies. It appears to be independent of sex, age, ethnicity, type of dialysis, and underlying renal disease. Despite evidence that pruritus is associated with poorer patient outcomes, many physicians and healthcare professionals continue to fail to ask their patients whether they have this symptom and try different management plans as suggested later in this topic.

Clinical characteristics

- Varies over time and between patients—some patients experience pruritus for a few minutes each day, others report it continuously throughout the day.
- Skin appearance ranges from the normal to severe xerosis with or without secondary skin changes from repeated scratching.
- Pruritus can appear daily, weekly, or monthly, but tends to be more severe at night.
- Most common on the back, but arms, head, and abdomen also commonly affected.
- Common exacerbating factors are rest, dry skin, heat, sweat, and stress.
- Major alleviating factors are activity, cold ambient temperature, and hot or cold showers.
- Some patients find that their pruritus improves with dialysis, whereas in others the dialysis procedure makes it worse.

Impact on patient

- Pruritus is a disabling and distressing symptom with significant impact on mental and physical capacity of patient.
- Profound negative impact on sleep.
- In the international Dialysis Outcomes and Practice Patterns Study (DOPPS), pruritus was associated with 17% greater mortality risk; after adjustment for measures of sleep quality, this was no longer significant.
- Contributes to daytime fatigue, agitation, and depression.

Pathophysiology

Pruritus is a subjective sensation and therefore strongly influenced by the patient's psychological state. The cause is probably multifactorial.

- Hypercalcaemia, particularly in the presence of hyperphosphataemia, causes skin calcification and stimulates local mast cells with consequent release of histamine. This is independent of PTH level, as pruritus also occurs with iatrogenic hypercalcaemia after parathyroidectomy.
- Although the skin is often dry in patients on dialysis, this does not appear to be directly related to pruritus.
- In some patients, the pruritus may improve after increasing dialysis adequacy—suggests a role for some undefined uraemic toxin.
- Low-grade hypersensitivity to products used in the dialysis procedure.
- Related to the generalized proinflammatory state of patients with ESKD.
- Many other factors have been considered—abnormalities in afferent pain fibres, alterations in number of skin mast cells, inadequate removal of middle MW uraemic toxins, PTH.

Management
As the pathophysiology is so poorly understood, development of effective treatment has been particularly difficult.

General measures
- Take a history and examine the skin to exclude other dermatological problems. If pruritus has begun acutely, drugs and allergies should be considered, as well as rarer possibilities such as chicken pox.
- Ensure that the patient is well dialysed.
- Check plasma calcium and phosphate levels are normal.
- Parathyroidectomy in patients with tertiary hyperparathyroidism can provide dramatic relief, paralleling the rapid decline in plasma calcium concentration.
- Exacerbating factors such as hot baths should be avoided.
- *Moisturizing creams* and lotions should be used as first-line treatment to maintain skin moisture. Emulsifying agents should also be used in the bath, and soap is best avoided.
- Light clothing.
- Discourage scratching—short nails and consider gloves at night.

Specific measures (in order of relative usefulness)
- *Antihistamines* (e.g. hydroxyzine) can be useful. They do, however, cause drowsiness, but may be useful at night for patients whose sleep is otherwise disturbed.
- *Ultraviolet B phototherapy* can be effective, but is inconvenient as treatment is given 2–3 times per week. A number of trials support its use as the treatment of choice for moderate to severe uraemic pruritus. Mechanism of action unknown.
- *Topical capsaicin cream* (0.025%) can be effective, particularly if pruritus is localized, but initially can cause significant feeling of burning
- *Gabapentin*—found coincidentally to improve pruritus when given to patients for peripheral diabetic neuropathy. This has subsequently been confirmed in an RCT. Doses used have started at 100mg after each HD session titrating up to 300mg.
- *Topical tacrolimus ointment* 0.03% bd has also been used (case reports).
- If pruritus occurs only during HD, then the following can be tried:
  - change formulation of heparin
  - change type of dialysis membrane or mode of sterilization.

Pain

Pain is very common in patients with ESKD. Surveys of dialysis patients generally show that ~50% of patients will complain of pain. In symptom surveys, bone and joint pain are the most common, but there are many other causes of pain in these patients. This is not surprising; many patients on dialysis are elderly and will therefore have the musculoskeletal problems related to ageing. Significant numbers of patients are on no analgesics despite significant pain. This can be due to the patient not being asked specifically about presence of pain, and due to the physician being reluctant or not knowing how to prescribe analgesia in ESKD.

Causes of pain

Pain can be caused by co-morbidities, complications of ESKD, renal disease per se, and the dialysis procedure.

Co-morbidities

- Peripheral vascular disease—claudication, ischaemic ulcers, ischaemic toes, feet, fingers etc.
- Ischaemic heart disease—chest pain precipitated by exercise or dialysis
- Osteoarthritis—back, hips, knees, etc.; can also contribute to impaired mobility
- Osteoporosis—vertebral fractures, other fractures
- Malignancy—metastatic disease, myeloma
- Peripheral neuropathy—neuropathic pain most commonly in feet.

Complications of ESKD

- Renal bone disease—hyperparathyroidism, soft tissue calcification, fractures
- Gout
- Dialysis amyloid arthropathy
- Calciphylaxis.

Renal disease

- Polycystic kidney disease—bleeding into cysts
- Retroperitoneal bleeds from acquired cystic disease
- Urinary infection.

Dialysis related

- HD:
  - limb ischaemia secondary to vascular access
  - steal syndrome on dialysis
  - discitis or septic arthritis related to line infections
  - exacerbation of arthritic pains from immobility during HD session or during transport to/from HD
  - headaches and/or cramps during HD
- PD:
  - Abdominal discomfort
  - Peritonitis
  - EPS.

Impact on patient

- Poorly managed pain has major negative impact on quality of life—studies have shown that patients with persistent pain are more likely to want to withdraw from dialysis
- Disturbed sleep patterns
- Increased depression
- Impaired dialysis adequacy if patient unable to tolerate full session.

Management

General measures

- Determine cause of pain and treat appropriately.
- Encourage patient to mobilize—refer to physiotherapy if necessary. This will reduce risk of pressure ulcers, pain related to immobility, etc.
- Explore physical factors that may improve arthritic pain.
- Educate patient about taking analgesia regularly rather than waiting for pain to build up.
- Consider home-based dialysis therapy to avoid transport.

Drug treatment

This is discussed in ➲ Chapter 16 on end-of-life management.

Sleep disorders

Various questionnaires can be used to characterize sleep patterns. Around 50% of patients with ESKD using such questionnaires will admit to sleep disorders but very few complain about them to their physicians. The disorders include:
• daytime sleepiness
• insomnia
• sleep apnoea.

Daytime sleepiness

Several reasons for daytime sleepiness in ESKD patients have been proposed. These include:
• subclinical uraemic encephalopathy
• retention of melatonin
• tyrosine deficiency causing reduced neurotransmitters with arousal
• altered body temperature rhythm with associated changes in sleep–awake cycle
• release of sleep-inducing inflammatory cytokines during dialysis
• co-existent sleep apnoea syndrome.

Insomnia

Many patients complain of insomnia in various surveys (>60% in some).
• One large Italian survey of >800 HD patients suggested that insomnia is more common in patients dialysing on morning shift—could be due to psychological factors or interference with metabolic factors able to modify circadian rhythms.
• Age, excessive alcohol intake, cigarette smoking, and polyneuropathy also related to insomnia.
• Behavioural treatments include sleep restriction, sleep hygiene, and cognitive behavioural therapy; exercise programmes can also help.
• Effective medications include benzodiazepines (e.g. temazepam, triazolam, etc.) or newer non-benzodiazepines (e.g. zolpidem). Melatonin (3mg) has also shown short and medium-term benefits.
• Many other medications used are not generally effective, e.g. antihistamines, tricyclic antidepressants.

Medication-induced insomnia

Medications known to cause insomnia and used in ESKD population include phenytoin and steroids.

Sleep apnoea

Although only ~3% patients complain of sleep apnoea, use of a standardized questionnaire in centres linked to the DOPPS study has shown that ~30% patients have symptoms suggestive of the diagnosis. This is much higher than in the general population where the prevalence is 2–4%. The conditions are different—in the general population, sleep apnoea is predominantly the obstructive type, whereas in ESKD, the aetiology is a mixture of obstructive and central sleep apnoea. As a result, classical symptoms such as snoring are less common.

Various causes for sleep apnoea in ESKD have been proposed:
- Accumulation of uraemic toxins
- Respiratory adaptation to chronic metabolic acidosis causing low arterial pCO_2 levels with alterations in chemosensitivity during sleep
- Fluid overload leading to upper airway oedema contributing to reduced upper airway patency
- Uraemic neuropathy causing reduced upper airway muscle tone.

Clinical implications
- Cycles of apnoea, hypoxia, hypercapnia, and arousal.
- Abrupt generation of negative intrathoracic pressure in patients with upper airway obstruction, resulting in changes in cardiac output.
- Daytime sleepiness resulting in decreased quality of life, impaired cognitive ability, and negative effects on ability to work and socialize.
- Linked with development of hypertension, heart failure, and cerebrovascular disease in general population.
- Sleep apnoea therefore potentially a potent cardiovascular risk factor in ESKD, though this needs to be studied further.

Management
- Non-pharmacological strategies—weight loss, avoiding sedating medications, avoiding alcohol.
- Continuous positive airway pressure is mainstay of treatment in general population, but few reports of its use in ESKD.
- Nocturnal HD reported to be of benefit.
- Nocturnal APD reported to be of benefit compared with CAPD.
- Improves after transplantation.

Restless leg syndrome

A persistent uncomfortable feeling in the legs, most prominent at night, and only relieved by movement (akathisia). This can interfere with sleep, both of the patient and of his/her partner, and may be very distressing. Occurs in 20–60% of dialysis patients.

Clinical implications

- Diminished quality of life due to interference with sleep.
- Associated with increased mortality possibly due to sympathetic overactivity secondary to recurrent arousals from sleep.

Pathophysiology

- Potential risk factors include anaemia, iron deficiency, calcium–phosphate imbalance, low PTH levels, and peripheral neuropathy.
- In general population, iron deficiency associated with restless leg syndrome (RLS) as iron is a cofactor of dopamine production in brain.
- Alterations in dopamine and opioid synthesis associated with uraemia may explain high prevalence of RLS.

Management

- Non-pharmacological treatments include:
  - trial of abstinence from caffeine, nicotine, and alcohol
  - stopping medications that could make RLS worse, e.g. antidepressants
  - changing dialysis time or frequency; increasing frequency of dialysis may reduce symptoms
  - massages, warm baths or compresses before sleeping
  - exercise both during and between dialysis sessions.
- High-dose IV iron and correction of anaemia with EPO have been shown to improve RLS in patients with ESKD.
- Conventional treatment has been with clonazepam (0.5–2.0mg at night). Frequently this just makes patient drowsy without improving symptoms.
- Trials have shown that the newer anti-Parkinsonian drugs are effective, such as pergolide (starting at 25mcg at night) or pramipexole (starting at 88mcg at night). As starting doses are much lower than doses used in Parkinson's disease, side effects are minimal, though drowsiness or nausea can occur.
- First-line treatment should therefore be a dopamine agonist, e.g. pramipexole, pergolide, levodopa, bromocriptine, or ropinirole.
- Second-line agents, if RLS is associated with pain, are opiates, e.g. oxycodone, but watch for sedation.
- Antiepileptics also helpful, e.g. gabapentin or carbamazepine.
- Patients commonly become resistant to drug treatment. If symptoms recur, they should be changed to a different drug; the patient will typically respond to the first agent again in the future.

Anorexia

Many patients on dialysis have poor appetite, resulting in poor nutrition. Anorexia is a non-specific symptom, and is more common in the elderly and patients with multiple co-morbidities.

Causes

- Inadequate dialysis
- Anaemia
- Depression
- Constipation
- Nausea
- Diabetic gastroparesis
- Drugs, e.g. codeine-containing analgesics causing nausea, amitriptyline, and protein pump inhibitors (e.g. omeprazole) causing dry mouth
- Lack of taste
- Restricted diet limiting food options
- Dry mouth with or without mouth infection
- Hypokalaemia resulting from poor food intake
- Social isolation—eating alone can lead to reduced intake

Management

Treatment of anorexia is difficult, but strategies include:

- ensuring that patient is well dialysed
- treating anaemia with EPO and iron
- looking for and treating depression
- using antiemetics before meals, if patient has nausea
- looking for and treating gastroparesis
- reviewing drug prescription, polypharmacy, and use of over-the-counter drugs
- treating constipation
- if dry mouth, using saliva substitute every 1–2h, or chewing gum
- treating mouth infections, particularly thrush
- small tasty meals that patient has chosen or known to like
- reducing fatigue during eating by thoughtful presentation or help with eating.

Constipation

Common complaint in dialysis patients, particularly the elderly.

Causes

Often multifactorial:
- Low-fibre diet because of dietary restriction of fruit and vegetables
- Fuid restriction
- Poor appetite
- Physical inactivity
- Drugs, e.g. calcium and aluminium phosphate binders, codeine-containing analgesics, and oral iron supplements.

Management

Aimed at addressing these factors, before using laxatives:
- Increasing dietary fibre intake and physical activity, if possible
- Changing analgesia
- Change from oral iron supplements to IV iron
- If the patient remains constipated, then laxatives can be started.

Laxatives containing magnesium, citrate, or phosphate should be avoided. but the following are safe in dialysis patients:
- Stool softeners such as docusate
- Bisacodyl
- Lactulose
- Senna.

Nausea and vomiting

Causes
- Inadequate dialysis
- During HD commonly caused by IDH
- Peptic ulcer disease or gastritis with or without *Helicobacter* infection
- Hiatus hernia, gastro-oesophageal reflux, and/or oesophagitis
- Gastroparesis
- Drugs such as opioids or other analgesics containing codeine
- Rare complications such as EPS.

Management
- Ensure good dialysis and avoid hypotension on HD
- Stop non-essential drugs (such as vitamins)
- Review analgesia (opiates accumulate in renal failure and are potent emetics)
- Endoscopy if symptoms persist
- Treatment of peptic ulcer disease and elimination of *Helicobacter*
- Use of drugs such as ranitidine, omeprazole, or lansoprazole if oesophagitis or gastritis found on endoscopy, and antibiotic treatment of *Helicobacter* if confirmed
- Treatment of any gastroparesis with metoclopramide, and subsequently ondansetron if no improvement.

Patients with recurrent vomiting are at risk of developing hypokalaemia; oral potassium supplements and/or use of a higher potassium dialysate (if on HD) should then be used.

Cramps

Muscle cramps are very common, particularly in elderly—worse at night and during HD sessions.

Pathophysiology

Associated with imbalances of water and electrolytes, hypovolaemia, hypotension, and carnitine deficiency. Exact aetiology of cramps in relation to dialysis not fully understood, but worse with more rapid removal of fluid. In people with normal renal function, cramps are associated with muscle fatigue.

Management

- Non-pharmacological—muscle stretching and application of warmth
- Adjustment of rate of sodium and fluid removal on HD (see ➜ Chapter 2)
- Avoidance of IDH

These three are the most important, especially avoidance of hypotension on HD.

Other treatments:

- Quinine sulfate
- Levocarnitine supplementation IV (20mg/kg) on HD
- Vitamin E (400IU) has been shown beneficial to in small studies.

Fluid overload and oedema

Can be symptomatic, asymptomatic but clinically detectable, or covert (usually manifesting solely as hypertension).

Symptoms and signs

- Dyspnoea
- Orthopnoea
- Cough
- Peripheral oedema
- Abdominal distension
- Chest crepitations
- Raised JVP
- Hypertension.

Many are indistinguishable from those of primary cardiac failure, although BP almost always raised (unless heart failure also present when BP low). Echocardiography will exclude functional ventricular impairment.

Asymptomatic patients may have raised CVPs, ankle oedema, and chest signs, but not complain of breathlessness, especially if volume overload has developed insidiously, e.g. with progressive loss of flesh weight from malnutrition but no change in dry weight during HD, or with loss of UF in PD. Oedema may also be a feature of hypoalbuminaemia in patients with euvolaemia. Such patients are frequently relatively hypotensive, and require aggressive nutritional support.

Large numbers of patients are not considered fluid overloaded because they have no symptoms or signs, become hypotensive on dialysis if their dry weight is reduced further, but remain hypertensive. This cohort almost certainly is fluid overloaded, as units using long slow dialysis techniques are able to withdraw antihypertensive drugs in almost all patients. Persistent hypertension despite being on an ACEI or ARB is also suggestive of fluid overload. Fluid overload may be driven by salt intake. Non-invasive monitoring techniques may help achieve true dry weight in patients dialysed for shorter times (BVM).

Patients must be educated about:

- the importance of restricting salt (sodium) intake (most important)
- restricting fluid intake according to urine output (maximum 1L/day)
- the necessity of achieving a true dry weight to minimize the long-term risks of volume overload (LVH).

Management is discussed in the appropriate sections on HD and PD and nutrition for strategies to achieve fluid restriction.

Diuretics (high doses) are often used to maintain urine output in patients with ESKD. This can be useful in some patients on both HD and PD, as the extra urine volume reduces the patient's fluid restriction. Diuretics should be stopped after loss of residual function. Diuretics do not alter the rate of change of solute clearance in ESKD (neither slow nor hasten the decline), and hence do not preserve residual function, but simply maintain additional urine output in some patients.

Other complications of ESKD

Dialysis amyloid

It is tragic to see a patient survive the rigours of dialysis for many years only to succumb to a crippling arthritis due to β_2m amyloidosis (β_2mA) and the associated dialysis-related arthropathy. With the increasing use of more biocompatible membranes for HD, this major complication of long-term dialysis is now seen less frequently.

Clinical features

- Carpal tunnel syndrome occurs first after ~7 years on dialysis. All patients who have been on dialysis >20 years are affected and will have needed surgery. Usually affects both hands.
- Joint pains and stiffness, usually bilateral, start in shoulders, and extend to other joints. Pain is often worse at night and during HD.
- As the disease progresses, joint movements become restricted—particularly the shoulders.
- Chronic tenosynovitis of the finger flexors causes restricted movement, pain, and trigger fingers. Can become incapacitating.
- Very rarely extra-articular accumulation of amyloid results in lumps, e.g. in the tongue or subcutaneously near joints.
- Destructive spondyloarthropathy usually of the cervical spine causes remarkably few symptoms apart from mild pain. MRI may be needed to exclude the possibility of infectious discitis.
- Rarely, amyloid may be deposited in the epidural space, causing spinal cord compression.
- Pathological fractures occur, particularly of the femoral neck, due to amyloid cysts weakening the bone.

Pathogenesis and risk factors

β_2m has a MW of 11,800Da, and is usually filtered through the glomerulus, reabsorbed, and metabolized by proximal tubule cells. Approximately 1500mg is produced each week, and only 400–600mg is cleared even with high-flux dialysers. It therefore accumulates in patients on dialysis. Residual renal function is protective. β_2mA has a predilection for bone and collagen, resulting in accumulation in bones and joints. Modification of β_2m by AGEs may predispose to formation of amyloid and deposition on collagen.

Risk factors for β2mA

- *Years on dialysis:* β_2mA becomes more common the longer the time on dialysis; carpal tunnel problems after at least 7 years, joint problems after 10 years.
- *Age at onset of dialysis:* is an independent predictor of β_2mA. The older the patient at the onset of dialysis, the earlier they will develop β_2mA-related problems.
- *HD membrane:* β_2m blood levels are higher in patients dialysing on bioincompatible membranes such as cuprophane. Use of more modern biocompatible membranes leads to lower serum levels of β_2m and may delay the onset of β_2mA. Whether cellulose membranes stimulate the production of β_2m remains controversial. The inflammatory response associated with bioincompatibility may increase the risk of development

of β_2mA. Some membranes adsorb large quantities of β_2m and this can be affected by reprocessing.
- *Dialysis modality:* carpal tunnel syndrome and amyloid deposits have been described in PD patients, but less commonly as patients tend to remain on PD for less time than on HD. Less accumulation of β_2m occurs in patients on HDF, nocturnal dialysis, and daily dialysis.

Diagnosis

Diagnosis is often clinical as histology is difficult to obtain (joint biopsy is invasive and not without risk). Confirmation of the diagnosis usually depends on a combination of history (many years on dialysis), pattern of joint distribution, X-ray findings, and radioisotope scans.

X-rays

Bone cysts are the hallmark of β_2mA. The following criteria differentiate β_2mA from other causes of bone cysts:
- Cysts >10mm in the hip and shoulder, or 5mm in the wrist (classically the scaphoid bone).
- Cysts in areas other than those prone to developing cysts, such as the femoral neck or the weight-bearing area of the acetabulum; cysts in these areas should increase in diameter >30% per year to be considered due to β_2mA.
- Joint space adjacent to the bone defect should be normal (excludes osteoarthritic cysts).
- At least two joints should be involved.

Other radiology

- CT and MRI can detect lesions too small to be seen with plain X-rays.
- Ultrasound can be used to estimate rotator cuff thickness.

Radioisotope scanning

Amyloid scans (SAP, serum amyloid protein P) and [131I] β_2m scans have been used as successful research tools but are not widely available.

Management

The only successful 'treatment' is renal transplantation. After a transplant, joint pains virtually disappear and joint mobility gradually improves. Amyloid deposits remain, but may get smaller slowly with time. Patients who return to HD after a failed transplant, even of many years duration, can develop severe β_2mA-related arthropathy after a comparatively short period of time. Most patients who survive long enough on HD to develop β_2mA either cannot be transplanted or have had to return to HD after a transplant has failed. Lixelle columns, containing porous cellulose beads and hydrophobic organic compounds, adsorb β_2m (>1mg/mL column volume) but are only used in Japan.

The best management of β_2mA is therefore prevention. Other treatments are palliative.

Prevention of β₂mA

High-flux biocompatible synthetic membranes should be used in patients who are likely to be long-term survivors but have little or no chance of being transplanted (increased clearance of β₂m occurs, lower serum levels, and some evidence for reduced complications). Reprocessing of polysulfone may enhance β₂m clearance, but only when done with bleach and formaldehyde (peracetic acid may reduce adsorption of β₂m). Longer hours of dialysis increase clearance (including daily dialysis and nocturnal dialysis), and haemofiltration or HDF. But even HDF with polysulfone only removes ~1g/week β₂m.

Supportive treatment

- Analgesics: codeine/paracetamol combinations or NSAIDs if tolerated.
- Intra-articular steroid injections into an acutely painful single joint can be very effective.
- Low-dose prednisolone, starting with 10–20mg daily, may reduce symptoms, but does not affect progression of disease. The use of prednisolone, however, should be considered carefully in patients who may already have osteopenia, and are at high risk of infection.
- Changing HD membrane to a high-flux biocompatible type may improve joint pains, and using haemofiltration or HDF.
- Carpal tunnel decompression when needed. Symptoms often recur, but may take 2–3 years.

Renal cysts and retroperitoneal bleeding

Acquired renal cystic disease and renal cell carcinoma are both complications of long-term dialysis.

Acquired renal cystic disease

This is the development of renal cysts in a patient with non-cystic kidney disease. Most of the cysts are very small, <0.6cm diameter (below the sensitivity of CT scanning). Prevalence increases with the duration of dialysis from ~10% pre-dialysis, to 40% after 3 years and 90% after 10 years on dialysis. More common and more severe in men than women. Incidence is the same on HD and PD. Usually asymptomatic. The two major complications are retroperitoneal haemorrhage and renal cell carcinoma (uncommon). One 'benefit' is increased synthesis of EPO resulting in an improvement in anaemia—some patients can discontinue EPO therapy and a few may become frankly polycythaemic requiring venesection.

Diagnosis
US or CT scan showing four or more cysts in each kidney.

Management
No specific management unless retroperitoneal bleeding occurs.

Retroperitoneal bleeding

Spontaneous retroperitoneal haematoma can be a major catastrophe with a significant mortality. The presenting symptom is loin pain, which can be severe. Hypotension and tachycardia also occur. Haematuria is often absent. Severe hyperkalaemia may occur as potassium is absorbed from altered blood in the haematoma.

Diagnosis
Ultrasonography or CT scan.

Management
Circulatory support, blood transfusion as needed, and analgesia. Heparin should be avoided on HD to minimize further bleeding. Embolization or nephrectomy should be considered if evidence of continued bleeding. Repeat imaging should be done 6–8 weeks after the bleed to look for a possible tumour that could have been missed on the initial scan done in the presence of haemorrhage.

Renal cell carcinoma

Information about renal tumours in ESKD comes predominantly from Japanese surveys. The ratio of observed to expected renal tumours in the dialysis population varies from 3- to 10-fold depending on the length of time on dialysis. Tumours are more common:
- in younger patients
- with longer time on dialysis.

Tumours in patients who have been on dialysis for a long time compared with those that occur early in dialysis are:
- more common in men (~90%)
- more likely to metastasize (~30%)
- more likely to cause cancer death (~13%).

Tumours are usually painless, but can present with loin pain and/or haematuria. Only 5% are associated with a spontaneous rise in Hb. About 80% are associated with acquired renal cystic disease.

Diagnosis

By US or CT scan. False-negative rate is 10% with each technique, so both may be needed.

Prognosis

Survival has been reported to be the same or better than with renal tumours in the general population. Sites of metastases seem to be the same and can occur years after removal of the original tumour. As the renal tumour is usually symptomless, metastases may be present at the time of diagnosis.

Screening

There is no consensus about which patients should be screened or how often. The following plan is a useful guide:
- Patients with low life expectancy are not at high risk of developing a renal tumour and do not need to be screened.
- A predicted survival of >5 years may be a sensible arbitrary selection process for screening, though this will be governed by local economic and resource issues.
- Screening needs to be repeated but, as metastasis is less likely during early stages of dialysis, screening can be less frequently.
- Initial screening could therefore be every other year and then annually after being on dialysis for 10 years.
- If other illnesses intervene changing overall prognosis, screening should be discontinued.
- Symptoms are not a guide; <1 in 15 will have symptoms at time of diagnosis.
- Presence of acquired renal cystic disease not a guide; 10% of patients on dialysis for >20 years who develop renal tumours do not have cysts.

Neurological complications

Neurological complications can be due to:
- renal failure itself, with improvement on starting dialysis or increasing dialysis adequacy
- accumulation of toxins, such as $\beta_2 m$ or aluminium
- direct effect of dialysis process
- cerebrovascular disease.

Peripheral polyneuropathy

Develops in advanced renal failure or in patients who are underdialysed. More common in men and affects mostly the legs.

Symptoms
- Sensory symptoms (paraesthesiae, burning sensations, pain) occur before motor symptoms.
- Sensory symptoms improve rapidly on starting or increasing dialysis.
- Motor involvement resulting in muscle atrophy, myoclonus, and eventual paralysis is not reversible.

Management
The development of neuropathy is an indication for starting dialysis urgently.
- Ensure patient is adequately dialysed.
- Consider using high-flux membrane for HD.
- Neuropathic pain is difficult to treat and various medications can be used:
  - amitriptyline starting at 25mg at night and increasing dose gradually according to efficacy and side effects
  - carbamazepine starting at 100mg bd; blood levels should be monitored as dose is increased
  - gabapentin starting at 100mg od or 300mg post HD; dose is limited by drowsiness and dizziness. Pregabalin may be better tolerated.

Carpal tunnel syndrome

A complication of long-term dialysis usually directly related to the accumulation of $\beta_2 mA$. Management is surgical.

CNS disorders

Uraemic encephalopathy
This is an acute or chronic brain syndrome found in severe AKI or CKD. Principal features are cognitive (difficulties with attention, mental tasks, memory), neuromuscular (myoclonus, asterixis, hiccoughs, easy fatigability), somatosensory (hallucinations, decreased libido, paranoia, impaired sleep pattern), or autonomic (feeling cold, hypothermia). If not started on dialysis, fits and then coma will develop. The degree of improvement of these symptoms on starting dialysis depends on the adequacy of dialysis achieved.

Dialysis disequilibrium syndrome

Headache, confusion, blurred vision and, if severe, fits and coma developing during or immediately after the first HD session, particularly if the patient is severely uraemic, elderly, or has a history of fits. Probably caused by an osmotic imbalance between blood and brain causing cerebral oedema during solute clearance from the vascular compartment. The best management is prevention—uraemic patients should start dialysis gently by making the first few dialysis sessions short and frequent, e.g. 2h on consecutive days, using low blood flows (<200mL/min) and small surface area dialysers. Symptoms usually resolve spontaneously over a day or so.

Dialysis headaches

Many patients experience headache on dialysis. These are usually frontal and, if severe, can be accompanied by nausea and vomiting. Visual disturbances do not occur. Most commonly due to solute disequilibria effects (sodium or urea, calcium or phosphate), excess UF requirements, and hypotensive or other drugs. Frequency of headaches can be reduced by limiting interdialytic weight gains (thereby reducing the amount of fluid removed during each session), and careful control of all potential exacerbating factors. The use of bicarbonate dialysate is also beneficial as the vasodilatation induced by acetate dialysate may also contribute. In some patients, said to be due to caffeine or cocaine withdrawal.

Seizures on dialysis

Most common when dialysis commenced in patients who are severely uraemic. Incidence reduced over years as dialysis is initiated earlier.

Causes specific to dialysis
- Uraemic encephalopathy
- Disequilibrium syndrome
- Rapid rise in Hb after starting EPO
- Hypotension
- Cerebrovascular disease
- Electrolyte disorders, e.g. hypocalcaemia, hypoglycaemia, hypo- or hypernatraemia
- Air embolism.

Depression

Depression is the most common psychiatric illness in patients with ESKD, affecting 20–30% patients on dialysis, with 10% having a major depressive disorder. Even so, depression has proved remarkably difficult to assess and quantify in the dialysis population for various reasons:
• Wide variety of assessment tools have been used in different studies.
• Somatic characteristics of depression are very similar to uraemia, e.g. anorexia, sleep disturbances, fatigue.

Screening for depression

Various screening tools for depression have been developed; these include the BDI, HADS, and Geriatric Depression Score. They are mostly used for research studies, but some renal units use them routinely to detect patients at risk of depression. Subsequent psychiatric evaluation is needed to confirm the diagnosis. When these tools are used, around 30% of patients on dialysis are found to be at risk of depression; the majority of at risk patients are not recognized clinically.

Implications of depression

• Depression affects outcomes through a variety of mechanisms:
  • compliance
  • nutrition
  • immune status
  • interpersonal relationships
  • differential access to care.
• Depression is associated with adverse outcomes in many studies:
  • increased hospitalization
  • independent risk factor for peritonitis on PD
  • increased mortality.

Factors affecting diagnosis

Demographic and social factors affect degree of depression in chronic disease, including:
• age
• gender
• ethnicity
• socio-economic status
• marital status and satisfaction
• family interactions
• recent bereavement
• interactions between patients, doctors, healthcare team
• alcohol and recreational drugs
• dialysis modality
• transplant status and history.

Treatment

There is a lack of information about efficacy of treatment of depression in ESKD and outcomes. Various treatments are used with variable success. ERBP guidelines have suggested an 8–12-week trial of an antidepressant in patients who meet DSM criteria for moderate major depression. Caution should be used since many drugs commonly used have side effects which may be worse in patients with CKD, e.g. effects on cardiac rhythm and hypotension, GI effects (nausea and vomiting), and increased bleeding risk (SSRIs):

• *Selective serotonin re-uptake inhibitors*, e.g. sertraline, fluoxetine, have been shown to improve symptoms markedly in short-term studies. Patients, though, are often resistant to starting them and compliance rates with their use are poor. These are the preferred antidepressants. Paroxetine may have increased anticholinergic side effects.
Citalopram and escitalopram are also well tolerated in ESKD. Tricyclic antidepressants have an increased risk of anticholinergic side effects in ESKD and should be avoided. Venlafaxine has active metabolites which accumulate and may cause cardiac toxicity and constipation.

• *More frequent HD* has also been suggested to improve depressive symptoms.

• *Cognitive behavioural therapy* in selected patients can be efficacious and a practical treatment option. Has shown significant benefits in RCTs.

• *Exercise programmes* have also been shown to improve BDI scores and symptoms of fatigue.

Symptoms suggestive of depression

• Depressed mood most of the time
• Loss of interest or pleasure in most activities for most of the time
• Loss of weight
• Change in sleep pattern
• Psychomotor change
• Fatigue or loss of energy most days
• Feelings of worthlessness or guilt
• Decreased ability to think or concentrate
• Suicidal ideation
• Thoughts of death.

Cognitive impairment

High prevalence of risk factors for cognitive impairment in patients with ESKD—cardiovascular risk factors, hypertension, cerebrovascular disease, periodic episodes of hypotension. General awareness of cognitive problems remains low and there are remarkably few studies about the risk of cognitive dysfunction in patients on dialysis.

Implications

- Negative impact on quality of life
- Difficulty in making financial decisions
- Poor awareness of needs regarding social care
- Poor understanding of information so difficult to make decisions about:
  - choice of dialysis modality
  - transplantation
  - advanced directives related to future treatment
- Poor concordance with drug therapy, fluid, and dietary restrictions.

Prevalence

- Increased prevalence shown in elderly patients with CKD with 2- to 3-fold increase in patients with eGFR <45mL/min/1.73m^2 compared with >60mL/min/1.73m^2.
- Surveys suggest that 50–80% patients on HD have some degree of cognitive impairment.
- Risk factors included lower level of education, and prior stroke.
- Cognitive function has been shown to be related to HD session, with worse performance during HD and immediately afterwards.

Cognitive function testing

Because of the high prevalence and clinical implications of developing cognitive impairment, many nephrologists are now recommending that older patients should have regular cognitive function testing. There are a large number of tests available; elderly care physicians locally will have a favoured tool. It is important to select tests that detect executive dysfunction as well as memory problems.

Management

There are no studies specifically about management of cognitive dysfunction in patients with ESKD. The information that a patient has cognitive dysfunction should therefore be passed to their primary care physician so that appropriate community support can be provided, including referral to memory clinics and social services.

Prognosis

Development of dementia is a predictor of poor survival. Once cognitive impairment is detected, or found to be declining, patients and families should be told so that they can plan for future care, and make necessary arrangements for financial planning. Many patients will want to arrange powers of attorney for healthcare and/or finances.

Gastrointestinal bleeding

GI blood loss is common among patients on dialysis. It can be of varying severity but tends to be more frequent and more severe among patients on HD, presumably related to the use of heparin.

Presentation

Not always clinically obvious and should always be considered when the Hb level unexpectedly drops, there is resistance to EPO therapy, or evidence of iron deficiency.

Diagnosis

Can be surprisingly difficult (see Table 15.1). In many patients (even those requiring blood transfusions) the source of bleeding is never determined. This is partly due to the increased incidence of angiodysplasia, which often occurs in parts of the bowel not reached by endoscopy. Common investigations include:

• *Faecal occult bloods* are not particularly useful if bleeding is intermittent. They are frequently positive in HD patients in the absence of any overt bowel pathology.
• *Gastroscopy* is usually the first investigation. However, many dialysis patients have mild gastritis or duodenitis that is not considered severe enough to cause bleeding.
• *Colonoscopy*—preparation is difficult, as the bowel needs to be cleaned out. The patient must swallow large volumes of a solution that acts as an osmotic laxative. Although little absorption from the gut occurs, preparation is best done as an inpatient because there is a small risk of the patient developing pulmonary oedema, or volume depletion as some patients used to a strict fluid restriction find it difficult to drink the large volumes of fluid required. An enema may be necessary.
• Further investigations for haemodynamically unstable patients, or those needing multiple transfusions, include arteriography and radioisotope studies.

Management

• Treatment of specific lesions is the same as in the general population, including *Helicobacter* eradication.
• Use of heparin on HD should be reduced long term as much as possible for patients with no obvious diagnosis. Bleeding tends to be intermittent and can recur.
• HD in patients with overt bleeding is difficult. Dialysis should be heparin free (or with regional anticoagulation), if possible.
• Blood transfusions should be given during dialysis (to avoid the risk of hyperkalaemia), unless the patient is haemodynamically unstable (and then potassium levels need to be closely monitored).
• As altered blood in the gut is absorbed, there is a high risk of hyperkalaemia, which may need to be treated with insulin and dextrose if the patient is too unstable for dialysis.
• Other treatments to reduce bleeding times may be useful, e.g. desmopressin.

Table 15.1 GI bleeding: causes

Causes increased in dialysis patients	Causes similar to the general population
Gastritis	Oesophageal tears
Duodenitis	Gastric carcinoma
Oesophagitis	*Helicobacter* related
Oesophageal varices (e.g. hepatitis C liver disease)	Colonic polyps
Peptic ulceration	Diverticular disease
NSAIDs	Inflammatory bowel disease
Gastric erosions	Colonic/rectal carcinoma
Angiodysplasia	Aortoenteric fistula (after aneurysm repair)
Ischaemic bowel	

Acidosis

Acidosis is a feature of severe renal failure and poor dialysis, due to the failure to excrete hydrogen ions and accumulation of acidic waste products. The biochemical features are:

- low plasma bicarbonate
- low plasma pH if uncompensated, as in AKI or in situations of acute deterioration of CKD; low pCO_2 if severe and the patient hyperventilates
- plasma pH is normal if acidosis is compensated, as in CKD
- hyperkalaemia in presence of low pH—for each drop in pH of 0.1, the plasma potassium rises by 0.7mmol/L as hydrogen ions are buffered by uptake into cells in exchange for potassium.

Clinical consequences of chronic acidosis

Bone

Acidosis has an adverse effect on skeletal structure. Bone buffering of hydrogen ions increases release of calcium and phosphate. Acidosis may also play a part in the genesis of hyperparathyroidism by making the parathyroid gland less sensitive to feedback from plasma calcium, resulting in higher PTH levels for a given plasma calcium level. Acidosis may also stimulate parathyroid cell proliferation.

Muscle catabolism

Acidosis increases muscle breakdown. This increases serum urea and other protein breakdown products, thereby exacerbating uraemic symptoms. Increased muscle breakdown increases the protein intake needed to maintain nitrogen balance. Acidosis therefore worsens the poor nutritional state often associated with renal failure.

Treatment

Pre-dialysis patients

Are at special risk of chronic acidosis. Sodium bicarbonate (starting at 500–600mg bd) should be given in an attempt to maintain the plasma bicarbonate in the normal range. This is often poorly tolerated because the increased sodium intake causes fluid overload and makes BP control difficult. There is therefore a tendency by many nephrologists not to correct acidosis, although trials now suggest a significant benefit on the rate of decline of renal function in CKD. High doses may be needed.

HD patients

Often have low plasma bicarbonate levels pre-dialysis. This is less frequent with the use of bicarbonate dialysate, but a significant proportion of patients remain acidotic pre-dialysis, despite having adequate dialysis (as judged by current standards) and using bicarbonate dialysate. Oral sodium bicarbonate is rarely used in HD patients, as the sodium load will increase the patient's thirst thereby increasing interdialytic weight gains and worsening BP control. Daily or nocturnal dialysis improves control of acidosis.

PD patients

The introduction of reduced calcium concentration (1.25mmol/L), increased lactate concentration (40mmol/L) dialysate has meant that virtually all PD patients using standard dialysate have normal, and some even elevated, plasma bicarbonate levels. Patients using bicarbonate-based biocompatible dialysate also have normal, though lower, plasma bicarbonate levels. Oral sodium bicarbonate should be given to patients with consistently low plasma bicarbonate.

Sexual dysfunction

Sexual dysfunction is a very common problem in patients with CKD.

Men

The most frequently reported symptoms of sexual dysfunction in male patients include:
- decreased libido
- difficulty with sexual arousal
- erectile dysfunction (ED)
- premature or delayed ejaculation
- difficulty achieving orgasm.

These symptoms are associated with testicular damage and impaired spermatogenesis that may lead to infertility.

Women

Symptoms of sexual dysfunction in female patients include:
- reduced libido
- difficulty with sexual arousal
- lack of vaginal lubrication
- pain during intercourse
- difficulty achieving orgasm.

Most women with ESKD are amenorrhoeic and infertile. Various medical and psychological factors underlie this high level of sexual dysfunction.

Psychosocial factors

Common, and include:
- depression and anxiety
- fear of failure
- marital discord tends to be more common in dialysis patients
- changes in body image and self-esteem.

Medical factors

- *Hormonal abnormalities in men* including reduced testosterone levels, raised prolactin levels, and co-morbidities such as malnutrition, obesity, diabetes mellitus (DM), and hypertension have all been associated with low testosterone levels.
- *Hormonal abnormalities in women* include hypothalamic, pituitary, and ovarian dysfunction. Failure to ovulate and other menstrual irregularities in women are often related to hypothalamic and pituitary dysfunction.
- *ED* is more common with increasing age, but also increased in renal disease:
  - usually caused by a combination of organic and psychological factors
  - often the result of multisystem disease processes involving the hypothalamic–pituitary–gonadal axis, autonomic nervous system, vascular supply to the penis, and penile tissue damage from either infection or trauma
  - exacerbated by anaemia because of low oxygen delivery to the corpora cavernosa.

- *Drug therapy:*
  - diuretics, antihypertensive, and antidepressant medications and H$_2$ blockers can contribute to ED
  - spironolactone and cimetidine block androgen receptors
  - glucocorticoids reduce testosterone synthesis directly via gonadal steroid receptors and centrally at the hypothalamic level
  - tricyclic antidepressants, benzodiazepines, and opiates may induce secondary hypogonadism through central mechanisms.
- *Zinc deficiency:*
  - associated with testicular failure in animal studies
  - replacement of zinc in dialysis patients with sexual dysfunction and low zinc serum levels failed to result in any significant improvement in their sexual experiences. Use of oral zinc supplements has variable results in terms of sperm counts, testosterone levels, and decrease in impotence.
- *Autonomic neuropathy:*
  - decreases sensation and arousal stimuli during sexual activity
  - interferes with the complex neurological axis that is necessary for achievement of an adequate erection.
- *Vascular disease*—peripheral or ischaemic heart disease.
- *Anatomic and related to cause of renal failure*—congenital lower urinary tract problems requiring surgery, often repeated, are often associated with difficulties in achieving erection.

Management

A challenge! Causes of sexual dysfunction are frequently multifactorial and it is often difficult to distinguish the primary factor(s) responsible. Involves trying to optimize the medical and psychosocial environment for the patient.
- *Optimize dialysis* to limit endocrine dysfunction. Sexual dysfunction is less common in patients performing daily or overnight dialysis.
- *Psychosocial factors*—take a careful history and assess for depression. Consider counselling and medication.
- *Medications*—review carefully, e.g. β-blockers can affect sexual function.
- *Anaemia*—correct with EPO. Often dramatically improves sexual dysfunction.
- *Hyperparathyroidism*—control PTH levels with appropriate medical treatment.
- *Hyperprolactinaemia*—treat with dopaminergic agonists, e.g. bromocriptine or lisuride.
- *Endocrine abnormalities*—consider oestrogen (± progesterone) in women and testosterone in men. Testosterone may be useful to improve libido in women.
- *ED*—may be related to autonomic dysfunction and/or vascular disease. Maximize dialysis adequacy, minimize progressive vascular disease (BP control). Consider sildenafil, intracavernosal injections alprostadil, intraurethral alprostadil, vacuum devices.

Use of phosphodiesterase inhibitors
- Most reports are based on using sildenafil which has been shown to be effective in HD and PD patients.
- Improve erectile functioning in men with ED by sustaining guanosine 3´,5´-cyclic monophosphate (cGMP)-mediated smooth muscle relaxation in the corpus cavernosum.
- Safe to use provided patient does not have angina, is not taking nitrates, and is not hypotensive.
- Response rates to sildenafil have varied in different studies, probably because of the use of sildenafil in isolation, without consideration being given to the other factors that may contribute to sexual dysfunction.
- Newer inhibitors, e.g. vardenafil, can also be effective.

Aluminium toxicity

Aluminium accumulation comes from two sources:
- dialysate (in HD) prepared from water with a high aluminium concentration
- aluminium preparations used as phosphate binders.

Water treatment is now much improved with the generalized use of RO, so that dialysate aluminium concentration is now low even in areas where aluminium levels in the general water supply are high. Aluminium preparations are very rarely used as phosphate binders and, when they are, plasma aluminium levels are carefully monitored. The devastating consequences of aluminium toxicity, aluminium bone disease and dialysis encephalopathy, are therefore now rarely seen in dialysis patients. One recent outbreak of aluminium poisoning was caused by aluminium leaching from water pipes feeding a dialysis unit.

Aluminium bone disease

This is a 'low turnover' bone disease. The clinical manifestations are severe diffuse bone pain, muscle weakness, and spontaneous fractures. The plasma calcium is normal or slightly elevated and may rise dramatically with vitamin D therapy. Alkaline phosphatase levels are normal. Serum aluminium levels will be increased.

Anaemia and resistance to EPO therapy

Aluminium causes a microcytic anaemia; plasma ferritin levels are normal. Aluminium affects porphyrin and haem synthesis, erythroid maturation, and causes haemolysis. Plasma aluminium levels should always be determined in patients who are resistant to EPO treatment.

Dialysis encephalopathy/dementia

The initial findings are intermittent speech disturbances and dyspraxia. Twitching, myoclonic jerks, motor apraxia, fits, and personality changes develop as the disease progresses. In severe cases, the speech disturbances become more marked and eventually the patient becomes completely mute.

Diagnosis

Serum aluminium should be <20mcg/L (0.7μmol/L) in dialysis patients. Patients with serum aluminium >60mcg/L (2.2μmol/L) frequently have aluminium overload. Plasma aluminium levels reflect recent exposure and not total body aluminium. Single high levels can occur after single episodes of acute exposure. Sequential levels will suggest whether aluminium overload is starting to develop. It is important to consider the iron status as bone aluminium accumulation can occur despite low plasma aluminium levels in iron-overloaded patients.

Desferrioxamine test

The desferrioxamine (DFO) test is a valuable, non-invasive test to detect aluminium overload.

- Baseline serum aluminium is obtained before a dialysis session.
- 5mg/kg DFO in 100–150mL 5% dextrose is infused into the venous line over the last 60min of dialysis.
- A second serum sample is taken at the start of the next dialysis session.
- An increase in serum aluminium >50mcg/L suggests overload.
- Patients with PTH >65pmol/L are not prone to the effects of aluminium. Those with PTH <15pmol/L are at risk of aluminium toxicity.

Management

Prevention

Prevention is the best management as much of the damage induced by aluminium is irreversible.

- Use aluminium phosphate binders only when other phosphate binders are not tolerated, or provide inadequate control of serum phosphate levels.
- Dialysate aluminium concentration should be maintained at <10mcg/L.
- Measure serum aluminium levels every 3–6 months in patients taking aluminium phosphate binders. These should be stopped if serum levels are consistently >1.0μmol/L.
- A DFO test should be performed if serum aluminium levels are elevated (>2.2μmol/L) or if there is a clinical suspicion of aluminium toxicity.
- A DFO test should not be performed if serum levels of aluminium are >7μmol/L to avoid DFO-induced neurotoxicity.
- If possible, a bone biopsy should be performed to confirm diagnosis of aluminium bone disease.
- Sources of aluminium should be identified and stopped if aluminium toxicity occurs.

Treatment

- Treatment is by regular infusion of DFO (5mL/kg) at the end of dialysis, once per week, for 2–4 months, and often for >1 year. For patients with a large rise in plasma aluminium after the DFO test, DFO treatment is given 5h before dialysis.
- Care is needed. DFO is itself toxic, and the transient increase in plasma aluminium after DFO can induce fits, and cerebral, visual, and auditory neurotoxicity.
- Patients receiving DFO have an increased incidence of mucormycosis, which can be fatal.
- Side effects are due to ferrioxamine and aluminoxamine, and can be reduced by using lower doses of DFO (0.52–2.5mg/kg) and possibly by high-flux dialysis or haemofiltration (better removal of aluminium–DFO complexes).

Nephrogenic systemic fibrosis

Also known as nephrogenic fibrosing dermopathy. It was first recognized in the late 1990s. It is found in patients with renal failure, mostly on dialysis. Pathogenesis is still not well understood but appears to be linked to exposure to gadolinium (Gd)-containing contrast agents.

Clinical features

- Starts with swelling of distal parts of extremities followed by thickening, indurations and hardening of the skin over a few weeks. Sometimes trunk also involved but face almost never.
- Can be progressive with skin stiffness, pain, and serious physical disability as flexion of adjacent joints inhibited.
- Systemic involvement of lungs, myocardium, and striated muscles has been reported in some patients.
- Skin biopsy needed to confirm diagnosis and to differentiate from other fibrosing skin disorders.
- Specific histopathological features include:
  - thickened dermis with bundles of collagen and mucin deposition
  - proliferation of fibroblasts and elastic fibres
  - absence of inflammation—this makes this disorder a distinct entity.

Role of gadolinium

- Skin changes can occur with 2–4weeks of receiving Gd-containing contrast agents for MRI scans.
- Half-life of these agents is prolonged from 1.3h in healthy volunteers to 30–120h in CKD.
- Gd particles found in skin biopsies—highly supportive of pathogenic role of Gd.
- Details of various Gd agents in clinical use are shown in Table 15.2:
  - Majority of cases of nephrogenic systemic fibrosis have been reported after use of gadodiamide.
  - Gadodiamide is less stable than other forms so more likely to release free Gd ion.
  - A few cases reported with gadopentate and gadoversetamide.

A common feature of most affected patients has been use of high-dose Gd-containing contrast (2- to 3-fold greater than dose usually used).

Table 15.2 Gadolinium-containing contrast agents

Generic name	Brand	Elimination route
Gadobenate-dimeglumine	MultiHance®	Biliary/renal
Gadodiamide	Omniscan®	Renal
Gadopentate-dimeglumine	Magnevist®	Renal
Gadoteridol	ProHance®	Renal
Gadoversetamide	Optimark®	Renal

Gadolinium: recommendations

Nephrogenic systemic fibrosis is a new condition whose pathophysiology is still far from established. Recommendations from European and US regulatory agencies were different and are summarized here:

- Affected patients should be reported to national medical agencies and international registries with their history of Gd exposure.
- The European Medical Agency has stated that use of gadodiamide is contraindicated in patients with a eGFR <30mL/min/1.73m^2 and that use of other Gd-containing contrast agents has to be carefully thought about against possible risks.
- In the USA, the Food and Drug Agency (FDA) has stated that use of Gd-containing agents has to be carefully considered if eGFR is 15–60mL/min/1.73m^2 and that alternative investigation should be performed where necessary.
- The FDA also advises up to four HD sessions to eliminate Gd in patients with eGFR <30mL/min/1.73m^2.
- Where Gd-containing contrast has to be used, as low a dose and non-toxic a form as possible should be used.

All these recommendations have to be viewed in perspective. Many nephrologists and renal units have never seen a case of nephrogenic systemic fibrosis, particularly when using safer forms of Gd and avoiding high doses. Worldwide, ~300 cases were reported in registries by 2011 and fewer cases subsequently.

Blood biochemistry in ESKD

Many serum enzymes and proteins are elevated in ESKD due to reduced renal or dialysis clearance, and patient co-morbidity. (See Table 15.3.)

Acute myocardial infarction

The pattern of enzyme rises is unchanged in ESKD. Combination of troponin I and CK-MB provides best markers of myocardial damage. Troponin T (more than troponin I) can be raised in asymptomatic patients with CKD. Elevated levels, even if not associated with acute myocardial damage, are associated with increased risk of cardiac events and cardiac death.

Liver disease

ESKD patients have low or low-normal AST and ALT levels (cause unknown). A rise to the upper limit of normal may be a marker of hepatocellular damage and should provoke investigation. Interpretation of ALP requires isoenzyme measurement, and assessment of GGT, ALT/AST, and PTH levels.

Pancreatitis

Can be difficult to diagnose in ESKD as amylase levels often raised, but never more than 3-fold. P3 amylase isoenzyme may be specifically raised in pancreatitis. Heparin can increase apparent lipase levels. Use of icodextrin CAPD fluid can cause false-negative assays for serum amylase, by interfering with the assay.

Table 15.3 Blood biochemistry in ESKD

Enzyme	% of ESKD population with change in enzyme level	Change inserum level
Creatinine kinase	↑ in 30–70%	To × 3 normal
CK-MB	↑ in 5%	↑ by 50% at most
Lactic dehydrogenase	↑ in 35%	To × 3 normal
Troponin I	↑ in <25%	Slight increase in some patients only
Troponin T	↑ in 10–80%	Up to × 14 normal
Brain natriureticpeptide (BNP)	↑ in most	To × 2–3 normal
AST	↓ in 10–90%	↓ by 20–50%
ALT	↓ in 10–90%	↓ by 20–50%
ALP	↑ in 50%; increases in bone and liver isoenzymes may have underlying causes; intestinal ALP also ↑ in 50% patients	↑ by 50%
GGT	↑ in 10–15% (in those without liver disease, alcohol, or drugs)	To × 3 normal
Amylase	↑ in 50%	To × 3 normal (patients using icodextrin CAPD fluid can have falsely low amylase levels as routinely measured)
Lipase	↑ in 50%	To × 2 normal

Tumour markers in ESKD

Variably affected by ESKD or dialysis. (See Table 15.4.)

Table 15.4 Tumour markers in ESKD

Marker	Effect of renal failure
Prostate-specific antigen (PSA)	Free PSA slightly ↑ in ESKD (reference range does not need adjustment)
	Total PSA unchanged by dialysis
	Free PSA may be cleared by some high-flux membranes
Carcinoembryonic antigen (CEA)	↑ in ~1/3 patients with ESKD (but not consistently)
CA 19.9	↑ in ESKD
CA 125	Not significantly ↑ in ESKD
	↑ in CAPD patients after peritonitis
α-Fetoprotein (AFP)	Unchanged
Cytokeratin fragment 19 (CYFRA)	↑ in most patients with ESKD by ~25%
CA 72.4	Unchanged
ProGRP	↑ in most patients with ESKD by ~25%
βHCG	Unchanged

Quality of life

Measures of health-related quality of life (HRQL) in renal disease are increasingly important both for research and for clinical management.

- There is increasing awareness that any comprehensive evaluation of health outcomes should assess patient-based outcomes, in addition to traditional clinical indicators such as mortality and morbidity.
- Traditional health indicators provide a very limited picture of outcome when evaluating non-curative treatments for chronic diseases.
- There is increased demand for evidence of the cost-effectiveness of new treatments, in which both the costs and benefits (including those to a patient's well-being) must be weighed.

There are two main approaches to measuring HRQL: generic and disease-specific measures.

Generic measures

- Applicable across different diseases, enabling comparison, e.g. between ESKD and other chronic diseases such as arthritis.
- Include well-known and widely used measures such as the Medical Outcomes Study Short Form-36 (SF-36), Nottingham Health Profile, Sickness Impact Profile (SIP), and World Health Organization Quality of Life assessment (WHOQOL). Using the SF-36, most studies in ESKD show that physical quality of life, as to be expected, is lower than that found in healthy people. Mental quality of life, however, does not appear to be so impaired and is similar to that of other groups of individuals with other types of chronic disease.

Disease-specific measures

- Used to evaluate HRQL in specific conditions such as ESKD, HIV/AIDS, hypertension, dementia, etc.
- Designed to tap specific areas of the target condition not covered by generic measures, so are generally more responsive in detecting clinically important change and/or treatment effects.
- Kidney Disease Quality of Life (K/DQOL) Questionnaire is an example of a renal-specific measure of HRQL.

Although HRQL is a useful tool for research studies or audit, caution is needed when used in clinical practice for individual patients:

- Collecting HRQL data can be time-consuming.
- Patients with disabilities or who cannot communicate in the language of the HRQL tool are at a disadvantage and may be excluded.
- Most importantly, the precision of HRQL instruments is not sufficiently high to make reliable decisions based on the performance of a single individual.

Compliance and concordance

Medical staff often talk about the 'compliance' of patients with dialysis regimens, prescribed medications, and dietary restrictions. The situation is often completely different when viewed from the patient's perspective. In reality, non-compliance is a basic human trait! And the complex medical regimens imposed on patients with ESKD engender non-adherence.

From compliance to concordance

Although widely used and accepted, the term compliance is suggested to have a negative effect on patient care. In terms of a definition, compliance is seen as the degree to which a patient's behaviour corresponds to the recommendations of the healthcare provider. In this case, failure to comply suggests that the patient is at fault. Another term frequently used is adherence: the extent to which a patient's behaviour and or lifestyle changes correspond with agreed recommendations from the healthcare provider. One implication of this viewpoint is that a patient can make a rational decision to carry out or, more importantly, not to carry out a procedure which will impact on health and well-being. The controversial nature of this discourse has led to the evolution of a preferred concept, concordance, which is defined as an agreement between persons and suggests an equal partnership between a patient and the healthcare provider which involves joint decision-making.

Non-concordance is prevalent in dialysis patients, with an incident rate of up to 86% in many cases. Relevant areas include drug therapy, fluid and dietary allowance, dialysis regimen, and lifestyle changes, e.g. managing obesity and smoke cessation. Irrespective of the area, non-concordance is a costly behaviour which carries a huge financial burden on any health service. For example, non-concordance is seen to be associated with patients having more frequent hospitalizations and increased carer input. Knowledge of this suggests the need for healthcare providers to look at ways in which patients can be supported to enhance concordance and so promote better patient outcomes.

Factors to be considered when faced with a patient who is non-concordant include:
- a non-confrontational approach
- the mental competence of the patient
- does the patient understand the issues?
- are they too sick to understand?
- the use of relatives, friends, and counsellors to help explain.

There is no single solution. All patients should be treated regardless of their previous or current behaviour. concordance can be enhanced by a patient-centred, multi- and inter-professional approach with empathy.

Employment and rehabilitation

The ultimate aim of dialysis is to give the patient as normal a lifestyle as possible. This includes enabling patients to remain at work. Patients should not simply live for dialysis. Such patients understandably become depressed, and their heavy dependence on social benefits greatly increases the cost of dialysis. Starting dialysis is psychologically a devastating event in a patient's and their family's life. Although a few will be resilient enough to continue life as normal, the majority will need the full support of their healthcare team. The process of rehabilitation involves assessing the patient's goals and desires, understanding their physical and mental capacities, appraising the resources available to provide support, and optimizing medical care.

Dialysis as a disability

The physical limitations and disability of the dialysis patient occur because of effects of renal failure itself, co-morbid disease, the treatment regimen, and psychosocial problems. Many patients continue feeling tired and therefore find physical work difficult. Patients who find it difficult to comply with salt and fluid restrictions are limited by shortness of breath associated with fluid overload.

Ability to work

Apart from the patient's well-being, there are various factors limiting the ability of the dialysis patient to work:
- Some employers are prejudiced, particularly if the patient has missed a lot of work before starting dialysis. Other employers are helpful and will provide flexible hours around dialysis.
- HD: the regular hours plus transport time can interfere with work. Attempts should be made to select dialysis times that fit with the patient's work. HD in hospital is difficult to organize round a variable shift pattern. Some patients find it easier to dialyse at night or at home.
- CAPD: four exchanges a day can be difficult to fit in with work unless one exchange can be done at work (e.g. in a medical area or separate room), the patient lives close enough to go home, or the patient only works part-time.
- APD: this is possibly the easiest form of dialysis to undertake and continue work as it is mostly done at night. Any extra manual exchange can be done on return home from work. APD is difficult to fit round a variable shift pattern.

Despite all the above, many patients do manage to continue in full-time employment.

Death in dialysis patients

Survival rates

Mortality rates for patients with ESKD are worse than most cancers with an overall median survival of <6 years, though this does vary with age. UK Renal Registry data shows that 5-year survival after starting renal replacement treatment is:
- >90% for 18–34-year-olds
- 70% for 45–54-year-olds
- 30% for 65–74-year-olds
- <20% for >75-year-olds.

These rates are much lower than in the general population. Mortality rate for 45–54-year-olds is ~18 times that for people of the same age in the general population. This is also true for the elderly: mortality rate for >75-year-olds with ESKD is 4-fold higher than age-matched controls.

Predictors of increased mortality risk

Both co-morbidity and complications of ESKD affect survival. The key predictors of poor survival are age, co-morbidity, and poor nutrition. Many individual predictors have been identified and are listed here:
- Being on dialysis compared with having a functioning transplant
- Age
- Vascular co-morbidity:
    - Peripheral vascular disease has been shown to be best predictor of poor survival in many studies
    - Ischaemic heart disease
    - Cerebrovascular disease
- Diabetes
- Poor nutrition
- Malignancy
- Low plasma albumin
- Poor control of calcium and phosphate levels:
    - Hyperphosphataemia
    - Hypercalcaemia
    - Raised Ca–P product
- Impaired cardiac function:
    - LVH
    - Left ventricular dilatation
    - Hypotension
- Anaemia:
    - EPO resistance
- Infection:
    - Chronic viral infections, e.g. hepatitis B, C, HIV
    - Recurrent dialysis-related infections
- Poor compliance
- Poor vascular access
- Lack of pre-dialysis renal care
    - 30–40% patients are referred <1 month before needing to start dialysis—so-called crashlanders; mortality rate for such patients increased by 15–30%
    - Detrimental effects of late referral are summarized in Box 16.1

Box 16.1 Detrimental effects of late referral
- Lack of interventions which might slow progression of renal failure
- Failure to plan for RRT
- Failure to plan vascular access with consequent increased reliance on CVCs and risk of infection
- Failure to provide psychological and social support
- Increased hospitalization rate
- Lower quality of life.

Causes of death

Causes of death are related to pre-existing co-morbidity and complications of ESKD.

- Cardiac causes account for >50% of deaths:
  - MI accounts for <10% of these
  - Heart failure with left ventricular dilatation is more common—often related to chronic fluid overload
  - About 60% of cardiac deaths are sudden due to arrhythmias related to electrolyte disorders or impaired cardiac function
- Peripheral vascular disease:
  - Amputation
  - Sepsis—gangrene, osteomyelitis
  - Often associated with poor nutrition
  - Associated cardiac disease
- Cerebrovascular disease:
  - Stroke
  - Complications of stroke—poor nutrition, depression
  - Associated cardiac disease
- Infection—accounts for ~20% of deaths:
  - General infections, e.g. pneumonia
  - Dialysis related—septicaemia (HD), peritonitis (PD)
  - Transplant related—general + opportunistic infections
- Malignancy:
  - One-sixth less common than cardiac disease
  - More common in transplant recipients
- Stopping dialysis:
  - Usually in association with one or more of the above.

Cardiac arrest during dialysis

Cardiac arrest is not uncommon in dialysis patients and occurs outside the hospital as well as on dialysis. All medical and nursing staff should be trained in advanced (cardiac) life support, and resuscitation equipment should be available. Ideally all patients should have had discussions about their wishes in the event of cardiac arrest, and these documented clearly. In general, doctors regard resuscitation as futile for most patients with ESKD and its associated co-morbidities (outside of clearly defined situations such as post MI), while most patients perceive it to be a useful intervention. Patients need education as to the role and likely outcome from resuscitation after cardiac arrest.

Causes

Sudden death has many causes and cannot be simply ascribed to 'cardiac' causes:

- Large electrolyte swings (particularly potassium)
- Volume overload
- Arrhythmias
- Aortic dissection
- Intracerebral haemorrhage
- Subdural haematoma
- Cerebrovascular disease
- Infection.

Outcomes

A number of studies have looked at outcome of cardiac arrest in dialysis patients:

- Outcome worse than general population: only 8% of resuscitated dialysis patients leave hospital compared with 12% general population.
- In one study, 80% of patients who initially responded to cardiopulmonary resuscitation (CPR) were dead within 4 days.
- Patients and families have a much more optimistic attitude towards CPR. Education and advanced planning are therefore important.

Decisions relating to cardiopulmonary resuscitation

- Decisions about CPR must be made on the basis of an individual assessment of each patient's case.
- Advance care planning, including making decisions about CPR, is an important part of good clinical practice for those at risk of cardiorespiratory arrest.
- It is not necessary to initiate discussion about CPR if there is no reason to believe that the patient is likely to suffer a cardiorespiratory arrest.
- Where no explicit decision has been made in advance, there should be an initial presumption in favour of CPR.
- If CPR would not re-start the heart and breathing, it should not be attempted.
- Where the expected benefit of attempted CPR may be outweighed by the burdens, the patient's informed views are of paramount importance. If the patient lacks capacity, those close to the patient should be involved in discussions to explore the patient's wishes, feelings, beliefs, and values.
- If a patient with capacity refuses CPR, or a patient lacking capacity has a valid and applicable advance decision refusing CPR, this should be respected.
- A Do Not Attempt Resuscitation (DNAR) decision does not over-ride clinical judgement in the unlikely event of a reversible cause of the patient's respiratory or cardiac arrest that does not match the circumstances envisaged.
- DNAR decisions apply only to CPR and not to any other aspects of treatment.

Taken from the joint statement by the British Medical Association, the Resuscitation Council (UK), and the Royal College of Nursing (October 2007).

Management of cardiac arrest during dialysis

Should follow standard guidelines and protocols, unless of course patient has expressed a wish not to be resuscitated, and ensuring episode is true cardiac arrest rather than the much more common IDH:

- Check responsiveness
- Open airway
- Check breathing
- Give two effective breaths if needed
- Check circulation
- Precordial thump if witnessed arrest
- Start CPR (but do not delay defibrillation if available and appropriate)
- Attach defibrillator
- Assess rhythm
- Defibrillate for ventricular fibrillation or tachycardia
- Continue CPR for asystole/electromechanical dissociation
- Repeat defibrillation and continue CPR as necessary, with normal doses of adrenaline (epinephrine), amiodarone, or atropine as necessary.

In HD patients, particular care should be taken to exclude hyperkalaemia as a cause. For patients who arrest prior to their dialysis session, it may be worthwhile to rapidly institute dialysis to ensure that hyperkalaemia is not a contributing factor. An ECG and urgent serum biochemistry should always be performed. For patients on a machine at the time of arrest it is usual to stop UF and give a bolus of saline immediately. Full cardiac investigations are almost always required (if successfully managed). There is no contraindication to the subsequent use of an automatic implantable defibrillator if clinically indicated.

A cardiac arrest on a dialysis unit, whether the outcome is successful or unsuccessful, is very traumatic for staff and the other patients. It is almost impossible to conduct the resuscitation in private, it will be obvious if the patient lives or dies, and all present in the unit will have known each other from weeks, months, or years of regular dialysis. The patients in the unit at the time must not be ignored, but should be told the outcome, and given time to discuss the episode with a nurse or staff member they know. Nursing staff will also need to cope with the event, which may be especially shocking if it occurred while the patient was on a machine. The nursing staff may feel responsible, and should be appropriately counselled.

End-of-life issues

End of life is often not well managed in patients on dialysis for a variety of reasons:

- The end-of-life phase of a chronic illness is often not recognized by the patient or healthcare team.
- Dialysis patients have many other co-morbid conditions making end-of-life management complex.
- Many patients have pain, e.g. due to arthritis, vascular disease, immobility, and its management is often poor.
- Dialysis itself can be difficult to deliver.
- Inpatient care is frequently under a medical team that does not know the patient well.

Table 16.1 summarizes many of the clinical features observed at the end of life.

Difficulties in continuing PD at end of life

- Patient is often too sick to carry out self-care treatment.
- May no longer be able to live independently.
- Poor nutrition.
- Increased risk of peritonitis.
- Patient technique often impaired.
- PD may be being performed by ward nurses.

Difficulties in continuing HD at end of life

- Vascular access may be problematic requiring frequent (and often, unpleasant) catheter insertions.
- Patients become more dependent:
  - need transport to and from HD unit
  - may no longer be able to manage at home.
- Increasing problems of hypotension on dialysis with risk of cardiac arrest.
- Increasing dementia or confusion may make patient less able to cope with dialysis procedure.

Table 16.1 Clinical features of end of life

Function	
General	Answer of 'No' to 'Would you be surprised if patient died in next 12 months?
	Intractable infections
	Increasingly severe symptoms needing more complex management
	Multiple admissions with complications of treatment
	Patient withdrawing from world around them, e.g. refusing tablets, food and drink, or basic nursing care (*but* must exclude obvious clinical depression)
Debility	Unintentional weight loss >10% over last 3 months
	Decline in performance status over last 6 months so that now requires aid for ≥3 activities of daily living
	Spending most of time in bed as a result of above
	Presence of progressive deep decubitus ulcers (bedsores)
	Dysphagia resulting in poor nutrition and/or recurrent chest infections
Disease-related	
Dialysis-related	Increasing difficulty with access for HD with multiple failures and few or no options, and PD or transplantation not feasible
	Persistent and problematic hypotension on HD, and PD not feasible
	Loss of UF on PD, and HD or transplantation not options
	Patient frequently refuses dialysis or states that they want to stop
Cardiovascular	Recurrent chest pain at rest or on dialysis with no options of cardiac intervention and not responding to medical therapy
	Recurrent arrhythmias and/or hypotension necessitating shortening of time on HD
	Unable to carry out any physical activity without chest pain or shortness of breath (New York Heart Association class IV)
	Worsening peripheral vascular disease not amenable to corrective surgery and leading to amputations
	Recurrent cerebrovascular events with increasing functional impairment
	Development of gut ischaemia
Other co-morbid conditions	Malignancy—progressing or difficult to treat in renal patient
	Chronic obstructive airways disease with disabling shortness of breath at rest and persistent hypoxaemia
	Progressive dementia with increasing functional impairment
	Presence of any other condition with <6-month prognosis and no treatment possible

Palliative care

Supportive care should be offered to patients throughout their lifetime with ESKD. Patients with renal failure have symptoms and pain related directly to their renal disease and to their multiple co-morbid conditions. Although many dialysis patients die suddenly, an end-of-life phase can be recognized in many, particularly the elderly, those who withdraw from dialysis, and those who choose conservative treatment and no dialysis.

It is not possible to provide 'end-of-life protocols' as individual patients, families, and healthcare teams need to be involved. Various ground rules, however, are helpful (see Box 16.2):

- Discussions should take place with the patient, family, and healthcare team, that the focus of care is the comfort of the patient and not the prolongation of life.
- Patient and family should be asked where they wish end of life to take place—hospital, hospice, home, etc.
- Unnecessary investigations, including blood tests and routine monitoring, e.g. BP, should be stopped.
- Review prescription chart—continue drugs that provide symptomatic relief but others should be stopped.
- Ensure that comfort care, particularly care of mouth and skin, is in place.
- For good symptom control, 'as required' medication should be prescribed for all likely symptoms, in addition to regular medication for ongoing symptoms.
- Patient and family should be enabled to meet their spiritual and religious needs.

Box 16.2 UK Renal National Service Framework: markers of good practice at end of life

- Patients with ESKD should have access to expertise in discussion of end of life issues.
  - This emphasizes the importance of communication and shared decision making between healthcare team, patient, and family
- Renal healthcare workers should be trained in symptom relief relevant to this group of patients.
  - This is key to good end-of-life care
- Prognostic assessment based on available data should be available to all patients.
- Patients and families can only make informed choices if they know the possible outcomes from the particular actions under consideration.
- Information about treatment choices.
  - This includes non-dialytic therapy or stopping renal replacement therapy once started
- Jointly agreed care plan in line with palliative care principles.
  - This will mean joint working with primary care and palliative care teams.
- Ongoing medical care for those who choose not to dialyse.
  - Patients are reassured to know that the no dialysis option is not a no treatment option but rather a maximal supportive care option with full medical care to maintain function as long as possible.
- Support to die with dignity.
  - It is beholden on the physician to ensure the quality of care is maintained to death and into bereavement.
- Culturally appropriate bereavement support to family, carers, and staff.

Failure to do this will impact on the care families and professional carers are able to provide.

Information taken from British Medical Association and the UK Resuscitation Council.

Palliative care: management of symptoms

Pain
- Common—usually related to co-morbid conditions, such as vascular disease, arthritis, or immobility.
- Dying patients have the right to be pain free, and this should be the principal aim of management.
- Strong opioids are often needed; they should be given continuously and intermittently as needed to keep the patient pain free (see also ➔ Pain management in ESKD, p. 549).

Nausea and vomiting
- Antiemetics, e.g. metoclopramide, cyclizine, or haloperidol should be given with opioid analgesia.
- If patient remains symptomatic, levomepromazine 5mg SC prn up to 8-hourly or 5–10mg SC/24h as a continuous infusion can be useful.

Shortness of breath
- There are many causes of shortness of breath at the end of life.
- Pulmonary oedema due to fluid overload is unusual as dying patients tend not to drink much.
- Main cause is anxiety and the following may be helpful:
  - cool fan on the face
  - oxygen
  - reassuring presence of family or staff
  - explanation to family and patient.
- Strong opioids such as fentanyl and alfentanil, used at doses of 50–100% of that used for pain, can be used if needed.
- Cheyne–Stokes respiration is usually a terminal event and the patient is often unconscious. Important to explain this to relatives so that they are reassured that the patient is not suffering.

Retained respiratory tract secretions
- Hyoscine butylbromide 20mg 4-hourly prn or as a 24h infusion(40–120mg) can be useful.
- Suction may be needed.

Terminal restlessness and agitation
- Try midazolam 2.5–5mg SC up to hourly prn.
- If symptoms persist after two doses, consider a syringe driver with midazolam 10–20mg/24h + prn dose as needed.

Withdrawal of dialysis

It is not uncommon for patients or family to feel that the quality of life on dialysis is so poor that they would rather die. Dialysis is a medical treatment and not a natural way of being kept alive—withdrawal of dialysis is therefore ethically distinct from stopping feeding (for example). Stopping dialysis is also not the same as euthanasia; the patient is being allowed to die naturally and is not being given a toxic dose of a drug. Withdrawal of dialysis accounts for >20% of mortality among American dialysis patients. Although the proportion is less in the UK and many other countries, it is important to have a system that helps the patient come to the correct decision and support them through the process. Withdrawal of dialysis will lead to death within 7–14 days in most cases but this is very dependent on residual renal function. Withdrawal of dialysis is not the same as withholding dialysis.

Patient autonomy and the right to self-determination will inevitably lead to some patients refusing treatment. This may be appropriate and should engender a full and honest discussion between the care team and the patient, but may also be the result of incorrect beliefs. Advance directives (living wills) will become increasingly common in medical practice.

Discussions about withdrawing dialysis should include:
- an assessment of the patient's ability to make a decision must be made (are they mentally fit?)
- reversible factors should be addressed
- full discussion with the dialysis team
- full involvement of the family
- and full care and support of the patient after withdrawal.

The *Mental Capacity Act (2005)* gives guidance about healthcare decisions for patients who lack capacity in England.
- If the patient's wishes are not known and/or the patient had not appointed a healthcare proxy, the senior clinician has the responsibility to make a decision about what course of action would be in the patient's best interests.
- The aim should be to reach a consensus, enabling all relevant people to contribute, but ultimately the responsibility lies with the consultant.
- Where there is difficulty reaching a consensus, despite multidisciplinary clinical discussion, independent or ethical review should be considered, using legal advice where necessary.

Withdrawal of dialysis: case histories

Case history 1

BJ was a 52-year-old man who had started dialysis 25years previously. He had developed GN after leaving university, leading to ESKD. During this time he married and started a successful career. He continued this during 15 years of home HD. Unfortunately his marriage did not survive, leading to divorce. He then had a successful renal transplant, but, after 7 years, presented with oesophageal varices. Investigations revealed portal hypertension secondary to hepatitis C. Around this time, transplant function declined and he had to recommence dialysis. His second wife left him. Over the next few years, his health declined—he was hypotensive secondary to calcific mitral valve disease, had periodic bleeding from his varices, and became harder to transfuse as he had developed red cell antibodies. At his own request, he started to see the counsellor to discuss withdrawing from dialysis, and then met his consultant to discuss what would happen when dialysis was withdrawn. He decided that he would take this step after the summer, as he had found the last winter particularly difficult. That autumn, during one of his many admissions for transfusion, he announced he no longer wanted further transfusions or dialysis. He was transferred to a single room and was given appropriate end-of-life care. He died peacefully 48h later.

Case history 2

SM was a 67-year-old blind, diabetic woman who had started dialysis 2 years earlier. She had been maintained on APD managed by her husband, who also had to help her with most activities of daily living. They came to see the counsellor together, with the wish to stop dialysis, as they felt that SM's quality of life was so poor. They were seen several times, allowing discussion about whether quality of life could be improved socially or medically. They were also seen by the consultant to discuss her existing medical condition, the option of hospital HD to ease the burden on her husband, and what would happen were dialysis to be withdrawn. The decision was made to discontinue dialysis. The couple continued to be seen by the counsellor and their PD nurse to discuss whether SM wanted to die in hospital or at home. The GP was informed when the decision was made for home. The couple selected the date for the last night of APD. Regular visits were made by the GP, district nurse, and PD nursing team, and SM died peacefully 1 week later.

Withdrawal of dialysis: discussion of cases

Both of the preceding scenarios (➜ Withdrawal of dialysis: case histories, p. 606) illustrate important features of the process involved in helping patients wanting to discontinue dialysis:

- recognition of the patient's right to stop dialysis—it is the patient's wishes that are paramount
- identification of an individual to whom patients can turn and who is not an immediate member of their healthcare team—many patients feel that they are letting down their carers
- time for numerous discussions when patients and their families can explore their feelings as to why they want to stop dialysis and their thoughts about dying—it is important that possible medical options are also mentioned during this process
- involvement of the medical and nursing carers who have been most closely involved with the patient
- discussion about the dying process, whether it will be painful, how long it will take, and where the patient wants to die
- provision of support and pain relief both at home and in hospital
- recognition that withdrawal from dialysis does not mean withdrawal from the close contacts made with staff on a dialysis unit.

Both of the patients discussed in the previous topic (➜ Withdrawal of dialysis: case histories, p. 606) were able to make their own decisions and raised the topic of withdrawal themselves. There are occasions when it is the healthcare team who feel that dialysis should be withdrawn, e.g. increasing dementia, dense stroke, or a patient unable to cope with the simplest of activities. Again, the process is based on multiple discussions with the patient (if he/she is mentally competent) and the family. The patient and family need to be helped to understand that there is not going to be any medical improvement. It is often unrealistic to expect the family to make the decision, particularly if they view this step as a kind of euthanasia.

Quality of death

Principles of a good death include anticipating that the end of life is close, choosing where death occurs, having time to say goodbyes, spiritual and emotional support, and control of pain and other symptoms. The best way to illustrate this is by case histories:

Case 1: a good-quality death

Harry Smith was 63 years old when he developed ESKD due to diabetes. He had retired when 60 and lived with his wife who still worked as a teacher. He had many of the complications of diabetes—IHD requiring coronary angioplasty when age 59, retinopathy requiring laser treatment, and evidence of peripheral neuropathy. He had been referred to the renal clinic a couple of years previously when his plasma creatinine was 220µmol/L. His BP was difficult to control with systolic pressures usually between 150 and 170mmHg. His renal function continued to decline. He and his wife were also worried about his increasingly poor short-term memory. Following discussions about dialysis, he and his wife opted for PD. He was admitted for insertion of a PD catheter when his plasma creatinine was 520µmol/L. He became very agitated during his short inpatient stay and it proved impossible to train him to do his own dialysis. His wife therefore arranged to take time off work so she could help him and hoped that with dialysis he would improve. However, Harry's dementia continued to progress and she could not even leave him at home on his own as he became very agitated. A brain CT scan done round this time confirmed the diagnosis of generalized small vessel disease. After 4 weeks at home on PD, Harry and his wife were seen on the PD unit by the consultant and his named nurse. The options of continuing PD, organizing help at home, converting to HD, or stopping dialysis were discussed. Unfortunately, Harry was no longer competent enough to take part in the conversation. His wife made the decision to stop dialysis and have the catheter removed. This was done the following week after she had time to reflect with her family. The GP was informed and the community palliative care team organized home visits. As Harry had just started dialysis, he still had some residual renal function. He survived at home for another few weeks, but without the added stress of dialysis, and died at home with his wife and family around him.

Case 2: a poor-quality death

Mr Black was an 82-year-old man who had been on HD for 2 years after developing ESKD due to renovascular disease. He was a retired company director and lived with his second wife who was ~20 years younger and still worked as a lawyer. He had one daughter. He had originally coped well with HD but then developed an ischaemic foot and had to be admitted for antibiotics and pain control. After vascular investigations, a femoral–popliteal bypass was performed, but this was not successful and he required a below-knee amputation and was eventually discharged after a 3-month hospital admission. One month later, his other foot became ischaemic and he was readmitted. The options were discussed and he was advised about the high risk of further surgery. He and his family decided to go ahead and he had another below-knee amputation with no immediate post-operative complications. His general state, however, remained poor; he was often in pain and rehabilitation was not possible. Ten days post-op, he was seen on the ward round by a different consultant as the renal consultants rotated every 2 weeks. He was on HD, was in pain, and was moaning 'take me off, take me off'. The dialysis session was terminated and he was given pain relief. Later that day the wife, daughter, and son-in-law met with the consultant who explained the poor prognosis and suggested that it would be in the patient's interest to recognize that he was at the end of life and keep him as comfortable as possible. The family were taken aback at this and said that no one had explained that even if he survived the operation, his chance of survival was poor. They insisted on full management with nasogastric feeding, antibiotics, and continued dialysis. Mr Black eventually died a few weeks later and throughout this time was confused, became increasingly weak, and was in intermittent pain. Some weeks after his death, the wife wrote a long letter complaining about nursing issues and commenting on the fact that the regular changing of the consultant in charge resulted in changing treatment plans and little consistency in the information being given to the family.

Transplantation for dialysis patients

Assessment for transplant suitability

All patients with ESKD should be considered for transplantation. Patient survival is better in transplant recipients than those remaining on a transplant waiting list matched for time on dialysis. Quality of life is also better (although patients need to be shepherded through the initial post-transplant period). All patients should be carefully counselled as to the potential availability of living related or unrelated (especially spousal) donors. Blood group or HLA incompatibilities between unrelated donors should not now preclude the ability to donate, as this can be achieved by desensitization programmes, antibody removal strategies, or by transplanting through shared pools (crudely the donor of patient A giving kidney to patient B, and vice versa).

Absolute contraindications for transplant include:
- current or recent malignancy (excluding basal or cutaneous squamous cell carcinomas)
- active infection
- severe cardiac or respiratory failure
- positive HLA cross-match with potential recipient.

Relative contraindications include:
- extensive peripheral vascular disease
- coronary artery disease (unless fully treated)
- urological abnormalities
- advanced age (>70 years—but biological age more important than chronological age, and increasingly good outcomes reported in those >65 years)
- high risk for peri-operative mortality
- active systemic illness
- active liver disease (hepatitis B or C)
- HIV (only contraindication if uncontrolled HIV or active opportunistic infection, malignancy, etc.)
- coagulopathy
- psychosis or dementia
- non-compliance
- renal diseases with high risk of recurrence (oxalosis, HUS, FSGS).

For most of these relative contraindications, appropriate investigations, pre-transplant interventions, and careful counselling may allow successful transplantation.

Once patients have been accepted on to a transplant programme it may be many years before they actually receive a deceased donor graft (average wait in the UK ~3 years). Patients should receive intermittent re-education about the procedure. Co-morbidity should be regularly re-assessed, especially cardiac disease. Blood transfusions should be avoided, and cytotoxic antibodies measured regularly.

Living donor transplantation

Increasing use should be made of living related or unrelated donors as all countries have a large shortfall in deceased donor organs. Outcomes for the recipient are significantly better than for deceased donor grafts. Donors require extensive screening to ensure complete health and absence of renal disease. Assuming the donor is fit there is little evidence of long-term morbidity in donors. Unrelated living donors are usually spouses or biologically unrelated siblings, and rarely close friends. Live donor exchange schemes are increasingly being developed whereby a donor of a donor–recipient pair provides a kidney for a second recipient whose donor gives their kidney to the recipient of the first pair. An altruistic donor starting this process can make such exchanges into an extended chain. Payment for organ donation is illegal in most countries.

Advantages
- Better graft survival over cadaveric transplantation.
- Allows planning of transplant operation to suit recipient and donor.
- Generally allows pre-emptive transplantation (prior to need for dialysis).
- Shorter time on dialysis (associated with better graft outcomes).
- Primary graft function more common as there is reduced ischaemic time.
- Potential psychological benefit and better compliance.
- Expands donor pool.
- Donors report major psychological benefit even if graft does not survive a prolonged time.

Disadvantages
- Peri-operative mortality risk to donor (~1 in 3000).
- Donor morbidity (wound, pneumonia, deep-vein thrombosis).
- Late complications, although rare, are reported, most commonly hypertension.
- Potential for coercion and lack of freely given consent. Crucial to ensure as much as possible donors are acting freely.

Contraindications to living donation
- Age <18 or >75 years
- Type 2 diabetes, abnormal glucose tolerance
- Hypertension (relative contraindication; if controlled on single agent may be a candidate under some circumstances and if other cardiovascular risks low)
- Malignancy
- Other significant co-morbidities
- Proteinuria
- Haematuria needs full urological investigations and renal biopsy
- Reduced GFR
- Transmissible infection (HIV, hepatitis).

Pre-transplant management

Patients should be well dialysed (if already on dialysis) prior to transplant surgery to minimize post-operative complications.

Donor details should be documented:
- whether cadaveric, donation after circulatory (non-heart beating) or brain death, or living
- age, gender, cause of death (deceased donors), and side (left or right)
- co-morbidities, ICU complications, BP and urine output pre-retrieval
- renal function at time of surgery
- virology (CMV especially), infection risks, tissue type, blood group of donor.

The recipient should be carefully examined pre-operatively, and a detailed history taken to ensure no new co-morbidities have developed since being placed on the transplant waiting list, especially cardiovascular or infectious, or the development of malignancy. (See Table 17.1.)

Note especially:
- recent ill health, virological tests (CMV especially)
- last cardiac assessment, current exercise capacity, ECG
- peripheral pulses especially in legs
- baseline urine output, urine dipstick (for proteinuria especially), and underlying primary renal disease
- detail of immunological cross-match with donor, and nature of HLA mismatches.

Patients should be carefully consented, and immunosuppression planned carefully based on perceived immunological risk (first or subsequent transplant; sensitization; previous immunosuppression for underlying renal disease; age).

Any pre-operative dialysis should have minimal or no anticoagulation. Patients on PD should be drained out prior to surgery. Patients taking aspirin and clopidogrel for cardiac disease may need platelet transfusion to cover enhanced bleeding risk during surgery.

Table 17.1 Assessment of patients prior to transplantation

Cardiac	ECG in all; invasive assessments in all with diabetes, hypertension, and smokers if any history of IHD, and patients >55 years. Non-invasive tests such as thallium radionucleotide scintigraphy and dobutamine stress echocardiography relatively insensitive in dialysis patients. Low-risk patients <50 years without diabetes do not need cardiac screening
Peripheral vascular disease	Dopplers ± angiography if absent foot pulses, arterial bruits, or symptoms of peripheral vascular disease. Consider carotid artery Dopplers in patients >55 years, those with diabetes or previous cerebrovascular disease
Respiratory	CXR in all; lung function testing as appropriate
Urinary tract	Formal urological assessment (with US, voiding cystourethrogram, cystoscopy as necessary) if previous UTIs, bladder outflow obstruction, history of reflux, or congenital abnormality
GI	Endoscopy if symptoms of ulcer disease. Consider liver biopsy if abnormal liver function or evidence of hepatitis viral infections
Systemic disease	Investigate for active systemic disease (ANCA, anti-GBM, SLE serology)
Infectious diseases	Ensure any previous TB adequately treated; screen for viral infections
Thrombophilia	Consider thrombophilia screen in all patients to minimize risk of post-transplant vascular thrombosis
Underlying renal disease	Document where possible for possible later recurrence; defer transplant if active
Laboratory investigation	Especially virology (HBV, HCV, HIV, CMV, varicella zoster virus), tissue typing, blood group, anti-HLA cytotoxic antibodies, thrombophilia screen
Psychological assessment	Requires full discussion with patient, including risks, complications, drug side effects (especially cancers), estimated graft survival rates, nature of home support, employment

The transplant operation

Care of the potential donor is crucial before organ retrieval, including management of acid–base status, ventilatory function, control of infection, haemodynamic stability and volume resuscitation, and control of potential endocrine insufficiency (adrenal, thyroid, vasopressin). The surgery of organ retrieval should be meticulous, and the kidney carefully examined once returned to the recipient team prior to placement (back-table preparation). Cadaveric organs will be retrieved with the renal artery usually on a cuff of aorta, and renal vein with a cuff of inferior vena cava. Living donated organs will have the renal artery and vein in isolation without cuff or patch of major vessels. Organs are perfused with iced saline, Marshall's, Ringer's lactate or University of Wisconsin solutions.

Surgery

- Kidney is carefully examined prior to surgery, and any preparation performed on the artery or vein.
- Accessory arteries are important to identify and ensure they will be anastomosed, or kidney will suffer a partial infarction.
- The organ is implanted into the iliac fossa into the external iliac artery and vein.
- Surgery is completely extraperitoneal in most cases.
- Native kidneys are not removed.
- Vascular anastomoses are usually end-to-side (end of the renal vessels onto the side of the iliac vessels).
- Recipient is well hydrated during the anastomosis surgery, and furosemide or mannitol often administered.
- Ureter is implanted into the bladder through a submucosal tunnel usually, with placement in most cases of a stent
- Patients usually have a drain placed in the peri-renal space.

Care should be taken of native fistulae.

PD catheters are sometimes removed at the time of surgery. This, however, prevents patients receiving PD if there is delayed graft function, and is often delayed until after successful engraftment and the patient is known to have good graft function.

Warm ischaemic time: time between circulatory arrest and time of cold storage. This is generally close to zero in cadaveric transplantation, slightly longer in living transplantation, but may be considerable from non-heart beating donors.

Cold ischaemic time: time that kidney is in cold storage between retrieval and transplantation. Can be up to 48h, though very rarely >36h.

Post-transplant management

Crucial that an experienced team manages patients after transplantation. Patients need review immediately after surgery, and frequently thereafter, with repeated testing of electrolytes, monitoring of urine output, and re-assessment of fluid balance. Patients can be oliguric especially if prolonged cold ischaemic time, or significantly polyuric, passing 1–2L of urine per hour. (See Table 17.2.)

Immediate post-transplant assessment (in recovery)

- Review operation and anaesthetic note (peri-operative complications? Fluids given? Hypotension? Immediate urine output? Warm ischaemic time? Bleeding?)
- Check all immunosuppression given as necessary
- Urine output (what was pre-transplant daily urine output?)
- Wound
- Drain content
- BP, pulmonary pressure, and central venous pressure (CVP)
- Clinical examination of chest for pulmonary oedema
- SaO_2 and arterial blood gasses
- Urea and electrolytes ((U&Es) especially potassium), full blood count (FBC (fall in Hb?)).

24h to 1 week post-transplantation

- Fluid balance review (continuously by nursing staff). Patients accumulate fluid in general despite diuresis and good graft primary function.
- CVP assessment in general for 24–48h.
- Urine output through catheter (leave in place for at least 5 days to protect vesico-ureteric anastomosis).
- Drain volumes (usually removed when minimal—after 2–3 days).
- Keep volume replete with 0.9% saline and 5% glucose: usually given as hourly rate of urine output + 30–100mL/h depending on CVP measurement.
- Daily or twice-daily U&Es and FBC initially; if oliguric, may have increased K. If polyuric, decreased K, Mg, or PO_4, especially. Hb can fall from blood loss and dilution.
- Daily blood glucose.
- Monitoring of blood immunosuppressive drug levels (ciclosporin, tacrolimus especially).
- Anticoagulation as necessary depending on risk of vascular thrombosis.
- Dialysis plan if no primary function.
- Early mobilization, chest physiotherapy, nil-by-mouth until gut ileus resolved.
- Prophylactic therapies for CMV (e.g. valganciclovir), osteoporosis (e.g. bisphosphonates or vitamin D), oral fungal infections (e.g. nystatin), *Pneumocystis* pneumonia (e.g. oral co-trimoxazole), TB (if at high risk using isoniazid and pyridoxine), aspirin, statins, and possibly heparin or LMWHs.
- Avoid NSAIDs. Watch for opiate accumulation if using patient-controlled analgesia and especially if poor graft function.
- US assessment of graft perfusion.

Table 17.2 Surgical complications

Vascular anastomotic leak	Presents with haemorrhagic shock, falling Hb, blood in drain, oliguria. Urgent return to theatre for exploration. Reverse clotting diatheses, cross-match, and transfuse
Vascular thrombosis (arterial or venous)	Especially in patients with thrombophilia or anticardiolipin antibodies. Presents with reduced urine output, graft pain or tenderness, graft swelling, macroscopic haematuria. Requires urgent diagnosis (Doppler US) or immediate surgical exploration. Rarely successful
Urinary leak	Most commonly from vesico-ureteric anastomosis. Presents as reduced urine output, pain, graft swelling, scrotal or labial swelling. US. Biochemical analysis of fluid leak or collection. May settle spontaneously if stent retained in ureter and with drain or require surgical re-implantation
Lymphocoele	Usually small. Swelling over kidney, collection on imaging, limb swelling, DVT, oliguria from obstruction. Diagnose by US and sometime fluid biochemistry (to exclude urine leak). Usually resolve spontaneously. May require percutaneous drainage or more rarely surgical intervention
Wound infection	Fever, pain, erythema, raised CRP or WBCs. Usually from Gram-positive organisms
Deep vein thrombosis, pulmonary embolism, pneumonia, ileus, etc.	As may occur after any surgery

Delayed graft function

- Patients requiring dialysis more than once after transplantation or with a serum creatinine >400µmol/L after 1 week.
- Occurs in 5–40% of kidney transplants.
- May be associated with poor longer-term graft function although may only be true in presence of concurrent rejection episodes.
- Biopsy shows ATN.
- Differential diagnosis includes early rejection, vascular thrombosis, obstruction, thrombotic microangiopathy.

Risk factors

- Non-heart-beating donor (donation after circulatory death)
- Long cold ischaemia time (>24h)
- Poor storage/perfusion
- ATN in donor
- Vascular disease or hypertension in donor
- Older donor age (>55 years)
- Vascular disease in recipient
- Intra- or post-operative hypotension
- Use of calcineurin inhibitors.

Diagnosed clinically or by renal biopsy having excluded surgical causes by imaging and clinical examination. Management depends on cause, but includes optimizing BP and fluid balance, and calcineurin inhibitor blood levels. Graft function usually recovers.

Dialysis during delayed graft function

Patients will need dialysis during a period of delayed graft function. Either HD or PD can be continued.

For patients undergoing HD, hypotension should be avoided at all costs to prevent further insults to the kidney, heparin use minimized or avoided early, electrolytes carefully monitored, and drug dosing adjusted as necessary.

Patients with PD catheters can continue PD if the transplant operation was completely extraperitoneal, and should ideally use low-volume APD. Scrupulous care should be taken to avoid infection (peritonitis) especially as ward nursing staff may be unfamiliar with PD connections, exchanges, etc.

Dialysis access after successful transplantation

Patients with tunnelled CVC lines should have these removed under sterile conditions before discharge from hospital with a functioning graft.

Fistulae should be left initially. They can be tied off if necessary at a later stage after graft function has stabilized.

PD catheters are sometimes removed at time of transplant surgery, or can be removed under local anaesthetic usually prior to discharge if graft function good, or (less commonly) at time of removal of ureteric stent a few weeks post-operatively. If PD catheters are left in place for a few weeks they should be managed very carefully to avoid infection.

Drug dosing

Contributors

Wendy Lawson
Lead Pharmacist, Imperial College Healthcare Trust, London, UK

Rania Betmouni
Clinical Pharmacist, Cromwell Hospital, London, UK

Drug handling in renal impairment

There are many ways that drug handling is affected in ESKD. Renal failure can alter both drug pharmacokinetics and pharmacodynamics. Patients are often taking multiple drugs, with increased risk of drug interactions. Dialysis itself may clear some drugs, and there may be differences between haemofiltration, PD, and HD. Drug doses should not be reduced blindly as this may result in inadequate therapy.

Bioavailability

Gastroparesis, nausea, vomiting, and anorexia may all reduce drug absorption. Advanced uraemia alkalinizes saliva, which reduces absorption of drugs preferring an acid environment. Phosphate binders can form insoluble products with some drugs and decrease their absorption.

Volume of distribution (Vd)

Represents the ratio of administered drug to the plasma concentration, and indicates the degree of distribution or binding of a drug to tissues. Will be increased in patients with oedema or ascites for water-soluble drugs, and decreased in muscle wasting or volume depletion. Drugs with a large Vd (e.g. >0.6 L/kg) are not confined within the circulation, tend to be lipid-soluble, and hence will not be cleared by HD.

Protein binding

Altered by acid–base balance, malnutrition, and inflammation.

Drug metabolism

May be altered unpredictably in renal failure (e.g. reduced hydrolysis reactions). Renally excreted and toxic metabolites may accumulate (e.g. metabolites of morphine or pethidine/meperidine).

Renal excretion

Will be dependent on the precise degree of renal dysfunction, and determined by the extent of filtration, tubular secretion, and reabsorption. Patients on dialysis may still have appreciable residual renal function.

Dialytic clearance

Depends on the molecular weight (MW) and degree of protein binding of a drug. Drug clearance will vary to a degree according to extent of haemofiltration during HD. Membranes (especially synthetic ones) will vary in their ability to adsorb drugs, but this can be considerable. PD does not usually clear drugs well, unless they have a low Vd, low protein binding, and no other route of excretion.

Loading doses

Do not usually need to be altered in stage 5 CKD.

Dosing of commonly used drugs

Tables 18.1–18.13 list the dose modifications for commonly used drugs in patients with stage 5 CKD, on HD. and PD. Definitions of severe renal failure given in prescribing information vary for different drugs and have not been clearly aligned with the CKD classification, and we have generally used data for patients with creatinine >350µmol/L, or Ccrea <10–15mL/min. Furthermore, there is controversy as to whether drug dosing using eGFR is appropriate for some drugs since the eGFR is normalized for BSA, and this may be incorrect when considering drug dosing, Vd, metabolism, etc. *We therefore do not recommend eGFR be used for drug dosing as it is currently not validated.* Published data are often conflicting on the precise doses to be used in patients with stage 5 CKD, and we have provided consensus data where possible. Doses are provided for oral drug use unless stated otherwise or if only available as one formulation, e.g. parenteral, then doses are for that formulation.

Much of the data on drug handling in HD were obtained historically using low-flux, cellulose, or modified cellulose dialysis membranes. Synthetic membranes often adsorb significant amounts of drug, and high-flux membranes may have significantly increased diffusive and convective clearance of drugs. Data are therefore often not available for drug dosing using current dialytic technologies. To avoid potential problems with underdosing, in general drugs should be given after dialysis, or into the venous line at the end of the session (if IV). Drugs that might be removed during dialysis should generally be given as soon after dialysis as possible, to avoid patients being undertreated for significant periods.

The lists provided here represent commonly used practical dosing schedules. All doses should be confirmed with manufacturers' recommendations prior to use.

Abbreviations

LD = loading dose
LMWH = low-molecular-weight heparin
ON = at night
PCP = *Pneumocystis carinii* pneumonia (now called *Pneumocystis jirovecii*)
PO = oral
q6h = every 6h
q12h = every 12h etc.
SC = subcutaneous
SL = sublingual
UFH = unfractionated heparin.

Table 18.1 Dosing of antimicrobials

Drug	Dosage for CKD stage 5	Dosage for HD	Dosage for PD
Amikacin	Titrate to levels	Titrate to levels. See text	Titrate to levels. See text
Amoxicillin IV/PO	025–1g q8h	As for CKD stage 5	As for CKD stage 5
Ampicillin IV/PO	0.25–1g q6h	As for CKD stage 5	As for CKD stage 5
Azithromycin	Standard dose	Standard dose	Standard dose
Aztreonam	25% standard dose	As for CKD stage 5	As for CKD stage 5
Benzylpenicillin	0.6–1.2g q6h	As for CKD stage 5	As for CKD stage 5
Cefaclor	250mg q8h	250–500mg q8h	250mg q8–12h
Cefalexin	250–500mg q8–12h	As for CKD stage 5	As for CKD stage 5
Cefotaxime	Up to 1g q8–12h	As for CKD stage 5	1g q24h
Ceftazidime	0.5–1g q24h	0.5–1g q24–48h	As for CKD stage 5
Ceftriaxone	1–2g q24h	As for CKD stage 5	As for CKD stage 5
Cefuroxime IV	750mg–1.5g q12–24h	As for CKD stage 5	As for CKD stage 5
Cefuroxime PO	Standard dose	Standard dose	Standard dose
Chloroquine	Treatment: 50% standard dose	As for CKD stage 5	As for CKD stage 5
Ciprofloxacin IV/PO	50% standard dose	IV: 200mg q12h; PO: 250–500mg q12h	IV: 200mg q12h; PO: 250mg q8–12h
Clarithromycin	IV: 250–500mg q12h: PO: standard dose	As for CKD stage 5	As for CKD stage 5
Clindamycin	Standard dose	Standard dose	Standard dose
Co-amoxiclav (amoxicillin/ clavulanic acid) IV/PO	IV: 1.2g stat, then 600mg q8h or 1.2g 12h; PO: 375–625mg q8–12h??	IV: 600mg q24h (post-HD) PO: As for CKD stage 5	As for CKD stage 5
Colistimethate IV	If >60kg, 1 million units q18–24h	As for CKD stage 5	As for CKD stage 5

(continued)

Table 18.1 (Contd.)

Drug	Dosage for CKD stage 5	Dosage for HD	Dosage for PD
Co-trimoxazole IV/PO sulfamethoxazole (SMX)/ trimethoprim (TMP)	PCP treatment:: 30mg/kg SMX/TMP q12h PCP prophylaxis: 50% standard dose q48–72h	PCP treatment: as for CKD stage 5 PCP prophylaxis: 50% standard dose q48–72h (post-HD)	PCP treatment: as for CKD stage 5
Daptomycin	4–6mg/kg q48h depending on indication	As for CKD stage 5 (post-HD)	As for CKD stage 5
Doxycycline	Standard dose	Standard dose	Standard dose
Ertapenem	50% standard dose	1g three times a week post-HD	As for CKD stage 5 or 1g three times a week
Erythromycin IV/PO	Standard dose	Standard dose	Standard dose
Fidaxomycin	Use with caution	Use with caution	Use with caution
Flucloxacillin IV/PO	IV: 1g q6h ; PO: max 1g q6h	As for CKD stage 5	As for CKD stage 5
Gentamicin	Titrate to levels	See text	See text
Imipenem/ cilastatin	250–500mg (or 3.5mg/kg whichever is lower) q12h	As for CKD stage 5	As for CKD stage 5
Levofloxacin IV/PO	When standard dose is 500mg, give 500mg stat then125mg q24h; when standard dose is 250mg, give 250mg stat then 125mg q48h	As for CKD stage 5	As for CKD stage 5
Linezolid	Standard dose	Standard dose	Standard dose
Meropenem	50% standard dose q24h	Standard dose post-HD on dialysis days only	As for CKD stage 5
Metronidazole IV/PO	Standard dose	Standard dose	Standard dose
Moxifloxacin IV?PO	Standard dose	Standard dose	Standard dose
Nitrofurantoin	Avoid	Avoid	Avoid
Phenoxymethyl-penicillin	Standard dose	Standard dose	Standard dose

Table 18.1 (Contd.)

Drug	Dosage for CKD stage 5	Dosage for HD	Dosage for PD
Piperacillin/ tazobactam	4.5g q12h	As for CKD stage 5, supplement with 2.25g post-HD	As for CKD stage 5
Quinine dihydrochloride IV	Treatment: 5–7mg/ kg q24h	As for CKD stage 5 (post-HD)	As for CKD stage 5
Teicoplanin	Day 1–3 standard dose, then from day 4 standard dose q72h or 33% of standard dose q24h	As for CKD stage 5	As for CKD stage 5
Temocillin	1–2g q48h	As for CKD stage 5	As for CKD stage 5
Ticarcillin/ clavulanic acid	1.6g q12h	As for CKD stage 5 (post-HD)	As for CKD stage 5
Tigecycline	Standard dose	Standard dose	Standard dose
Tobramycin	Titrate to levels	See text	See text
Trimethoprim	50% standard dose	As for CKD stage 5	As for CKD stage 5
Vancomycin IV PO	Titrate to levels Standard dose	See text Standard dose	See text Standard dose

Table 18.2 Dosing of antifungals

Drug	Dosage for CKD stage 5	Dosage for HD	Dosage for PD
Abelcet® (amphotericin lipid complex)	Standard dose	Standard dose (post-HD)	Standard dose
AmBisome® (liposomal amphotericin)	Standard dose	Standard dose (post-HD)	Standard dose
Anidulafungin	Standard dose	Standard dose	Standard dose
Caspofungin	Standard dose	Standard dose	Standard dose
Fluconazole IV/PO	50% standard dose	Standard dose post-HD on dialysis days only (assuming 3 times a week) or 50% standard dose daily	As for CKD stage 5

(continued)

Table 18.2 (Contd.)

Drug	Dosage for CKD stage 5	Dosage for HD	Dosage for PD
Flucytosine IV	50mg/kg stat, then adjust according to levels	50mg/kg stat post-HD; adjust according to levels	12.5mg/kg q6h; adjust according to levels
Fungizone® (Amphotericin sodium deoxycholate)	Standard dose q24–36h	As for CKD stage 5	As for CKD stage 5
Itraconazole IV	Avoid	Avoid	Avoid
Itraconazole PO	Standard dose	Standard dose	Standard dose
Micafungin	Standard dose	Standard dose	Standard dose
Posaconazole PO	Standard dose	Standard dose	Standard dose
Voriconazole IV	Not recommended	Not recommended	Not recommended
Voriconazole PO	Standard dose	Standard dose	Standard dose

Table 18.3 Dosing of antiretrovirals

Drug	Dosage for CKD stage 5	Dosage for HD	Dosage for PD
Abacavir	Standard dose	Standard dose	Standard dose
Amprenavir (avoid oral solution)	Standard dose	Standard dose	Standard dose
Atazanavir	Standard dose	No data	No data
Darunavir	Standard dose	Standard dose	Standard dose
Didanosine	≥60kg: 100mg q24h <60kg: 75mg q24h	As for CKD stage 5 (post-HD)	As for CKD stage 5
Efavirenz	Standard dose	Standard dose	Standard dose
Emtricitabine	200mg q96h	As for CKD stage 5 (post-HD) HD should be started at least 12h post dose	No data
Fosamprenavir	Standard dose	Standard dose	Standard dose
Indinavir	Standard dose	Standard dose	Standard dose

Table 18.3 (*Contd.*)

Drug	Dosage for CKD stage 5	Dosage for HD	Dosage for PD
Lamivudine HIV	Loading dose 150mg stat then 50mg stat, oral solution q24h	As for CKD stage 5 (post-HD)	As for CKD stage 5
Lamivudine Hepatitis B	Loading dose 35mg, then 10mg–15mg oral solution q24h	As for CKD stage 5 (post-HD)	As for CKD stage 5
Lopinavir	Standard dose	Standard dose	Standard dose
Nelfinavir	Standard dose	Standard dose	No data
Nevirapine	Standard dose	Standard dose (post-HD)	No data
Raltegravir	Standard dose	Standard dose	No data
Ritonavir	Standard dose	Standard dose	Standard dose
Saquinavir	Standard dose	Standard dose	No data
Stavudine	≥60kg: 20mg q24h <60kg: 15mg q24h	As for CKD stage 5 (post-HD)	No data
Tenofovir	245mg every 7days	As for CKD stage 5	No data
Tipranavir	Standard dose	Standard dose	Standard dose
Zidovudine (AZT)	100mg q8h	As for CKD stage 5	As for CKD stage 5

Table 18.4 Antiretroviral combination drugs

Drug	Dosage for CKD stage 5	Dosage for HD	Dosage for PD
Abacavir, lamivudine (Kivexa®)	Avoid combination product; use individual drugs	Use individual drugs	Use individual drugs
Abacavir, lamivudine, zidovudine (Trizivir®)	Use individual drugs	Use individual drugs	Use individual drugs
Efavirenz, emtricitabine, tenofovir (Atripla®)	Use individual drugs	Use individual drugs	Use individual drugs
Emtricitabine, tenofovir (Truvada®)	Use individual drugs	Use individual drugs	Use individual drugs
Lamivudine, zidovudine (Combivir®)	Use individual drugs	Use individual drugs	Use individual drugs
Lopinavir, ritonavir (Kaletra®)	Standard dose	Standard dose	Standard dose

Table 18.5 Dosing of antivirals

Drug	Dosage for CKD stage 5	Dosage for HD	Dosage for PD
Aciclovir IV	50% standard dose q24h	As for CKD stage 5 (post-HD)	As for CKD stage 5
Aciclovir PO	Standard dose q12h	As for CKD stage 5 (post-HD)	As for CKD stage 5
Adefovir	10mg 72h	10mg every 7 days post-HD (assuming 4h HD 3 times a week)	No data
Cidofovir	Avoid	Avoid	Avoid
Entecavir	50–100mcg q24h	As for CKD stage 5 (post-HD)	As for CKD stage 5
Famciclovir	Unit dose q24h depending on diagnosis and if immunocompromised	As for CKD stage 5 on dialysis days only	No data
Foscarnet	Avoid	Avoid	Avoid
Ganciclovir IV	1.25mg/kg q24h	1.25mg/kg q24h (post-HD)	As for CKD stage 5
Oseltamivir	Treatment and prophylaxis: avoid if CrCl <10mL/min; if CrCl 10–30mL/min Treatment: 30mg q24h Prophylaxis: 30mg q48h Treatment: 30mg after every HD session Prophylaxis: 30mg after every second HD session		Treatment: 30mg single dose Prophylaxis: 30mg weekly
Ribavirin PO	Avoid Avoid		Avoid
Tenofovir	245mg every 7 days As for CKD stage 5		As for CKD stage 5
Valaciclovir	*Treatment:* Herpes simplex/zoster: 500mg–1g q24h Herpes simplex: 500mg q24h *Suppression:* Herpes simplex immunocompromised: 500mg q24h; Herpes simplex immunocompetent: 250mg q24h *CMV prophylaxis:* 1g q24h As for CKD stage 5 (post-HD)		As for CKD stage 5

Table 18.5 (*Contd.*)

Drug	Dosage for CKD stage 5	Dosage for HD	Dosage for PD
Valganciclovir	Prophylaxis: 450mg twice a week Prophylaxis: 450mg 3 times a week post-HD on dialysis days only		
Zanamavir inhalation	Standard dose Standard dose	Standard dose	

Table 18.6 Dosing of antituberculous drugs

Drug	Dosage for CKD stage 5	Dosage for HD	Dosage for PD
Ethambutol	5–7.5mg/kg q24h or 15mg/kg q48h replace with 15–25mg/kg 3 times a week (maximum 2.5g)	15–25 mg/kg post-HD on dialysis days only (assume 3 times a week)	15mg/kg q48h
Isoniazid	Standard dose	Standard dose (post-HD)	Standard dose
Pyrazinamide	50–100% standard dose 25–30mg/kg 3 times a week	25–30mg/kg post-HD on dialysis days only (assume 3 times a week)	Standard dose
Rifampicin	50–100% remove this and replace with standard dose	As for CKD stage 5	As for CKD stage 5? May not get through PD membrane

Table 18.7 Dosing of cardiovascular drugs

Drug	Dosage for CKD stage 5	Dosage for HD	Dosage for PD
Amlodipine	Standard dose	Standard dose	Standard dose
Aspirin	Treatment: avoid Prophylaxis: standard dose	As for CKD stage 5	As for CKD stage 5
Atenolol	Start low dose, then titrate to BP and pulse. Metoprolol may be preferred	See text	See text
Atorvastatin	Standard dose	Standard dose	Standard dose
Bezafibrate (non-sustained release)	Avoid	200mg q72h	200mg q72h

(continued)

Table 18.7 (*Contd.*)

Drug	Dosage for CKD stage 5	Dosage for HD	Dosage for PD
Carvedilol	Standard dose	Start low dose, then titrate to response	Start low dose, then titrate to response
Digoxin	Complex kinetics: a lower LD is used 250–500mcg then 62.5mcg ad adjust according to levels	As for CKD stage 5	As for CKD stage 5
Diltiazem	Standard dose	Standard dose	Standard dose
Dipyridamole	Standard dose	Standard dose	Standard dose
Doxazosin	Standard dose	Standard dose	Standard dose
Enalapril	Start low dose, then titrate to BP and pulse	See text	As for CKD stage 5
Eplerenone	Avoid	Avoid	Avoid
Ezetimibe	Standard dose	Standard dose	Standard dose
Fosinopril	Start low dose, then titrate to BP and pulse	See text	As for CKD stage 5
Furosemide	If indicated, may require higher doses up to 500mg	As for CKD stage 5	As for severe CKD stage 5
Irbesartan	Standard dose	Standard dose	Standard dose
Isosorbide mono/dinitrate	Standard dose	Standard dose	Standard dose
Labetalol	Standard dose	Standard dose	Standard dose
Lisinopril	Start low dose, then titrate to BP and pulse	See text	As for CKD stage 5
Losartan	Start 25mg q24h, then titrate to response	As for CKD stage 5	As for CKD stage 5
LMWHs	Prophylaxis: controversy—either standard dose or 50% standard dose Treatment: prolonged anticoagulation use with caution; consider UFH	As for CKD stage 5	As for CKD stage 5
Metoprolol	Start low dose, then titrate to BP and pulse	See text	As for CKD stage 5
Nifedipine	Start low dose, then titrate to BP and pulse	As for CKD stage 5	As for CKD stage 5
Perindopril	Start low dose, then titrate to BP and pulse	See text	As for CKD stage 5
Pravastatin	Standard dose	Standard dose	Standard dose

Table 18.7 (*Contd.*)

Drug	Dosage for CKD stage 5	Dosage for HD	Dosage for PD
Propranolol	Start low dose, then titrate to BP and pulse	See text	As for CKD stage 5
Ramipril	Start low dose, then titrate to BP and pulse	See text	As for CKD stage 5
Rosuvastatin	Avoid	Avoid	Avoid
Simvastatin	Maximum 10mg q24h at night	As for CKD stage 5	As for CKD stage 5
Valsartan	Start 40mg q24h, then titrate to BP and pulse	As for CKD stage 5	As for CKD stage 5
Verapamil	Standard dose	Standard dose	Standard dose
Warfarin	Standard dose	Standard dose	Standard dose

Table 18.8 Dosing of oral hypoglycaemics

Drug	Dosage for CKD Stage 5	Dosage for HD	Dosage for PD
Exenatide	Avoid	Avoid	Avoid
Glibenclamide	Start with low dose and adjust	Start with low dose and adjust	Start with low dose and adjust
Gliclazide	Start with low dose and adjust	Start with low dose and adjust	Start with low dose and adjust
Glimepiride	Start with low dose and adjust	Start with low dose and adjust	Start with low dose and adjust
Glipizide	Start with low dose and adjust	Start with low dose and adjust	Start with low dose and adjust
Linagliptin	Dose as normal	Dose as normal	Dose as normal
Liraglutide	Avoid	Avoid	Avoid
Metformin	Avoid	Avoid	Avoid
Pioglitazone	Dose as normal	Dose as normal	Dose as normal
Repaglinide	Start with low dose and adjust	Start with low dose and adjust	Start with low dose and adjust
Saxagliptin	Low dose 2.5mg	Low dose (FDA licensing)	Avoid
Sitagliptin	Low dose 25mg	Low dose 25mg	Low dose 25mg
Vidagliptin	Low dose 50mg	Low dose 50mg	Low dose 50mg

Table 18.9 Dosing of analgesics

Drug	Dosage for CKD stage 5	Dosage for HD	Dosage for PD
Alfentanil	IV or SC: pre-procedure or breakthrough 50–100mcg	As for CKD stage 5	As for CKD stage 5
Amitriptyline	10mg ON	As for CKD stage 5	As for CKD stage 5
Buprenorphine SL	Reduce dose 25–50% initially and titrate	As for CKD stage 5	As for CKD stage 5
Transdermal	Standard dose	Standard dose	Standard dose
Clonazepam	Start low dose and titrate to response	As for CKD stage 5	As for CKD stage 5
Codeine phosphate IV/PO	15–30mg q6h	As for CKD stage 5	As for CKD stage 5
Diamorphine	SC or IM: 2.5mg q8h, titrate to response	As for CKD stage 5	As for CKD stage 5
Fentanyl			
SC	Pre-procedure or breakthrough 12.5–25mcg q1–4h	As for CKD stage 5	As for CKD stage 5
Transdermal	12–25mcg/h q72h	As for CKD stage 5	As for CKD stage 5
Gabapentin	100mg q24h and titrate (maximum 300mg)	200–300mg post-HD on dialysis days only	300mg q48h
Hydromorphone PO (non-modified release)	Start low and titrate to response	As for CKD stage 5	As for CKD stage 5
Levetiracetam	250–500mg q12h	LD: 750mg, then 500mg–1g q24h (post-HD)	As for HD
Morphine	Avoid	Avoid	Avoid
Oxycodone (non-modified release)	Start low dose 2.5mg q6–8h and titrate for short-term use	2.5mg q6h	As for HD
Paracetamol	500mg–1g q6–8h	As for CKD stage 5	As for CKD stage 5
Pethidine (meperidine)	Avoid	Avoid	Avoid
Pregabalin	Commence 25mg q24h, titrate to response (maximum 75mg)	As for severe RF (post-HD)	As for severe RF
Tramadol PO (non-modified release)/IV	50mg q12h	50mg q6–8h	50mg q6h

Table **18.10** Dosing of CNS drugs

Drug	Dosage for CKD stage 5	Dosage for HD	Dosage for PD
Amitriptyline	Start low and titrate	As for CKD 5	As for CKD 5
Carbamazepine	Standard dose	Standard dose	Standard dose
Chlordiazepoxide	50% of standard dose	50% of standard dose	50% of standard dose
Chlorphenamine	Standard dose	Standard dose	Standard dose
Citalopram	Start low dose and titrate	As for CKD 5	As for CKD 5
Clonazepam	Start low dose and titrate to response	As for CKD 5	As for CKD 5
Diazepam	Start low dose and titrate to response	As for CKD 5	As for CKD 5
Domperidone	Standard dose	Standard dose	Standard dose
Dosulepin	Commence 25mg ON	Standard dose	Standard dose
Fluoxetine	Standard dose q24–48h	Standard dose or q24–48h	Standard dose or q24–48h
Granisetron	Standard dose	Standard dose	Standard dose
Imipramine	Standard dose	Standard dose	Standard dose
Levetiracetam	250–500mg q12h	LD: 750mg, then 500mg–1g q24h (post HD)	As for HD
Lorazepam	Standard dose	As for CKD 5	As for CKD 5
Metoclopramide	50–100% standard dose	As for CKD 5	As for CKD 5
Mirtazapine	Reduce dose and titrate to response	As for CKD 5	As for CKD 5
Nitrazepam	Reduce dose and titrate to response	As for CKD 5	As for CKD 5
Ondansetron	Standard dose	Standard dose	Standard dose
Orlistat	Standard dose	Standard dose	Standard dose
Paroxetine	50% of standard dose	As for CKD 5	As for CKD 5
Phenytoin	Standard dose	Standard dose	Standard dose
Sertraline	Standard dose	Standard dose	Standard dose

(continued)

Table 18.10 (Contd.)

Drug	Dosage for CKD stage 5	Dosage for HD	Dosage for PD
Sodium valproate	Standard dose	Standard dose	Standard dose
Temazepam	Reduce dose and titrate to response	As for CKD 5	As for CKD 5
Venlafaxine (non-modified release)	50% standard dose q24h	As for CKD 5 (post-HD)	As for CKD 5
Zopiclone	3.75–7.5mg ON	As for CKD 5	As for CKD 5

Table 18.11 Dosing of gastrointestinal drugs

Drug	Dosage for CKD stage 5	Dosage for HD	Dosage for PD
Balsalazide	Avoid	Avoid	Avoid
Bisacodyl	Standard dose	Standard dose	Standard dose
Docusate sodium	Standard dose	Standard dose	Standard dose
Esomeprazole	Standard dose	Standard dose	Standard dose
Hyoscine butylbromide	SC: 20mg stat and q2h prn	As for CKD stage 5	As for CKD stage 5
Hyoscine hydrobromide	SC: 400mcg stat and q4h prn	As for CKD stage 5	As for CKD stage 5
Lactulose	Standard dose	Standard dose	Standard dose
Lansoprazole	Standard dose	Standard dose	Standard dose
Mebeverine	Standard dose	Standard dose	Standard dose
Mesalazine	Avoid	Avoid	Avoid
Omeprazole	Standard dose	Standard dose	Standard dose
Pantoprazole	Standard dose	Standard dose	Standard dose
Rabeprazole	Standard dose	Standard dose	Standard dose
Ranitidine IV/PO	50–100% standard dose	As for CKD stage 5 (post-HD)	As for CKD stage 5
Senna	Standard dose	Standard dose	Standard dose
Sucralfate	Avoid	Avoid	Avoid
Sulfasalazine	Avoid	Avoid	Avoid

Table 18.12 Dosing of immunosuppressants

Drug	Dosage for CKD stage 5	Dosage for HD	Dosage for PD
Ciclosporin	Standard dose titrate to levels	Standard dose titrate to levels	Standard dose titrate to levels
Mycophenolate	Up to 1g q12h, if outside transplant period; ideally titrate to levels	250–500mg q12h; ideally titrate to levels	250–500mg q12h.; ideally titrate to levels
Prednisolone	Standard dose	Standard dose (post-HD)	Standard dose
Sirolimus	Standard dose	Standard dose	Standard dose
Tacrolimus	Standard dose titrate to levels	Standard dose titrate to levels	Standard dose titrate to levels

Table 18.13 Miscellaneous drugs

Drug	Dosage for CKD stage 5	Dosage for HD	Dosage for PD
Alendronic acid	Avoid	Avoid	Avoid
Alfacalcidol	Standard dose	Standard dose	Standard dose
Allopurinol	100mg q24h and titrate	As for CKD stage 5	As for CKD stage 5
Colchicine	50% standard dose	As for CKD stage 5	As for CKD stage 5
Etidronate	Avoid	Avoid	Avoid
Ibandronic acid	IV: standard dose but infusion rate 2mg/h PO: 50mg once weekly	As for CKD stage 5	As for CKD stage 5
Methotrexate	Avoid	Avoid	Avoid
Pamidronate	Standard dose, but max infusion rate 20mg/h	As for CKD stage 5	As for CKD stage 5
Pioglitazone	Standard dose	Standard dose	Standard dose
Risedronate	Avoid	Avoid	Avoid
Rosiglitazone	Standard dose	Standard dose	Standard dose
Sildenafil	Commence with 25mg	As for CKD stage 5	As for CKD stage 5
Strontium	Avoid	Avoid	Avoid
Tadalafil	Commence with 10mg	As for CKD stage 5	As for CKD stage 5
Vardenafil	Commence with 5mg	As for CKD stage 5	As for CKD stage 5

Some drugs that do not require dosage alteration in CKD stage 5, haemodialysis, and peritoneal dialysis

Alfacalcidol
Amiodarone
Amitriptyline
Amlodipine
Amphotericin (all IV formulations)
Anidulafungin
Aspirin (prophylaxis)
Atorvastatin
Azithromycin
Bisacodyl
Budesonide
Buprenorphine (transdermal)
Calcitriol
Carbamazepine
Caspofungin
Cefuroxime axetil (PO)
Chlorambucil
Chlorphenamine
Ciclosporin
Clindamycin
Clonazepam
Clopidogrel
Cyclizine
Dexamethasone
Diazepam
Diltiazem
Dipyridamole
Disodium pamidronate
   (↓ rate of infusion)
Docusate sodium
Domperidone
Dosulepin
Doxazocin
Doxycycline
Erythromycin
Esomeprazole
Ezetimibe
Felodipine
Ferrous sulphate
Granisetron
Hydrocortisone
Irbesartan

Isoniazid
Isosorbide mono/dinitrate
Itraconazole PO
Labetalol
Lactulose
Lansoprazole
Labetalol
Levothyroxine
Linezolid
Mebeverine
Methylprednisolone
Metronidazole
Micafungin
Moxifloxacin
Omeprazole
Ondansetron
Orlistat
Pantoprazole
Phenoxymethylpenicillin
Phenytoin
Pioglitazone
Posaconazole
Pravastatin
Prednisolone
Quinine sulphate
Rabeprazole
Rifampicin
Senna
Sevelamer
Sertraline
Sirolimus
Sodium fusidate
Sodium valproate
Tacrolimus
Tamoxifen
Unfractionated heparin
Vancomycin PO
Verapamil
Voriconazole PO
Warfarin
Zanamivir inhalation
Zolpidem

Some drugs to be avoided in CKD stage 5, haemodialysis and peritoneal dialysis

Alendronic acid
Aspirin (treatment doses)
Balsalazide
COX-2 inhibitors
Cidofovir
Disodium etidronate
Eplerenone
Exenatide
Foscarnet
Gaviscon®
Itraconazole IV
Lithium carbonate
Liraglutide
LMWHs (prolonged treatment caution)
Metformin
Mesalazine

Methotrexate
Minocycline
Morphine
Nitrofurantoin
NSAIDs
Peptac®
Pethidine
Ribavirin (PO)
Risedronate sodium
Rosuvastatin
Saxagliptin
Sodium clodronate
Sucralfate
Sulfasalazine
Tetracycline
Voriconazole IV

Notes on specific cardiovascular drugs

ACEIs and ARBs

ACEIs effectively reduce BP in patients with CKD, and have beneficial effects on the progression of renal disease (especially proteinuric). They may cause a fall in GFR in patients with bilateral renal artery stenosis (or a single stenosed kidney), which is often unknown at the time of initiation of treatment, but relatively common given the prevalence of vascular disease in patients with CKD. They can impair renal function in the absence of artery stenosis in patients with hypoperfused kidneys. Patients with severe renal impairment must be started with a low dose, increasing slowly. GFR and serum potassium levels must be monitored closely (checked 1–2 weeks after starting therapy). Serum potassium may rise 0.5mmol/L. Dietary advice should be reinforced at the time.

Many ACEIs are excreted renally, and maintenance dosage should be as low as possible to produce the desired therapeutic effect. ACEIs excreted both by kidneys and hepatic metabolism (e.g. fosinopril) only require dosage reduction in severe renal failure. Probably applies to ARBs but fewer data available.

Patients can suffer severe hypotension when taking ACEIs or ARBs if they become volume depleted, as angiotensin-mediated vasoconstriction plays a crucial part in the cardiovascular response to volume depletion. They should be used with caution in patients on HD because of the risk of hypotension with fluid removal. ACEIs can also interact with some synthetic HD membranes, particularly AN69®, and cause anaphylactoid reactions.

β-Adrenoceptor antagonists

β-Blockers can reduce renal blood flow and adversely affect renal function in patients with severe renal impairment. Dosages should be reduced especially if eliminated renally, e.g. atenolol, sotalol. Renally excreted β-blockers (especially atenolol) may accumulate in ESKD and cause profound bradycardia and subsequent hypotension and collapse. Metoprolol may be preferred.

Calcium antagonists

Mainly eliminated by hepatic metabolism and can usually be administered in standard dosages in patients with severe renal impairment.

Digoxin

Due to its complex pharmacokinetics, loading dose should be reduced to 500mcg or 250mcg. Maintenance doses should be reduced to 62.5mcg daily or alternate days. Plasma digoxin concentration should be monitored closely and used to guide dosage.

Notes on specific opioid analgesics

Opioid analgesics
The major problem is accumulation of active (toxic) metabolites. Dosage reduction may be necessary, and patients should be observed for adverse effects (respiratory depression, drowsiness, coma, and neurological toxicity). These side effects are more pronounced when used concomitantly with CNS drugs

Codeine
Significant increase in half-life in CKD stage 5, and metabolites (e.g. norcodeine and codeine-6-glucuronide) can cause severe adverse effects (as above), and sometimes prolonged narcosis. Use with care.

Tramadol
Renally excreted. Requires 50% dose reduction (usual dose given 50mg bd or tds). Active metabolites such as O-desmethyl-tramadol accumulate.

Morphine
Metabolized to morphine-3-glucoronide and morphine-6-glucoronide. These active metabolites may produce prolonged analgesia and respiratory depression, and accumulate, or paradoxically inhibit the analgesic effects of morphine. Chronic dosing *not* recommended.

Pethidine (meperidine)
Converted to norpethidine, a potent active metabolite that accumulates in severe renal failure and can cause seizures. Should not be used.

Papaveretum
Not recommended in patients with severe renal disease.

Hydromorphone
More potent than morphine. Metabolized to active metabolites: hydromorphone -3 glucuronide and hydromorphone -6-glucouronide. Can accumulate in severe renal impairment but can be used with careful titration.

Fentanyl
Less toxicity in CKD than other opiates, but not available orally so must be given IV, SC, transdermally (by patches), or sublingually.

Oxycodone
Although hepatically metabolized, active metabolites can accumulate; watch for sedation.

Notes on NSAIDs

NSAIDs accumulate in CKD and may be nephrotoxic, cause hyperkalaemia, salt and water retention, and inhibit the action of many antihypertensive agents. They are primarily metabolized to an acyl glucuronide, which accumulates, and can deconjugate to act as a reservoir for the parent compound (increasing its level). They can cause a reduction in GFR which may be severe, usually reversible, and is still important in dialysis patients (especially PD) in whom loss of residual function is of great importance. Aspirin may not inhibit cyclo-oxygenase in the kidney, and does not usually cause renal impairment. NSAIDs increase the bleeding tendency in uraemic patients in addition to their ulcerogenic effects.

The use of NSAIDs and cyclo-oxygenase 2 inhibitors in severe CKD are not recommended.

Notes on specific antibiotics

Gentamicin

Predominantly renally excreted, and dosing is critically dependent on renal function. For patients with CKD and on dialysis single doses should be given based on adjusted dosing weight (ADW) (see Box 18.1), and subsequent doses guided by drug level monitoring.

Gentamicin is extensively cleared during dialysis, but the precise amount removed depends on the modality used and the nature of the membrane (e.g. increased binding to AN69®). Post-dialysis gentamicin levels provide the best guide to optimal dosing frequency (usually required after every dialysis session), while pre-dialysis levels indicate the actual dose required on each occasion. Gentamicin levels rebound particularly after high-flux dialysis, and an immediate post-dialysis level will underestimate true gentamicin level. Usual loading dose is 1.5–2mg/kg (use adjusted dosing weight if obese). Redose when random level <1mg/L.

Prolonged gentamicin use in particular may have a detrimental effect on residual function both in CKD and in PD patients, but this does not occur with short-term use. Vancomycin and gentamicin may have a synergistic ototoxic and nephrotoxic effect.

Vancomycin

Predominantly renally excreted, and dosing is critically dependent on renal function, but is not extensively cleared by dialysis, and weekly dosing usually provides prolonged therapeutic levels after an initial dose of 750mg–2g. Loading dose usually adjusted to actual body weight: 750 mg if <40Kg; 1g if 40–59Kg; 1.5g if 60–90Kg; 2g if >90Kg. Drug level should be monitored and subsequent doses administered when the target trough level is reached (usually after 5–8 days). Vancomycin clearance is greater with PMMA membranes than polysulfone or AN69®, and increased in high-flux dialysis and CRRT. In these circumstances, loading with 750mg–1g and supplementing with 500mg after each dialysis is effective at maintaining therapeutic levels. It is important to seek microbiology advice as the therapeutic level depends on indication. Patients with significant residual function will require more frequent dosing.

Box 18.1 Ideal body weight (IBW) and adjusted dosing weight (ADW)

Use IBW if patient weighs 20% more than IBW.

IBW male=50+1kg per cm over 152cm (or 50+2.3kg per inch over 5 feet)

IBW female=45+1kg per cm over 152cm (or 45+2.3kg per inch over 5 feet)

Then, adjusted dosing weight for obesity=IBW+0.4 (actual body weight − IBW).

Amikacin and *tobramycin* have similar pharmacokinetics:
- Amikacin loading dose: 5mg/kg (use adjusted dosing weight as above if obese). Re-dose when random level reaches <5mg/L.
- Tobramycin loading dose: 1–1.5 mg/kg (use adjusted dosing weight as above if obese). Re-dose when random level reaches ≤ 1mg/L.

Other antibiotics

Tetracyclines

Should be avoided, although doxycycline and minocycline can be used if necessary (no dose alteration).

Penicillins

Are generally renally excreted and moderately removed by dialysis. Neurotoxicity has been reported in renal failure with high-dose penicillins and carbapenems.

Trimethoprim

Will raise serum creatinine levels in patients with residual renal function by inhibiting tubular secretion of creatinine.

Factors affecting drug removal by continuous renal replacement therapy

Patients on CRRT are often critically ill and so correct drug dosing is particularly important.

Volume of distribution

Drugs with a large Vd (e.g. >0.6L/kg) are not confined within the circulation, and therefore are not removed by CRRT. Drugs with a low Vd may still be poorly removed by CRRT as they may have a lower blood concentration than peripheral tissue concentration (e.g. digoxin), thus total body clearance due to CRRT may be negligible.

Molecular weight

Small compounds rely more on diffusion for clearance and larger ones more on convection during CRRT. Most drugs have a MW <1500Da. The precise MW of a drug, and the balance of dialysis and haemofiltration during CRRT, will determine its clearance. The increased pore size of most haemofilter membranes (0.01μm compared with 0.001μm for most HD membranes) also allows increased clearance of drugs with MW below ~5000Da. Diffusion is more important in continuous HD rather than continuous haemofiltration.

Protein binding

Removal of drugs by convection can be affected by binding to plasma proteins, e.g. albumin. UF cannot remove drug–protein complexes that have MW >50kDa, but only free drug. Many factors may affect protein binding and thus alter the degree of drug removal by CRRT, e.g. serum protein concentration, pH, drug interactions, and bilirubin concentration.

Route of drug elimination

Drugs that are primarily eliminated unchanged by the kidneys will have increased clearance in AKI when CRRT is commenced. Drugs eliminated by non-renal routes may not have significantly enhanced clearance by CRRT.

Filter membrane

Synthetic membranes are usually used in CRRT, and may bind larger quantities of drugs than occurs during HD with modified cellulose membranes, e.g. AN69® binds aminoglycosides. Polysulfone, polyamide, and polyacrylonitrile also differ in their electrical charge, which may affect convective and diffusive clearance of charged drugs.

Timing of CRRT

CRRT is a continuous therapy, and drugs removed will be continually cleared. This can lead to problems if CRRT is stopped for a period of time, but the drug dosing schedule is not changed. During ongoing therapy though there is less of a problem in the timing of administration of drugs.

Modality of CRRT

The clearance of drugs will vary to a degree according to the extent of continuous dialysis and haemofiltration used during CRRT. In pure haemofiltration no drug is removed by diffusion, only by convection, and rate of drug clearance will be proportional to the UF rate. Overall the most important RRT-related factor affecting drug removal is effluent volume.

Total drug removal

Can be calculated from measurement of drug levels in ultrafiltrate (UF), and allow supplemental dosing to be more accurate: Only applicable when drug level can be measured:

$$\text{Amount removed (mg)} = \text{UF concentration (mg/L)} \times \text{UF rate (L/min)}$$
$$\times \text{time of CRRT (min)}.$$

Alternatively:

$$\text{Amount of drug required (mg)} = [\text{desired plasma level (mg/L)} -$$
$$\text{current level (mg/L)}] \times \text{Vd (L/kg)}$$
$$\times \text{body weight (kg)}.$$

Dosing of drugs commonly used during continuous renal replacement therapy

For simplicity only dosing for continuous venovenous haemodiafiltration (CVVHDF) has been shown. Drug elimination will be affected by the precise balance of filtration and dialysis. Table 18.14 is therefore only an outline. All are IV unless otherwise stated.

Table 18.14 Dosing for continuous venovenous haemodiafiltration (CVVHDF)

Drug	Dosage for CVVHDF
Aciclovir	5–10mg/kg q24h
Amikacin*	10mg/kg loading dose then 7.5mg/kg 24–48-hourly: adjust according to levels
Amphotericin (all formulations)	Standard dose; liposomal preparations should be infused into the venous return line, and not pre-filter, as they increase the risk of filter clotting
Anidulafungin	Standard dose
Benzylpenicillin	75% standard dose
Caspofungin	Standard dose
Cefotaxime	1–2g q12h
Ceftazidime	0.5–1g q12h or 1–2g q12h
	May be affected by flux of filter
Ceftriaxone	2g q12–24h
Cefuroxime	750mg q12h (high-flux filter)
Ciprofloxacin	200–400mg q12h
Clarithromycin	250–500mg q12h
Clindamycin	Standard dose
Co-amoxiclav	1.2g stat then 1.2g q12h
Co-trimoxazole IV/ PO: sulfamethoxazole/ (SMX)/trimethoprim (TMP)	PCP treatment: 60mg/kg SMX/TMP q12h for 3 days then 30mg/kg SMX/TMP q12h
Digoxin	125–250mcg. Monitor levels
Ertapenem	500mg q24h
Erythromycin	Standard dose
Flucloxacillin	Standard dose
Fluconazole	Standard dose

Table 18.14 (*Contd.*)

Drug	Dosage for CVVHDF
Flucytosine	37.5mg/kg IV q12–24h guided by drug level and FBC
Ganciclovir	2.5mg/kg q24h induction. Maintenance 1.25mg/kg
Gentamicin*	1–3mg/kg stat, then monitor levels daily—usual maintenance dose 2mg/kg 24–48-hourly
Imipenem/cilastatin	250mg q6h or 500mg q6–8h
Itraconazole	Contraindicated
Linezolid	Standard dose
Meropenem	1g q8h
Metronidazole	Standard dose
Morphine	50–75% standard dose
Moxifloxacin	Standard dose
Omeprazole	Standard dose
Pantoprazole	Standard dose
Piperacillin/tazobactam	4.5g q8h
Teicoplanin	Loading dose: standard dose according to indication; maintenance dose: reduce from day 4 using standard dose according to indication every 3 days or 33% standard dose q24h
Tigecycline	Standard dose
Vancomycin	500mg–1g stat, then monitor levels. Only give subsequent doses when vancomycin level reaches trough
Voriconazole IV	Contra-indicated
Voriconazole PO	Standard dose

*Use IBW for patients >120% IBW.

Standards and guidelines

Overview of UK guidelines

The UK Renal Association standards are defined in their clinical practice guidelines, with a major 4th edition being published in 2007, and further updates on selected topics since then. Guidelines cover:
- AKI
- Anaemia in CKD
- Assessment of potential kidney transplant recipients
- Blood borne viruses
- Cardiovascular disease in CKD
- CKD-mineral and bone disorders
- Detection monitoring and care of patients with CKD
- Haemodialysis
- Nutrition in CKD
- Peritoneal access
- Peritoneal dialysis
- Planning, initiation and withdrawal of RRT
- Post-operative care of kidney transplant recipients
- Water treatment facilities, dialysis water and dialysis fluid quality
- Vascular access for haemodialysis.

Full guidelines can be found at ℘ www.renal.org.

The British Transplant Society produces guidelines relevant to kidney transplantation: ℘ www.bts.org.uk.

The UK National Institute for Health and Care Excellence (NICE: ℘ www.nice.org.uk) and Scottish Intercollegiate Guidelines Network (SIGN: ℘ www.sign.ac.uk) produce guidelines covering many aspects of medicine but including many renally related topics.

K/DOQI and KDIGO guidelines

The US National Kidney Foundation-Dialysis Outcomes Quality Initiative (NKF-DOQI) was established in 1995 to improve patient outcomes and survival by providing recommendations for optimal clinical practices. This was achieved by structured review of the literature and development of evidence-based clinical practice guidelines. In 1999, the NKF re-examined the evidence for the existing recommendations, and expanded the project to include other aspects of CKD prior to the need for dialysis. Hence the new guidelines were renamed Kidney Disease Outcomes Quality Initiative (K/DOQI), and were originally published in 2000, with updates on various aspects of CKD published subsequently (⅌ www.kidney.org/professionals/KDOQI/guidelines_commentaries).

The most recent guidelines cover:
- Diabetes and CKD
- Anaemia in CKD
- CKD evaluation
- Bone metabolism and disease in CKD
- Hypertension in CKD
- Dyslipidaemia in CKD
- Nutrition in children with CKD
- HD adequacy
- PD adequacy
- Vascular access
- CV disease in dialysis patients.

More recently, clinical practice guidelines have been published by the kidney disease improving global outcomes (KDIGO) initiative (⅌ www.kdigo.org/home) covering:
- AKI
- Anaemia in CKD
- BP in CKD
- Care of kidney transplant recipients
- CKD evaluation and management
- CKD-MBD
- Glomerulonephritis
- Hepatitis C in CKD
- Lipids in CKD.

European Renal Best Practice

The ERA-EDTA started producing best practice guidelines in 2008, renamed subsequently as renal best practice. The specific aim was not to duplicate existing guidelines but to identify gaps in practice, and also produce guideline statements on those produced by other bodies such as the US NKF (⅊ www.european-renal-best-practice.org).

Current publications include:

- 'Diagnosis and treatment of hyponatraemia'
- 'Are there better alternatives than haemoglobin A1c to estimate glycaemic control in the chronic kidney disease population?'
- 'Management and evaluation of the kidney donor and recipient'
- 'Glucose-lowering drugs in patients with chronic kidney disease'
- 'ERBP position statement on the KDIGO Guidelines on Acute Kidney Injury'
- 'Measuring the quality of renal care'
- 'A systematic review regarding the association of illness perception and survival among end-stage renal disease patients'
- 'ERBP position statement on the KDIGO Guideline for the Management of Blood Pressure in Non-dialysis-dependent Chronic Kidney Disease'
- 'What guidelines should or should not be: implications for guideline production'
- 'Fabry nephropathy: indications for screening and guidance for diagnosis and treatment'
- 'Crush recommendations: a step forward in disaster nephrology'
- 'Endorsement of the KDIGO guidelines on kidney transplantation'
- 'When to start dialysis: updated guidance following publication of the Initiating Dialysis Early and Late (IDEAL) study.'
- Endorsement of the KDIGO CKD–MBD guidelines
- Target haemoglobin to aim for with erythropoiesis-stimulating agents
- Diagnosis, prevention and treatment of haemodialysis catheter-related bloodstream infections (CRBSI)
- Catheter-related blood stream infections (CRBSI): a European view
- Educating ESRD patients on dialysis modality selection
- Evaluation of peritoneal membrane characteristics
- High-flux or low-flux dialysis
- Endorsement of the KDIGO hepatitis C guidelines
- Anaemia management in patients with CKD

Kidney Care Australia has produced a set of guidelines on haemodialysis, biochemical targets, dialysis adequacy, peritonitis treatment and vascular access, and AKI, CVD in CKD, early CKD, nutrition, diabetes and CKD (⅊ www.cari.org.au/Dialysis/dialysis_guidelines.html).

International Society of Peritoneal Dialysis

The International Society of Peritoneal Dialysis (ISPD) produces internationally applicable guidelines specific to PD (℗ www.ispd.org) covering:

- Prevention and treatment of catheter related infections and peritonitis in children receiving PD
- Assessment of growth and nutritional status in children on PD
- Treatment of peritonitis in paediatric patients receiving PD
- AKI
- Reducing the risk of PD-related infections
- PD related infections: recommendations
- Peritoneal access
- Encapsulating peritoneal sclerosis
- Solute and fluid removal.

Useful websites

Associations

American Association of Kidney Patients	⌕ www.aakp.org
American Nephrology Nurse Association	⌕ www.annanurse.org
American Society of Nephrology	⌕ www.asn-online.com
American Society of Transplantation	⌕ www.a-s-t.org
Australia and New Zealand Society of Nephrology	⌕ www.nephrology.edu.au
Australian Kidney Foundation	⌕ www.kidney.org.au
European Kidney Patients' Federation	⌕ www.ceapir.org
European Renal Association	⌕ www.era-edta.org/
International Society of Nephrology	⌕ www.isn-online.org
International Society of Peritoneal Dialysis	⌕ www.ispd.org
National Kidney Foundation	⌕ www.kidney.org
National Kidney Research Fund (UK)	⌕ www.nkrf.org.uk
Renal Pathology Society	⌕ www.renalpathsoc.org
UK Renal Association	⌕ www.renal.org
UK Renal Registry	⌕ www.renalreg.org
USRDS	⌕ www.usrds.org
Vascular Access Society	⌕ www.vascularaccesssociety.com
World Kidney Fund	⌕ www.worldkidney.org/

Miscellaneous

Baxter ESRD information site	www.kidneydirections.com
Biomedical calculators	www.mdcalc.com
Cybernephrology	www.cybernephrology.org
Dialysis message boards	www.ihatedialysis.com
DOQI guidelines	www.kidney.org/professionals/ guidelines/guidelines_commentaries
Forum of End-Stage Renal Disease Networks	www.esrdnetworks.org
Hypertension, Dialysis and Clinical Nephrology (HDCN)	www.hdcn.com
Kidney disease community	www.ikidney.com
Kidney School	www.kidneyschool.org
Medical algorithms	www.medal.org
Kidney patient guide	www.kidneypatientguide.org.uk
Medscape	www.medscape.com
Nephron Information Center	www.nephron.com
Nephronline	www.nephronline.com
Renal Fellow Network	www.renalfellow.blogspot.co.uk
RenalNet	www.renalnet.org
Renal Web (dialysis site)	www.renalweb.com
Travel dialysis site	www.globaldialysis.com/search-for-dialysis-centres.html

Index